# Immune Checkpoint Inhibitors - New Insights and Recent Progress

*Edited by Afsheen Raza*

Published in London, United Kingdom

Immune Checkpoint Inhibitors - New Insights and Recent Progress
http://dx.doi.org/10.5772/intechopen.100958
Edited by Afsheen Raza

Contributors
Nabil E. Omar, Arwa O. Sahal, Hebatalla M. Afifi, Rana Mekkawi, Hazem Elewa, Jacob Zaemes, Muneeb Rehman, Ruth He, Coleman Smith, Juan Huang, Jiawen Huang, Ika Nurlaila, Shaimaa M. Bebars, Afsheen Raza, Monde Ntwasa, Bonnie L. Russell, Selisha A. Sooklal, Sibusiso T. Malindisa, Hongzhang Deng, Pei Huang, Hui Wang, Man Chen



First published in London, United Kingdom, 2023 by IntechOpen
IntechOpen is the global imprint of INTECHOPEN LIMITED, registered in England and Wales, registration number: 11086078, 5 Princes Gate Court, London, SW7 2QJ, United Kingdom

British Library Cataloguing-in-Publication Data
A catalogue record for this book is available from the British Library

Additional hard and PDF copies can be obtained from orders@intechopen.com

Immune Checkpoint Inhibitors - New Insights and Recent Progress
Edited by Afsheen Raza
p. cm.
Print ISBN 978-1-80356-590-3
Online ISBN 978-1-80356-591-0
eBook (PDF) ISBN 978-1-80356-592-7

For EU product safety concerns:
IN TECH d.o.o., Prolaz Marije Krucifikse Kozulić 3, 51000 Rijeka, Croatia,
info@intechopen.com or visit our website at intechopen.com.

# Meet the editor

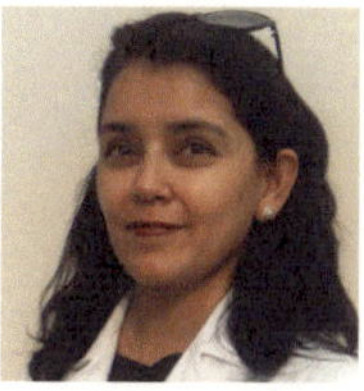

Dr. Afsheen Raza is a research scientist with extensive experience in cutting-edge molecular biology/immunology research and cancer clinical trials. She is currently working at the Translational Cancer Research Institute of the National Center of Cancer Care and Research (NCCCR), Hamad Medical Corporation, Qatar. She has more than 15 years of research experience with a prolific output of more than forty peer-reviewed publications in high-impact journals, international and national grants, and clinical trials research. Dr. Afsheen has also mentored and supervised master's and Ph.D. students as part of her academic training. She is internationally recognized for her scientific contribution to cancer immunology and immunotherapy and serves as editor for *Frontiers in Immunology* and *PLOS One* and is a reviewer for *Cells, Cancers*, and *Frontiers in Medicine*.

# Contents

# Preface

This book provides updated information on immune checkpoint inhibitors and their role in disease dynamics, especially in cancers. The chapters discuss the mechanisms of action of immune checkpoint inhibitors, the role of novel immune checkpoint inhibitors in therapeutics/immune-related adverse events, and immune checkpoint inhibitors as predictors of response. Furthermore, the chapters also focus on current clinical trials being carried out on several novel immune checkpoint molecules and their utility in therapeutics, overall response rates, and survival. The book delves into critical topics such as the advances and challenges of immune checkpoint molecules with respect to their use in clinical practice. The insights from this book serve as a foundation for preclinical and clinical studies to identify unexplored pathways that need attention at a global scale to improve the role of immune checkpoint inhibitors in cancers.

**Dr. Afsheen Raza**
Associate Professor,
Molecular Biology,
College of Health Sciences,
Abu Dhabi University,
Abu Dhabi, UAE

Section 1

# Immune Checkpoint Inhibitors - Mechanisms and Current Advances

**Chapter 1**

# Introductory Chapter: Introduction to New Insights and Recent Progress in Immune Checkpoint Inhibitors

*Afsheen Raza*

## 1. Introduction

Immune checkpoint inhibitor (ICI) is an established therapeutic strategy for various cancers. ICI comprises mainly of monoclonal antibodies that block immune regulatory checkpoint molecules, cytotoxic T-lymphocyte-associated protein 4 (CTLA-4), Programmed cell death protein-1 (PD-1) and Programmed Death Ligand-1 (PD-L1) [1]. To date, FDA has approved ICIs for various cancer types including anti-CTLA-4 (Ipilimumab, Tremelimumab), anti-PD-1 (Pembrolizumab, Nivolumab, Cemiplimab) and anti-PD-L1 (Atezolizumab, Avelumab, and Durvalumab) [2].

The main mechanism of action of immune checkpoint inhibitors is to target and augment host CD4+ and CD8+ T cell responses. Briefly, CTLA-4 is a T-cell surface receptor that binds costimulatory factors (CD80, CD86) on antigen-presenting cells. This activation transmits inhibitory signal to T cells thus, reducing Interleukin 2 (IL-2) production and T-cell proliferation. Moreover, PD-1 is a cell surface receptor expressed on B cells, T cells and NK cells. Its main function is to promote self-tolerance/ prevent autoimmunity via apoptosis of antigen-specific T-cells, suppression of T cell inflammatory activity and downregulation of the immune system. PD-1 has strong binding affinity to its ligands, PD-L1/PD-L2 and this binding delivers a strong inhibitory signal to suppress T cell receptor (TCR) mediated activation of IL-2 production and T cell proliferation for immune regulation [3].

## 2. Novel immune checkpoint inhibitors/combinatorial therapeutic regimens

Recently, many studies and clinical trials have focused on various aspects of immunotherapy including novel immune checkpoint inhibitors, combination therapeutic regimens, identification of predictive and prognostic biomarkers, management of immune related adverse events etc. The insights from these pre-clinical and clinical studies indicate unexplored pathways that need attention at a global scale to improve the role of these ICIs in cancers. Importantly, the novel immune checkpoint inhibitors, apart from anti-CTLA-4, anti-PD-1 and anti-PD-L1, can serve as a paradigm


IntechOpen

shift for patients, giving them a chance for additional treatment options. For e.g. recently, FDA approved anti-LAG-3 (Relatlimab) monoclonal antibody, that targets Lymphocyte-activation gene 3 (LAG-3) immune checkpoint and recommended it for untreated unresectable or metastatic melanoma in patients ≥12 years of age. Relatlimab is approved to be given in combination with anti-PD-1 (Nivolumab) as patients on this combination demonstrate better progression free survival than on Nivolumab alone. However, higher incidence of immune-related side effects have been associated with this combination indicating that new and novel immune checkpoint inhibitors need efficient monitoring for patient management [4]. On the other hand, many novel immune checkpoints are still under still investigation in clinical trials with promising results [5]. Some of these include

- T cell immunoglobulin and mucin domain-containing protein 3 (TIM-3) for advanced solid tumors/lymphomas

- B7 homolog 3 protein/B7 homolog 4 protein (B7-H3/B7-H4) for advanced solid tumors/B7-H4 positive solid tumors

- Adenosine A2A receptor (A2AR) for advanced solid tumors

- Cluster of differentiation 73 (CD73) for advanced solid tumors

- Natural Killer Cell receptor NKG2A, for Platinum-resistant, recurrent, or metastatic, head and neck squamous cell carcinoma (HNSCC)

- Poliovirus receptor related immunoglobulin domain (PVRIG)

- Poliovirus receptor-related 2 (PVRL2) for Advanced Solid tumors

In addition to novel immune checkpoints, several studies are also focusing on finding optimal combination therapeutic regimens of ICIs with other biomolecules to augment the immune response for better progression free and overall survival [5]. Some of these include:

- Tyrosine Kinase inhibitor, Focal adhesion kinase (FAK) in combination with Pembrolizumab and chemotherapy gemcitabine for advanced pancreatic adenocarcinoma

- Anti-CD-147-Signal regulatory protein α (SIRPα) fusion drug, ALX148, in combination with pembrolizumab, nivolumab, trastuzumab, rituximab, ramucirumab, 5FU, paclitaxel, or cisplatin for advanced solid tumors or refractory Non-Hodgkin's Lymphoma (NHL)

- Colony stimulating factor 1 (CSF-1 (M-CSF)/CSF-1R) Inhibitor in combination with durvalumab for advanced solid tumors

- B cell activator, Semaphorin 4D (SEMA4D), in combination with avelumab for advanced stage Non-small cell lung cancer (NSCLC)

- Angiopoietin-2 (Ang-2) in combination with pembrolizumab for advanced solid tumors

It is postulated that with the advent of novel and combinatorial immune checkpoint therapies, improved overall survival for solid, hematological, rare, and hard-to-treat cancers will improve the prospect of improved cancer management.

## 3. Predictive and prognostic biomarkers

In addition to novel therapeutic regimens, another area of immense importance is the identification of predictive and prognostic biomarkers for immune related adverse events/treatment dynamics. This is a vastly growing field, particularly due to the limited response rates (20–40%) observed in patients on ICI treatment. Finding predictive and prognostic biomarkers can not only help stratify patients for optimal treatment regimen but will also reduce the economic cost on patients. Furthermore, it can help to avoid the generation of drug resistance as the use of ICI for a specific cohort (such as responding patients) will control excess use of this precious drug. In lieu of this, soluble biomarkers (secreted in plasma, serum, urine, ascitic fluids etc.) are gaining a lot of attention. This is due to major advantages including ease of sampling, longitudinal monitoring, and less heterogeneity (as compared to tissue biomarkers). Several studies investigating the role of soluble CTLA-4 (sCTLA-4), soluble PD-1 (sPD-1), soluble PD-L1 (sPD-L1) and soluble PD-L2 (sPD-L2), especially in melanoma and NSCLC patients have shown promising results. The studies observed that soluble markers can exert enhancement and inhibitory effects on the immune system including early activation of CD8+lymphocytes, increased lytic activity of macrophages, up regulation of pro- and anti-inflammatory cytokines/chemokines, inhibition of IL-2 production/T cell activation and reverse signaling on dendritic cells (DC) leading to reduction in DC maturation. These soluble markers have also been postulated to bind and block the active site of ICI monoclonal antibodies, thus making the treatment regimen inefficient [6–16]. On the other hand, several predictive biomarkers such as C-Reactive proteins (CRP), Blood cell counts, IL-5, IL-6, IL-8, CXCL9, 10, 11, 13, CCL3, CCR3, sPD-L2 etc. have been associated as predictors of immune related adverse events in ICI treated patients indicating the importance of soluble markers [8, 17, 18]. However, this is still an untapped area with limited studies and larger prospective clinical trials are warranted to fully understand their role in immunotherapy.

Last, but not the least, the gut microbiome is an area of immense interest for their role in ICI treatment dynamics. Emerging evidence/clinical trials suggest that gut microbiota influences clinical response to immunotherapy [19]. For e.g., a study on fecal microbiota transplant (FMT) in metastatic melanoma from responding patients (on anti-PD-1 treatment) to non-responding patient lead to improved response rates [20]. In addition to this, various studies have documented the microbes *Blautia obeum, Collinsella aerofaciens, Enterococcus faecium, Klebsiella pneumonia, Parabacteroides merdae, Roseburia intestinalis, Veillonella parvula, Ruminococcaceae* to be associated with enhanced/inhibitory effects on anti-PD-1 treatment mainly due to their interaction with the cells of the tumor microenvironment [19, 21–23]. Therefore, the value of assessing the gut microbiome in immunotherapy is an area of significant interest and randomized controlled trials, examining modulatory effects of the gut microbiome in ICI treated patients, is recommended for better understanding of treatment dynamics.

In summary, a vast avenue of areas can be explored with regards to immune checkpoint inhibitors to provide novel insights into this emerging field. The above-mentioned areas are just the tip of the iceberg and exploration of other aspects such as genomics, transcriptomics, proteomics, metabolomics etc. can serve valuable for treatment management and better overall survival for ICI treated patients.

## Author details

Afsheen Raza
Hamad Medical Corporation, Qatar

*Address all correspondence to: araza@hamad.qa

## References

[1] Sharma P, Hu-Lieskovan S, Wargo JA, Ribas A. Primary, adaptive, and acquired resistance to cancer immunotherapy. Cell. 2017;**168**(4):707-723

[2] Twomey JD, Zhang B. Cancer immunotherapy update: FDA-approved checkpoint inhibitors and companion diagnostics. The AAPS Journal. 2021;**23**(2):39

[3] Iranzo P, Callejo A, Assaf JD, Molina G, Lopez DE, Garcia-Illescas D, et al. Overview of checkpoint inhibitors mechanism of action: Role of immune-related adverse events and their treatment on progression of underlying cancer. Frontiers in Medicine. 2022;**9**:875

[4] Institute NC. Opdualag Becomes First FDA-Approved Immunotherapy to Target LAG-3 2022. 2022. Available from: https://www.cancer.gov/news-events/cancer-currents-blog/2022/fda-opdualag-melanoma-lag-3

[5] Marin-Acevedo JA, Kimbrough EO, Lou Y. Next generation of immune checkpoint inhibitors and beyond. Journal of Hematology & Oncology. 2021;**14**(1):45

[6] Li Y, Xiao Y, Su M, Zhang R, Ding J, Hao X, et al. Role of soluble programmed death-1 (sPD-1) and sPD-ligand 1 in patients with cystic echinococcosis. Experimental and Therapeutic Medicine. 2016;**11**(1):251-256

[7] Zhu X, Lang J. Soluble PD-1 and PD-L1: Predictive and prognostic significance in cancer. Oncotarget. 2017;**8**(57):97671-97682

[8] Costantini A, Julie C, Dumenil C, Helias-Rodzewicz Z, Tisserand J, Dumoulin J, et al. Predictive role of plasmatic biomarkers in advanced non-small cell lung cancer treated by nivolumab. Oncoimmunology. 2018;**7**(8):e1452581

[9] Gu D, Ao X, Yang Y, Chen Z, Xu X. Soluble immune checkpoints in cancer: Production, function and biological significance. Journal for Immunotherapy of Cancer. 2018;**6**(1):132

[10] Okuma Y, Wakui H, Utsumi H, Sagawa Y, Hosomi Y, Kuwano K, et al. Soluble programmed cell death ligand 1 as a novel biomarker for nivolumab therapy for non-small-cell lung cancer. Clinical Lung Cancer. 2018;**19**(5):410-417

[11] Abu Hejleh T, Furqan M, Ballas Z, Clamon G. The clinical significance of soluble PD-1 and PD-L1 in lung cancer. Critical Reviews in Oncology/Hematology. 2019;**143**:148-152

[12] Nixon AB, Schalper KA, Jacobs I, Potluri S, Wang IM, Fleener C. Peripheral immune-based biomarkers in cancer immunotherapy: Can we realize their predictive potential? Journal for Immunotherapy of Cancer. 2019;**7**(1):325

[13] Raza A, Merhi M, Relecom A, Fernandes Q, Inchakalody V, Gul ARZ, et al. Evolving dynamic biomarkers for prediction of immune responses to checkpoint inhibitors in cancer. Advances in Precision Medicine Oncology. 2020

[14] Tiako Meyo M, Jouinot A, Giroux-Leprieur E, Fabre E, Wislez M, Alifano M, et al. Predictive value of soluble PD-1, PD-L1, VEGFA, CD40 ligand and CD44 for nivolumab therapy in advanced non-small cell lung cancer: A Case-Control Study. Cancer. 2020;**12**(2)

[15] Han B, Dong L, Zhou J, Yang Y, Guo J, Xuan Q, et al. The clinical implication of soluble PD-L1 (sPD-L1) in patients with breast cancer and its biological function in regulating the function of T lymphocyte. Cancer Immunology, Immunotherapy. 2021;**70**(10):2893-2909

[16] Ohkuma R, Ieguchi K, Watanabe M, Takayanagi D, Goshima T, Onoue R, et al. Increased plasma soluble PD-1 concentration correlates with disease progression in patients with cancer treated with anti-PD-1 antibodies. Biomedicines. 2021;**9**(12)

[17] Jia XH, Geng LY, Jiang PP, Xu H, Nan KJ, Yao Y, et al. The biomarkers related to immune related adverse events caused by immune checkpoint inhibitors. Journal of Experimental & Clinical Cancer Research. 2020;**39**(1):284

[18] Schalper KA, Carleton M, Zhou M, Chen T, Feng Y, Huang SP, et al. Elevated serum interleukin-8 is associated with enhanced intratumor neutrophils and reduced clinical benefit of immune-checkpoint inhibitors. Nature Medicine. 2020;**26**(5):688-692

[19] Oh B, Boyle F, Pavlakis N, Clarke S, Eade T, Hruby G, et al. The gut microbiome and cancer immunotherapy: Can we use the gut microbiome as a predictive biomarker for clinical response in cancer immunotherapy? Cancers (Basel). 2021;**13**(19)

[20] Baruch EN, Youngster I, Ben-Betzalel G, Ortenberg R, Lahat A, Katz L, et al. Fecal microbiota transplant promotes response in immunotherapy-refractory melanoma patients. Science. 2021;**371**(6529):602-609

[21] Erdman SE, Rao VP, Poutahidis T, Rogers AB, Taylor CL, Jackson EA, et al. Nitric oxide and TNF-alpha trigger colonic inflammation and carcinogenesis in Helicobacter hepaticus-infected, Rag2-deficient mice. Proceedings of the National Academy of Sciences of the United States of America. 2009;**106**(4):1027-1032

[22] Erdman SE, Poutahidis T. The microbiome modulates the tumor macroenvironment. Oncoimmunology. 2014;**3**:e28271

[23] Vetizou M, Pitt JM, Daillere R, Lepage P, Waldschmitt N, Flament C, et al. Anticancer immunotherapy by CTLA-4 blockade relies on the gut microbiota. Science. 2015;**350**(6264):1079-1084

Chapter 2

# Immune Checkpoints: The Rising Branch in Cancer Immunotherapy

*Ika Nurlaila*


## Abstract

In the cancer therapy realm, concepts of immunotherapy rose as a response to emerging adverse effects caused by conventional therapies, which to some cases even more quality-of-life-reducing than the cancer itself. Immunotherapy is aimed to systematically enhance immunity to eradicate cancerous cells without harming healthy neighbor cells. In this platform, immune checkpoint molecules are under massive explorations and have been thought to be bringing excellent outlook clinically. These molecules hinder anticancer immunity. As a result, cancer growth is favored. Therefore, inactivation of immune checkpoint by blocking engagement of checkpoint receptors and their cognate ligands will restore the anticancer functions of immune system elements; hence, they can reclaim their power to eradicate cancers. Each checkpoint possesses specific downstream mechanism for which the inhibitors are formulated. In this chapter, we discuss four major checkpoints in the context of general characteristics, structures, and their roles in some cancers. Relevant recent progress in respective checkpoint molecules is also discussed to broaden our horizon on how cancers and immune checkpoint molecules are at interplay.


**Keywords:** immunotherapy, cancer, immunity, checkpoint, inhibitors, CTLA-4, LAG-3, TIGIT, PD-1

## 1. Introduction

Cancer immunotherapy is a course of treatments by which the anticancer immunity is restored. This has transformed plethora in curing cancers [1] and rapidly evolving field of oncology. There are two primary therapeutic strategies employed in cancer immunotherapy. Immune checkpoint inhibitors, cytokines and vaccines, are principally aimed at enhancing the patient's own antitumor immunity. The other approach is administration of tumor-reactive immune cells which can be as chimeric antigen receptor (CAR) T cells, or T-cell receptor-engineered T cells. Excellent results have already been achieved in cancers including melanoma, leukemias, and lymphoma for which immunotherapy is now employed as a standard care [2]. Of these, immune checkpoint inhibitor approach has received much growing attention, especially after ipilimumab was first approved by FDA to treat melanoma [3]. Several immune checkpoints have been investigated for various types of cancers in the past decades, including but not limited to CTLA-4, PD-1, LAG-3, and TIGIT. They are named after "immune checkpoints" to indicate their function as gatekeepers of immune responses in physiological condition [4]. In order to deliver inhibitory signals, the receptors use mono-tyrosine signaling motifs such as immunoreceptor tyrosine-based inhibitory motif (ITIM) and immunoreceptor tyrosine-based switch motif (ITSM). As surface molecule, their activity can be inhibited by blocking antibodies to prevent ligation of ligand receptor. This is the big idea of developing immune checkpoint blockade [5]. Application of anti-PD-1/PD-L1 as checkpoint inhibitors has achieved success therapeutically as well as commercially [6]. This encourages much more exploration on other identified checkpoints, and they also show potential in animal models. Highlights in this chapter are the four major checkpoint molecules: CTLA-4, LAG-3, PD-1, and TIGIT, in regard with their structures, signaling pathways, and progress reports on their respective implementation clinically.

## 2. CTLA-4: the god father of immune checkpoint molecules

### 2.1 General description

Although immune responses are needed to assure protection against any harmful agents, excessive response potentiates damage. Therefore, an effective control must be warranted. Cytotoxic T-lymphocyte antigen-4 (CTLA-4), known as CD152, is constitutively expressed on regulatory T cells (Tregs) and conventional T cells after activation [7]. Often, this particular subset is overexpressed on exhausted T cells [8]; hence, it is used as one of prominent markers for T cell exhaustion. Mostly, CTLA-4 is situated within intracellular vesicles and expressed only transiently following activation of the immunological synapse prior to being endocytosed [9]. CTLA-4 is a pivotal brake system in immune responses. Its genetic ablation, which causes fatal lymphoproliferative diseases, renders it unique among other checkpoints [10, 11].

CTLA-4 is a member of the CD28 family receptors. It has a significantly higher affinity to ligands B7.1 or B7.2 than that seen for CD28. Consequently, CTLA-4 abrogates co-stimulatory signal which is elicited by CD28 [12, 13], In the context of recognition of tumor antigens, CTLA-4 is highly expressed in FOXP3-expressing regulatory T cells (Tregs) which leads toco-stimulatory prevention, braking the T cells response and facilitation of cancer cells immune escape [11]. Therefore, prohibiting negative regulation via binding of CTLA-4 is seen to be a plausible way to repromote stimulation and potentiation of T cell activation. CTLA-4 blocking antibodies have been reported to regress tumor growth and improve disease-free survival in various murine malignancy models [14].

There have been two antibodies which have been developed to inhibit the binding of CTLA-4, namely ipilimumab (known previously as MDX-010) and tremelimumab (known previously as ticilimumab). While ipilimumab is a fully IgG1 ƙ mAb, tremelimumab is an IgG2 mAb. Compared to ipilimumab, tremelimumab's half-life is twofold longer. However, it was ipilimumab that received approval from FDA to be harnessed as a checkpoint-based anticancer therapy [15].

CTLA-4is used for the treatment of metastatic melanoma and is undergoing clinical trials for lung, colorectal, gastric, kidney, pancreatic,ovarian, and prostate which commenced Phase III thereof [7]. Initially, the overall strategy of blocking CTLA-4 appeared to invite doubts, since there is no tumor specificity on which CTLA-4 ligands can bind. Moreover, lethal autoimmune and hyperimmune phenotype in CTLA-4-knockout mice seems to be positively correlated with immune toxicity caused by the blockade of this receptor [16]. This was not until Allison et al. showed a therapeutic window of this inhibitor. Harnessing mouse model, the team demonstrated that anti-CTLA-4 negatively affect the growth of colon carcinoma as well as fibrosarcoma. Intriguingly, anti-CTLA is able to exert its robust after effect palpable tumors are stably established [17].

### 2.2 Signaling pathway of CTLA-4

The first mechanism is coupling CD28 to its ligands CD80 (B7-1) and CD86 expressed on the surface of APCs. TCR ligation induces conformational changes in the CD28 molecule by which bivalent enhanced avidity binding to CD80 is mediated. Although these conformational changes are yet to be clearly addressed, the higher affinity of CTLA-4 as monovalent compared to that seen for CD28 is widely thought to be the reason. With no TCR stimulation, CD28 might still be able to bind to its ligands yet at low affinity. However, CTLA-4, which structurally is close to CD28, may initiate its bivalent binding before CD28. Accordingly, it is assumed that the high avidity of CTLA-4 for the shared ligands contributes to CTLA-4-mediated inhibition that overrides CD28-induced co-stimulation [18].

Following binding to either CD80 (B7-1) or CD86, CTLA-4 turns off APCs and then increases its activity upon TCR engagement. This culminates after 2–3 days of activation of conventional CD4+ and CD8+ T cells. As CD80 (B7-1) and CD86 elicit a co-stimulatory signal via CD28, a competitive role showed by CTLA-4 is vital for T cell attenuation to fine-tune the immune response. Rapid binding kinetics of CTLA-4 and CD28 to CD80 has been seen approximately at $k_{off} \geq 1.6$ and $\geq 0.43\ s^{-1}$ which allows their instant competition [7]. CTLA-4 is upregulated on the surface of Treg cells with which the level of CD80/CD86 co-stimulatory molecules, including their cytoplasmic domains, on APCs is reduced in a trans-endocytosis manner [8]. Subsequently, this dampens proliferation of non-Treg T cells and the cytokine productions [19] to modulate immune suppression on bystander cells [8].

### 2.3 The interplay of CTLA-4 in cancer

As for dissecting more on CTLA-4 role in cancers, first we need to understand the architecture of the one particular T cell subset referred to as $T_{reg}$ cells. These are particular compartment in CD4+ T subset which co-express CD25, the α-subunit of the interleukin-2 (IL-2) receptor that is canonical marker for $T_{reg}$ cells and has been implicated in immune suppression in cancer [20]. These cells were identified to carry mutations of FOXP3, the master transcription factor that regulates Treg phenotypes and function as immunosuppressant, years later. Consequently, CD25 and forkhead box P3 (FOXP3) are used to probe if CD4+ T cells are $T_{reg}$ cells instead of conventional T helper ($T_H$) cells [19].

The role of Treg in cancers is well seen in inflammatory site, where they infiltrate in to inactivate different types of $CD4^+$ T helper ($T_H$) cells and $CD8^+$ cytotoxic T cells (CTLs). This is why reversing Tregs' activities could revive the immune system and help in combating cancer [19]. Antihuman CTLA-4 monoclonal antibodies (mAbs) can effectively exert agonist not antagonist effect for it is not capable of binding more than 50% of CTLA-4 molecules. This statement was firmly supported by findings that in homozygous human CTLA knock-in mice ($ctla^{h/h}$) anti-CTLA-4 mAbs induce B7 upregulation, but this is not observed in hetereozygous mice ($ctla^{h/m}$). Moreover, this demonstrates that functional blocking would be required to block more than 50% CTLA-4, probably due to trans-endocytosis, could be facilitated by leaving 50% of

CTLA-4 unoccupied. Therefore, upregulation of B7 on dendritic cells (DCs) is physiologically connected in the blockade of B7-CTLA-4 counteraction [21].

### 2.4 Potential use of CTLA-4 in cancer immunotherapy

Ipilimumab was the first FDA-approved anti-CTLA-4 blocking antibody [8]. It response is markedly different to that of traditional chemotherapy. While patients receiving conventional chemotherapy exhibit a quick reduction of baseline tumor without evidence of new lesions, patients receiving ipilimumab may see first increase in their tumor burden followed by a reduction or total eradication of all lesions. This is attributable to late activation of the immune system as infiltrating T cells may take some time to destroy the tumor [22].

As the advantage from ipilimumab takes place often after what previously has been defined as “progression” by World Health Organization (WHO) or “Response Evaluation Criteria in Solid Tumors (RECIST)” criteria, new immune response criteria have been proposed. Therapeutic response toward ipilimumab culminates between 12 and 24 weeks with slow response persists even beyond 12 months. The adverse effect, which was observed in 10–15% grade 3 or higher, is immune-related and consists of colitis, hypophysitis, thyroiditis, rash, and hepatitis [22]. The treatment with immunosuppressive agents such as corticosteroids, which are aimed at alleviating immune-related side effects, does not seem to weaken antitumor response [23, 24]. Taken all these together, ipilimumab is safe to administer if monitoring and management of the side effects are conducted properly [22].

A new design of anti-CTLA4-NF mAb referred to BMS986218 has commenced its Phase I/II clinical trial to evaluate its side effect either as monotherapy or combination therapy with nivolumab (PD-1 inhibiting antibody). This particular trial is still recruiting patients with solid cancers at advanced stages [25]. Although it is still under initial phase of clinical trials, it bulks up body of evidence of promising and safe use of checkpoint-based cancer immunotherapy.

## 3. Lymphocyte activation Gene-3 (LAG-3)

### 3.1 General description

Lymphocyte activation gene-3 (LAG-3), also known as CD233, is expressed on the various hematopoetic lineage ranges from natural killer (NK) cells, B cells, γδ T cells, and activated and regulatory CD4 and CD8 T cells. In addition, this is expressed on tumor-infiltrating lymphocytes (TILs) [26]. In humans, LAG-3 is situated in chromosome 12 (12p13.32), while in mice it lies in chromosome 6 encoding a 498-amino acid protein [27]. LAG-3 locus and CD-4 co-receptor-encoding gene are adjacent to each other with similar exon/intron architecture which indicate strongly that LAG-3 and CD4 genes have evolved from a preexisting common evolutionary ancestor IgSF domain encoding gene [27]. It is surprising that, unlike other checkpoint molecules that become a hindrance for activated T cell proliferation, T cells lacking LAG-3 precisely show defect expansion. This was observed *in vitro.* Given that LAG-3 has relatively a higher affinity for MHC class II than that of CD4, hence if LAG-3 is present, theoretically CD4:MHC class II complex is perturbed. However, this was not observed by an experiment by Workman and Vignali where a set of transgenic mice carrying a knockout mutation of LAG-3 were pre-crossed with OT-II-TCR mice [28]. The OT-II-TCR is defined as MHC class II-restricted TCR that responds to residues 323–339 of chicken ovalbumin [29]. Workman and Vignali figured out that LAG-3 did not interfere CD4:MHC class II interaction. This seems to oppose previous finding by Huard and colleagues a decade earlier where human LAG-3:Ig fusion proteins were shown to be disrupting CD4:MHC class II interaction although not in a CD4:MHC class II-dependent manner [30]. Discrepancy of these results probably caused by spatial separation between LAG-3 and CD4 in the immunological synapse which might not restrict the function of the soluble LAG-3:Ig fusion protein. Non-overlapping binding sites on MHC class II molecules by LAG-3 and CD4 might as well contributed to the limitedly disturbed CD4:MHC class II interplay in the presence of LAG-3. Or alternatively, it was due to subtle binding and function mode differences in murine and human [28].

As a homolog of CD4, LAG-3 binds non polymorphic MHC class II [26] that leads to the negative regulation of T lymphocytes activation and homeostasis. This checkpoint molecule has a direct role in maintaining the tolerogenic state of CD8+ T cells *in vivo* [31]. In the genetic level, LAG-3 and CD4 share similarity in less than 20%. However, both demonstrate a striking similarity structurally [32]. CD4 and LAG-3 belong to a distinct class of immunoglobulin super family- (IgSF-) related protein with four extracellular Ig-like domains and tryptophan (W) x cystein (C) signature motif in domain 2 and domain 4 [26]. Differ to that of CD4, the interaction of LAG-3 and MHC class II is initiated is mediated via proline-rich, 30 amino acid loop in D1 (motif domain). Other than this, LAG-3 has a longer connecting peptide spanning the fourth Ig domain and the transmembrane region because of which LAG-3 is susceptible to cell surface shedding by disintegrin and metalloproteinase domain containing protein (ADAM) [27]. LAG-3 function is activated through a conserved KIEELE motif in its cytoplasmic domain. Hence lacking of this motif leads to negative regulatory function and reverse negative modulation on the T cells [28].

### 3.2 Signaling pathway of LAG-3

LAG-3 expression is induced by activation of either TCR or various cytokines particularly interleukin-12 (IL-12). On the other hand, its transcription is regulated by interplay of inducing and regulating elements including transcription factor binding sites. There have been several transcription factors, reported to have inductive effects to LAG-3 expression, such as thymocyte selection-associated high mobility group box protein (TOX), nuclear factor of activated T cells (NFAT) [33], and nuclear receptor subfamily 4 group A (NR4A) [34]. In contrast, T-box transcription factor (T-bet) is inversely correlated with LAG-3 and leads to cytotoxic T cell differentiation. Thereby, it is a critical transcription factor in regulating immune exhaustion. However, the correlation between T-bet and LAG-3 is bidirectional. Deletion of either T-bet or LAG-3 enhances the expression of the other which suggests that LAG either promotes T cell exhaustion or vice versa [34]. LAG-3 interferes TCR:CD3 complex on the T cell surface; hence, TCR signal transduction is perturbed. As a result, cell proliferation as well as CD3-induced cytokine production are terminated. LAG-3 and CD3 engagement in the immunological synapse down-modulates TCR signal transduction which results in inhibition of TCR:CD3-dependent intracellular calcium fluxes to ultimately halt T cell responses [35].

### 3.3 LAG-3 inhibitor cancer therapy

Britstol Myers Squibb [36]. Bristol Myers Squibb has formulated opdualag which consists of anti-LAG-3 mAb relatlimab with Opdivo (nivolumab) for the first-line treatment for metastatic or unresectable melanoma [37]. It was previously reported that combination therapy of relatlimab and nivolumab increased PFS to 10.1 months compared with nivolumab monotherapy that shows PFS of 4.6 months only. Furthermore, 36% of patients treated with nivolumab monotherapy showed PFS of 12 months while in relatlimab combined with nivolumab, PFS was 47.7% [38]. In addition to this, Novartis has formulated a combination therapy targeting PD-1 and LAG-3, known as spartalizumab +LAG-525. It is now in a Phase II clinical trials to evaluate its role in unresectable or metastatic disease [39].

Tebolimab, manufactured by Macrogenic, is one of the first in class bispecific antibodies which is now undergoing Phase I clinical trials. This is composed of antigen binding fragments (Fab) targeting LAG-3 and PD-1. Pieris formulated PRS-332 which had two Fab regions targeting PD-1 and engineered lipocalins (anticalins) which was designed to target LAG-3. Similarly, F-star Therapeutics produced antibody FS118 that harbored a Fab targeting LAG-3 in its constant region and withPD-L1 targeting domains [34].

Although not all of these are approved yet, but various platforms that are offered to put more volumes in LAG-3-based cancer immunotherapy indicates that the pertinent checkpoint is clinically pivotal in cancers and hence an excellent target for therapy.

## 4. Programmed Death-1 (PD-1)

### 4.1 General description

PD-1 gene was first identified in two different types of lymphoid cell lines be that 2B4.11 (a murine T cell hybridoma) and LyD9 (a murine hematopoietic progenitor cell line) following manipulations using ionomycin/phorbol 12-myristate 13-acetate (PMA) and IL-3-deprivation, respectively. Given the two cell lines shared the same feature in common that was programmed cell death, it was plausible that PD-1 was a player in the death-inducing process in the two manipulated cell lines. In addition, in mRNA level PD-1 was deemed to be one of the molecules whose *de novo* synthesis induced death in the two cell lines. Owing to its patterns in death-increasing manipulation-induced augmentation as well as in thymus-restricted expression, PD-1 is enforced as a cell-death-associated gene [40].

PD-1 as a checkpoint molecule is a 55 kDa transmembrane protein consisting of 288 amino acids with a membrane-permeating domain, an extracellular N-terminal domain (IgV-like) and a cytoplasmic tail at N and C ends [41] containing two tyrosine-based signaling motifs, tyrosine-based inhibitory motif (ITIM), and an immunoreceptor tyrosine-based switch motif (ITSM) [42]. This is expressed on B cells, T cells, natural killer T (NKT) cells, activated dendritic cells (DCs), and monocytes. In resting T cells, PD-1 is not expressed, but this can be induced. In normal human lymphoid tissue, PD-1 is expressed on germinal center-associated T cells [43]. PD-1 can be both beneficial and harmful. In the context of physiological condition, PD-1 reduces ineffective immune responses and maintains immune tolerance, to prevent autoimmune reactions [44]. As oppose, the expression of this checkpoint molecule in a tumor microenvironment (TME) mediates dilation of malignant cells and silence of the immune surveillance. Therefore, blocking interaction of PD-1 and its ligands either PD-L1or PD-L2 was deemed to potentially augment endogenous antitumor responses [45].

### 4.2 Signaling pathway of PD-1 in cancers

The primary ligand of PD-1 is PD-L1 that is also known as CD279 or B7-H. This ligand is a 290 amino acid-containing 33 kDa type I transmembrane glycoprotein with Ig and IgC domains in its extracellular region [46]. PD-L1 is not only a ligand, but it also carries receptor functions. PD-1 could act as a ligand to mediate transmission of antiapoptotic signal to tumor cells via PD-L1. The second known counter receptor of PD-1 is PD-L2 or B7-DC which binds with RGMb (repulsive guidance molecule b). This interaction leads to induction of pulmonary tolerance [47].

PD-L1 is expressed by tumor cells as an immune escape strategy [48]. It is associated with production of Th1 cytokines and interferons. It has been demonstrated that IFN-γ causes PD-L1 upregulation in ovarian cancer cells, whereas the inhibition of this interferon leads to reduction of PD-L1 expression in acute myeloid leukemia in mouse models. Both have been reported to take mitogen-activated protein kinase kinase (MEK/extracellular signal-regulated kinase (ERK)) and MYD88/TRAF6 pathways [49].

The PD-L1 secreted-IFN-γ subsequently induces protein kinase D isoform 2 (PKD2); thus, inhibition of this PKD2 activity inhibits the expression PD-L1. NK and T cells produce IFN-γ via Janus Kinase (JAK)1, JAK2, and signal transducer and activator of transcription (STAT)1 pathways, to ultimately upregulate PD-L1 expression on the tumor cells' membranes [50]. PD-L1, therefore, acts as a pro-tumorigenic factor in cancer cells via binding to its receptors and activating proliferative and survival signaling pathways. This finding further indicates that PD-L1 is implicated in subsequent tumor progression. In addition, PD-L1 has been shown to exert nonimmune proliferative effects on a variety of tumor cell types [41]. These are the basis of PD-1/PD-L1 blocking antibody development, which is intended for downregulating these expressions, to allow functional immune cells to perform robust tumor surveillance [51].

### 4.3 PD-1/PD-L1 in cancer immunotherapy

When a T cell recognizes antigen:MHC complex, expressed on the surface of the target cell, inflammatory process begins which is marked by the secretion of inflammatory cytokines that subsequently induces the expression of PD Ligand-1 (PD-L1) in the affected tissue. This PD-L1 activates secretion of PD-1 protein on the T cells which causes immune tolerance, an event where the immune system is no longer capable of mounting an inflammatory response even in the presence of antigen [52].

In the tumor microenvironment (TME), PD-1 and its ligand PD-L1 play a fundamental role in tumor progression and survival by escaping immune surveillance. As aforementioned, while PD-1 is expressed on various subsets of immune cells, PD-L1 is expressed on tumor cells and APCs. Upon their engagement, T cells become dysfunctional and exhausted. Moreover, interleukin-10 (IL-10) is produced largely in the tumor [53]. This is known as the cytokine synthesis inhibitory factor which inhibits the productions of diverse pro-inflammatory cytokines including IL-1α, IL-1β, IL-6, IL-8, IL-12, IL-18, tumor necrosis factor-α (TNF-α), and granulocyte macrophage-colony-stimulating factor (GMSF) in T cells as well as in macrophages. Moreover, IL-10 diminishes the expression of interferon-γ (IFN- γ) in T helper (Th) cells and peripheral blood mononuclear cells (PBMCs). On the other hand, cytokines stimulate proliferation of mast cells [54], a particular subset of tissue-resident myeloid cells that contain coarse granules of inflammatory mediators like histamine that contribute to shaping of tumor cells and tumor microenvironment (TME) [55]. Foxp3+ CD4+ Tregs have recently been observed to maintain PD-1 expression on their surfaces in order to create a highly immunosuppressive TME [44]. The FDA-approved PD-1/PD-L1-based immune checkpoint inhibitor therapy apparently outnumbers CTLA-4. Like CTLA-4, PD-1/PD-L1 checkpoint can be administered as monotherapy or combination with CTLA-4 [56].

Nivolumab and pembrolizumab are antibodies designed to block binding of PD-1 to its ligands. First approval for nivolumab with brand name Opdivo was in December 2014 when nivolumab was evidently great for treating unresectable metastatic melanoma. Few months later, again nivolumab was approved to be harnessed to treat NSCLC which resulted in 23.7% of objective response rate (ORR) and 91 days of progression-free survival (PFS) [57]. It was also used for treating Hodgkin's lymphoma patients for which overall survival (OS) was observed at 3 years for 80% patients with median PFS between 12 and 18 months [58]. As nivolumab, pembrolizumab with brand name Keytruda was initially approved in 2014 for metastatic melanoma. The ORR obtained in this treatment was at 18%. In May 2017, it received its second approval for its use in locally advanced or metastatic urothelial carcinoma. In non-Hodgkin's lymphoma and head and neck squamous cell carcinoma (HNSCC), treatment using pembrolizumab resulted in ORR of 53% and 19%, respectively [51]. The other FDA-approved anti-PD-1 antibody is Cemiplimab, also known as Libtayo, which is the first checkpoint designed for advanced cutaneous squamous cell carcinoma (CSCC). It was shown that the effects of Cemiplimab was durable, and no recurrence was observed even after more than 16 months [59].

As anti-PD-L1 antibodies, Atezolimumab (Tecentriq), Avelumab (Bavencio), and Durvulumab (Imfinzi) were also approved for cancer type targets. Atezolimumab is widely used for urothelial carcinoma [60, 61] and differs to the other two as it is a phage-derived human IgG1, whereas Avelumab and Durvulumab are fully human anti-PD-L1-IgG1 [51]. Avelumab is used to treat patients with metastatic Merkel cell carcinoma and NSCLC with ORR values of 62.1% and 12%, respectively [62, 63]. Durvulumab is designed to directly target PD-L1, to prevent tumor immune escape and enhance immune responses. In head and neck squamous cell carcinoma (HNSCC) ORR of 9.2% was observed. Moreover, 6-month progression-free in HNSCC patients rose to 25% for those patients who were PD-L1+ [64]. For NSCLC patient cohort, the ORR was observed at 66.3% [65].

## 5. T Cell Immunoreceptor with Immunoglobulin and ITIM Domain (TIGIT)

### 5.1 General description

TIGIT, also known as V-set and transmembrane domain containing (Vstm), *Washington University cell adhesion molecule* (wucam) or *V-set and immunoglobulin domain-containing protein 9* (VSIG9), is a receptor of the Ig superfamily. It is an important player in adaptive as well as innate immunity regulation [66]. TIGIT is expressed on activated T cells, both in $T_H$ and CTL subsets, NK cells, Tregs, and follicular $T_H$ [67]. In cancer, TIGIT is often co-expressed with PD-1 on tumor-antigen-specific CD8+ T cells and C8+ tumor-infiltrating lymphocytes (TILs) in human and mice [68]. In addition, it is co-expressed with Tim-3 and LAG-3 on exhausted CTLs in tumors [66]. When homozygously knocked out, TIGIT -/- mice do not develop autoimmunity. But when compared with wild-type mice, TIGIT -/- mice suffer severe autoimmune encephalitis, after immunized with myelin oligodendrocyte glycoprotein. This supports the role of TIGIT as a negative regulator of T cell functions [69].

Structurally, TIGIT is composed of an extracellular immunoglobulin variable domain, a type I transmembrane domain, a short intracellular domain encompassing one immunoreceptor tyrosine-based inhibitory motif (ITIM) and one immunoglobulin tyrosine tail (ITT)-like motif. The immunoglobulin variable domain and members of poliovirus receptor (PVR)-like family such as DNAM-1, CD96, CD155, CD111, CD112 (PVR-related 2 (PVRL2), nectin-2, CD113 (poliovirus receptor-related 3 (PVRL3), nectin-3), and PVRL4 share sequence homology in common [70].

### 5.2 TIGIT signaling pathways

TIGIT has three ligands namely CD155, CD112, and CD113. These ligands belong to nectin and nectin-like (NECL) molecules that mediate cell adhesion, cell polarization, and tissue organization [71]. Among these, CD155 is the main receptor for TIGIT. Both homodimerize and upon engagement form heterotetramers. CD155 is mainly expressed on dendritic cells (DCs), T cells, B cells, and macrophages but also in non-haematopoietic tissues [72]. Following the ligation of TIGIT:CD155, inhibitory signaling is initiated via ITT-like motif. Amino acid tyrosine at position of 225 (tyr225) of the ITT-like motif is phosphorylated and coupled onto cytosolic adapter of growth factor receptor-bound protein 2 (Grb2) and β-arrestin 2 to facilitate recruitment of Src homology-2 (SH2)-containing inositol phosphatase-1 (SHP-1). This recruitment thwarts phosphoinositide 3 kinase and mitogen-activated protein kinase signaling, thus reducing killing capacity in NK cells [73]. SHIP-1 also impairs TRAF6 and nuclear factor ₭ light-chain-enhancer of activated B cells (NF-₭B) which impedes production of IFN-γ by NK cells [74].

Other than CD155 as the highest binding magnitude ligand, CD112 and CD113 are also reported to bind well to TIGIT, but at lesser magnitude . While CD112 shows a broad range of expression in both hematopoietic and non-hematopoietic tissues, CD113 is restricted to non-hematopoietic tissues. Their overexpression is observed in in several malignancies [70]. CD112R has recently been found as a receptor for CD112 other than TIGIT. It was reported that the combined CD112R and TIGIT blockade allowed diffusion of CD4+ T cells and increased the productions of cytokines such as IFN-γ, IL-2, IL-5, IL-10, and IL-13. Moreover, blockade to these two checkpoints led to restored cytotoxicity and expansion of CD8+ T cells [75].

### 5.3 TIGIT's bright future in cancer immunotherapy

TIGIT is relatively new discovered checkpoint molecule that seems to be a promising target in immune checkpoint-based cancer immunotherapy. This checkpoint was evidently shown to prevent tumor antigen release by CD8+ T cells and impair T cell priming by DCs or obstruct cancer cells killing by CD8+ T cells. And it is now under investigation in various clinical trials [72].

Recently, six human-anti-TIGIT monoclonal antibodies (mAbs) of the IgG1 isotype are being investigated in clinical trials. OncoMed Pharmaceuticals (US) produced Etigilimab (OMP-313M32). The mouse version of this 313R12 mAb was reported to function similar to etigilimab, i.e. suppression of syngeneic colon and kidney tumors in immune competent mice and improved $T_H1$-type response. Now, etigilimab commences its pharmacokinetics assessment in a Phase I trial. Furthermore,

Arcus Bioscience's AB154 and Merck's MK-7684 drugs, which are designed as monotherapy for advanced solid cancers and solid cancers, respectively, are in Phase 1 trials. Merck's MK-7684 is also being tested in combination with pembrolizumab (anti PD-1 mAb). Tiragolumab by Genentech/Roche is also in Phase II trial designed as combination therapy with atezolumab (anti-PD-1 mAb) for advanced or metastatic non-small cell lung cancer (NSCLC). Bristol-Myers Squibb bulks up the trials for TIGIT by producing BMS-986207 which is IgG1 mAb (FcγR-null) anti-TIGIT to target advanced or metastatic solid cancers. The Fc portion on the IgG of this mAb has been mutated to avoid ligating to Fcγ receptor (FcγR) because Fcγ-dependent mechanisms were found to inhibit antitumor activity of anti-PD-1 mAbs. With similar strategy (IgG1 mAb and FcyR-null), Astellas Pharma (Potenza Therapeutics) has also designed ASP 8374 [72].

## 6. Conclusions

Immune checkpoint molecules are promising for cancer immunotherapy. Each has specific structure and specific ligands that can be engineered in such a way that immune-suppressing activity is redirected into immune-activating activity either as monotherapy or in combination with other checkpoints to help in tumor growth reduction. PD-1 and CTLA-4 are the two most common checkpoints with FDA approvals for several cancers, years ahead of other checkpoints. TIGIT and LAG-3 are also known to show promising potential in cancer immunotherapy. As in the context of cancer immunity, immune checkpoint molecules favor cancers by facilitating mechanisms that may support cancer growth or help to negate the effects of checkpoint molecules via inhibitory mechanisms. Combination of checkpoint molecules has also been shown to outperform single checkpoint therapy. However, immune checkpoint-based immunotherapy requires proper monitoring and management for adverse effects and exudes minimum risk to patients.

## Author details

Ika Nurlaila
Research Center for Vaccine and Drugs, The National Research and Innovation Agency (BRIN), South Tangerang, Indonesia

*Address all correspondence to: ika.nurlaila@brin.go.id

## References

[1] Twomey JD, Zhang B. Cancer immunotherapy update: FDA-approved checkpoint inhibitors and companion diagnostics. The AAPS Journal. 7 Mar 2021;**23**(2):39. DOI: 10.1208/s12248-021-00574-0. PMID: 33677681; PMCID: PMC7937597

[2] Kuo AS, Dusan H, Aldrich JM. Critical care anesthesiology. In: Gropper MA, Miller RD, Cohen NH, Eriksson LI, Anesthesia M, Chapter B, et al., editors. Miller's Anesthesia [Internet]. 9th ed. California, USA: Elsevier, Inc.; 2020. pp. 2654-2670. Available from: https://www.clinicalkey.com/#!/content/book/3-s2.0-B9780323596046000833

[3] Fellner C. Ipilimumab (yervoy) prolongs survival in advanced melanoma: Serious side effects and a hefty price tag may limit its use. Pharmacy and Therapeutics. 2012;**37**(9):503-530

[4] He X, Xu C. Immune checkpoint signaling and cancer immunotherapy. Cell Research. 2020;**30**(8):660-669

[5] Ribas A, Wolchok JD. Cancer immunotherapy using checkpoint blockade. Science. 2018;**359**(6382):1350-1355

[6] Wu X, Gu Z, Chen Y, Chen B, Chen W, Weng L, et al. Application of PD-1 blockade in cancer immunotherapy. Computational and Structural Biotechnology Journal. 2019;**17**:661-674

[7] Kareva I. Cancer as a systemic disease that requires a systemic approach. In: Underst Cancer from a System Biological Point View. 2018. pp. 79-90

[8] Seidel JA, Otsuka A, Kabashima K. Anti-PD-1 and anti-CTLA-4 therapies in cancer: Mechanisms of action, efficacy, and limitations. Frontiers in Oncology. 2018;**8**(March):1-14

[9] Wherry EJ, Kurachi M. Molecular and cellular insights into T cell exhaustion. Nature Reviews. Immunology. 2015;**15**(8):486-499

[10] Peggs KS, Quezada SA, Chambers CA, Korman AJ, Allison JP. Blockade of CTLA-4 on both effector and regulatory T cell compartments contributes to the antitumor activity of anti-CTLA-4 antibodies. The Journal of Experimental Medicine. 2009;**206**(8):1717-1725

[11] Savoia P, Astrua C, Fava P. Ipilimumab (Anti-Ctla-4 Mab) in the treatment of metastatic melanoma: Effectiveness and toxicity management. Human Vaccines & Immunotherapeutics. 2016;**12**(5):1092-1101

[12] Engelhardt JJ, Sullivan TJ, Allison JP. CTLA-4 overexpression inhibits T cell responses through a CD28-B7-dependent mechanism. Journal of Immunology. 2006;**177**(2):1052

[13] Brzostek J, Gascoigne NRJ, Rybakin V. Cell type-specific regulation of immunological synapse dynamics by B7 ligand recognition. Frontiers in Immunology. 2016;7(Feb):1

[14] Grosso JF, Jure-Kunkel MN. CTLA-4 blockade in tumor models: An overview of preclinical and translational research. Cancer Immunity. 2013;**13**:5

[15] Callahan MK, Wolchok JD. At the bedside: CTLA-4- and PD-1-blocking antibodies in cancer immunotherapy. Journal of Leukocyte Biology. 2013;**94**(1):41-53

[16] Pardoll DM. The blockade of immune checkpoints in cancer immunotherapy. Nature Reviews. Cancer. 2016;**12**(4):252-264

[17] Leach DR, Krummel MF, Allison JP. Enhancement of antitumor immunity by CTLA-4 blockade. Science. 1996;**271**(5256):1734-1736

[18] Beyersdorf N, Kerkau T, Hünig T. CD28 co-stimulation in T-cell homeostasis: A recent perspective. ImmunoTargets Theraphy. 2015;**4**:111

[19] Sobhani N, Tardiel-Cyril DR, Davtyan A, Generali D, Roudi R, Li Y. CTLA-4 in regulatory T cells for cancer immunotherapy. Cancers (Basel). 22 Mar 2021;**13**(6):1440. DOI: 10.3390/cancers13061440. PMID: 33809974; PMCID: PMC8005092

[20] deLeeuw RJ, Kroeger DR, Kost SE, Chang P-P, Webb JR, Nelson BH. CD25 identifies a subset of CD4+FoxP3− TIL that are exhausted yet prognostically favorable in human ovarian cancer. Cancer Immunology Research. 2015;**3**(3):245-253

[21] Du X, Tang F, Liu M, Su J, Zhang Y, Wu W, et al. A reappraisal of CTLA-4 checkpoint blockade in cancer immunotherapy. Cell Research. 2018;**28**(4):416-432

[22] Wolchok JD, Hoos A, Day SO, Weber JS, Hamid O, Lebbé C, et al. Guidelines for the evaluation of immune therapy activity in solid tumors: Immune-related response criteria. Clinical Cancer Research. 2009;**15**(23):7412-7420

[23] Tang L, Wang J, Lin N, Zhou Y, He W, Liu J, et al. Immune checkpoint inhibitor-associated colitis: From mechanism to management. Frontiers in Immunology. 2021;**12**:800879

[24] Brahmer JR, Lacchetti C, Schneider BJ, Atkins MB, Brassil KJ, Caterino JM, et al. Management of immune-related adverse events in patients treated with immune checkpoint inhibitor therapy: American Society of Clinical Oncology Clinical Practice Guideline. Journal of Clinical Oncology: Official Journal of the American Society of Clinical Oncology. 2018;**36**(17):1714-1768

[25] Anti-CTLA4-NF mAb (BMS986218), Nivolumab, and Stereotactic Body Radiation Therapy for the Treatment of Metastatic Solid Malignancies [Internet]. clinicaltrials.gov. 2021. Available from: https://clinicaltrials.gov/ct2/show/NCT04785287

[26] Hannier S, Tournier M, Bismuth G, Triebel F. CD3/TCR complex-associated lymphocyte activation gene-3 molecules inhibit CD3/TCR signaling. Journal of Immunology. 1998;**161**(8):4058-4065

[27] Ruffo E, Wu RC, Bruno TC, Workman CJ, Vignali DAA. Lymphocyte-activation gene 3 (LAG3): The next immune checkpoint receptor. Seminars in Immunology. 2019;**42**:101305

[28] Workman CJ, Vignali DAA. The CD4-related molecule, LAG-3 (CD223), regulates the expansion of activated T cells. European Journal of Immunology. 2003;**33**(4):970-979

[29] Yang L, Qin XF, Baltimore D, Van Parijs L. Generation of functional antigen-specific T cells in defined genetic backgrounds by retrovirus-mediated expression of TCR cDNAS in hematopoietic precursor cells. Proceedings of the National Academy of Sciences of the United States of America. 2002;**99**(9):6204-6209

[30] Huard B, Prigent P, Tournier M, Bruniquel D, Triebel F. CD4/major

histocompatibility complex class II interaction analyzed with CD4- and lymphocyte activation gene-3 (LAG-3)-Ig fusion proteins. European Journal of Immunology. 1995;**25**(9):2718-2721

[31] Grosso JF, Goldberg MV, Getnet D, Bruno TC, Yen H-R, Pyle KJ, et al. Functionally distinct LAG-3 and PD-1 subsets on activated and chronically stimulated CD8 T cells. Journal of Immunology. 2009;**182**(11):6659-6669

[32] Workman CJ, Rice DS, Dugger KJ, Kurschner C, Vignali DAA. Phenotypic analysis of the murine CD4-related glycoprotein, CD223 (LAG-3). European Journal of Immunology. 2002;**32**(8):2255-2263

[33] Graydon CG, Mohideen S, Fowke KR. LAG3's enigmatic mechanism of action. Frontiers in Immunology. 2020;**11**:615317

[34] Lecocq Q, Keyaerts M, Devoogdt N, Breckpot K. The next-generation immune checkpoint LAG-3 and its therapeutic potential in oncology: Third time's a charm. International Journal of Molecular Sciences. 23 Dec 2020;**22**(1):75. DOI: 10.3390/ijms22010075. PMID: 33374804; PMCID: PMC7795594

[35] Chocarro L, Blanco E, Zuazo M, Arasanz H, Bocanegra A, Fernández-Rubio L, et al. Understanding LAG-3 signaling. International Journal of Molecular Sciences. 17 May 2021;**22**(10):5282. DOI: 10.3390/ijms22105282. PMID: 34067904; PMCID: PMC8156499

[36] Britstol Myers Squibb. U.S. Food and Drug Administration Approves First LAG-3-Blocking Antibody Combination, Opdualag™ (nivolumab and relatlimab-rmbw), as Treatment for Patients with Unresectable or Metastatic Melanoma news.bms.com. 2022. Available from: https://news.bms.com/news/details/2022/U.S.-Food-and-Drug-Administration-Approves-First-LAG-3-Blocking-Antibody-Combination-Opdualag-nivolumab-and-relatlimab-rmbw-as-Treatment-for-Patients-with-Unresectable-or-Metastatic-Melanoma/default.aspx. [Accessed: September 21, 2022]

[37] FDA approves anti-LAG3 checkpoint. Nature Biotechnolology. 2002;**40**(5):625

[38] Tawbi HA, Schadendorf D, Lipson EJ, Ascierto PA, Matamala L, Castillo Gutiérrez E, et al. Relatlimab and nivolumab versus nivolumab in untreated advanced melanoma. The New England Journal of Medicine. 2022;**386**(1):24-34

[39] Parra LM, Webster RM. The Malignant Melanoma Market. USA: Springer; 2022. pp. 489-490

[40] Ishida Y, Agata Y, Shibahara K, Honjo T. Induced expression of PD-1, a novel member of the immunoglobulin gene superfamily, upon programmed cell death. The EMBO Journal. 1992;**11**(11):3887-3895

[41] Han Y, Liu D, Li L. PD-1/PD-L1 pathway: Current researches in cancer. American Journal of Cancer Research. 2020;**10**(3):727-742

[42] Riella LV, Paterson AM, Sharpe AH, Chandraker A. Role of the PD-1 pathway in the immune response. American Journal of Transplantation. 2012;**12**(10):2575-2587

[43] Keir ME, Butte MJ, Freeman GJ, Sharpe AH. PD-1 and its ligands in tolerance and immunity. Annual Review of Immunology. 2008;**26**:677-704

[44] Francisco LM, Sage PT, Sharpe AH. The PD-1 pathway in tolerance and

autoimmunity. Immunological Reviews. 2010;**236**:219-242

[45] Salmaninejad A, Khoramshahi V, Azani A, Soltaninejad E, Aslani S, Zamani MR, et al. PD-1 and cancer: Molecular mechanisms and polymorphisms. Immunogenetics. 2018;**70**(2):73-86

[46] Sanmamed MF, Chen L. Inducible expression of B7-H1 (PD-L1) and its selective role in tumor site immune modulation. Cancer Journal. 2014;**20**(4):256-261

[47] Xiao Y, Yu S, Zhu B, Bedoret D, Bu X, Francisco LM, et al. RGMb is a novel binding partner for PD-L2 and its engagement with PD-L2 promotes respiratory tolerance. The Journal of Experimental Medicine. 2014;**211**(5):943-959

[48] Ohaegbulam KC, Assal A, Lazar-Molnar E, Yao Y, Zang X. Human cancer immunotherapy with antibodies to the PD-1 and PD-L1 pathway. Trends in Molecular Medicine. 2015;**21**(1):24-33

[49] Abiko K, Matsumura N, Hamanishi J, Horikawa N, Murakami R, Yamaguchi K, et al. IFN-γ from lymphocytes induces PD-L1 expression and promotes progression of ovarian cancer. British Journal of Cancer. 2015;**112**(9):1501-1509

[50] Chen J, Feng Y, Lu L, Wang H, Dai L, Li Y, et al. Interferon-γ-induced PD-L1 surface expression on human oral squamous carcinoma via PKD2 signal pathway. Immunobiology. 2012;**217**(4):385-393

[51] Jiang Y, Chen M, Nie H, Yuan Y. PD-1 and PD-L1 in cancer immunotherapy: Clinical implications and future considerations. Human Vaccines & Immunotherapeutics. 2019;**15**(5):1111-1122

[52] Alsaab HO, Sau S, Alzhrani R, Tatiparti K, Bhise K, Kashaw SK, et al. PD-1 and PD-L1 checkpoint signaling inhibition for cancer immunotherapy: Mechanism, combinations, and clinical outcome. Frontiers in Pharmacology. 2017;**8**:561

[53] Sun Z, Fourcade J, Pagliano O, Chauvin J-M, Sander C, Kirkwood JM, et al. IL10 and PD-1 cooperate to limit the activity of tumor-specific CD8+ T cells. Cancer Research. 2015;**75**(8):1635-1644

[54] Chang C-M, Lam HYP, Hsu H-J, Jiang S-J. Interleukin-10: A double-edged sword in breast cancer. Tzu chi Medical Journal. 2021;**33**(3):203-211

[55] Lichterman JN, Reddy SM. Mast cells: A new frontier for cancer immunotherapy. Cells. 21 May 2021;**10**(6):1270. DOI: 10.3390/cells10061270. PMID: 34063789; PMCID: PMC8223777

[56] Rotte A. Combination of CTLA-4 and PD-1 blockers for treatment of cancer. Journal of Experimental & Clinical Cancer Research. 2019;**38**(1):255

[57] Sato K, Akamatsu H, Murakami E, Sasaki S, Kanai K, Hayata A, et al. Correlation between immune-related adverse events and efficacy in non-small cell lung cancer treated with nivolumab. Lung Cancer. 2018;**115**:71-74

[58] Goldkuhle M, Dimaki M, Gartlehner G, Monsef I, Dahm P, Glossmann J-P, et al. Nivolumab for adults with Hodgkin's lymphoma (a rapid review using the software RobotReviewer). Cochrane Database of Systematic Reviews. 2018;7(7):CD012556

[59] Migden MR, Khushalani NI, Chang ALS, Lewis KD, Schmults CD,

Hernandez-Aya L, et al. Cemiplimab in locally advanced cutaneous squamous cell carcinoma: Results from an open-label, phase 2, single-arm trial. The Lancet Oncology. 2020;**21**(2):294-305

[60] Rosenberg JE, Hoffman-Censits J, Powles T, van der Heijden MS, Balar AV, Necchi A, et al. Atezolizumab in patients with locally advanced and metastatic urothelial carcinoma who have progressed following treatment with platinum-based chemotherapy: A single-arm, multicentre, phase 2 trial. Lancet (London, England). 2016;**387**(10031):1909-1920

[61] Ning Y-M, Suzman D, Maher VE, Zhang L, Tang S, Ricks T, et al. FDA Approval Summary: Atezolizumab for the treatment of patients with progressive advanced urothelial carcinoma after platinum-containing chemotherapy. The Oncologist. 2017;**22**(6):743-749

[62] Marciscano AE, Gulley JL, Kaufman HL. Avelumab: Is it time to get excited? Expert Review of Anticancer Therapy. 2018;**18**:815-821

[63] Walker JW, Lebbé C, Grignani G, Nathan P, Dirix L, Fenig E, et al. Efficacy and safety of avelumab treatment in patients with metastatic Merkel cell carcinoma: Experience from a global expanded access program. Journal of Immunotheraphy Cancer. Apr 2020;**8**(1):e000313. DOI: 10.1136/jitc-2019-000313. Erratum in: Journal of Immunotheraphy Cancer. May 2020;**8**(1): PMID: 32269140; PMCID: PMC7252959

[64] Zandberg DP, Algazi AP, Jimeno A, Good JS, Fayette J, Bouganim N, et al. Durvalumab for recurrent or metastatic head and neck squamous cell carcinoma: Results from a single-arm, phase II study in patients with ≥25% tumour cell PD-L1 expression who have progressed on platinum-based chemotherapy. European Journal of Cancer. 2019;**107**:142-152

[65] Botticella A, Mezquita L, Le Pechoux C, Planchard D. Durvalumab for stage III non-small-cell lung cancer patients: Clinical evidence and real-world experience. Therapeutic Advances in Respiratory Disease. 2019;**13**:175

[66] Chauvin JM, Zarour HM. TIGIT in cancer immunotherapy. Journal of Immunotheraphy Cancer. Sep 2020;**8**(2):e000957. DOI: 10.1136/jitc-2020-000957. PMID: 32900861; PMCID: PMC7477968

[67] Shibuya K, Shirakawa J, Kameyama T, Honda S, Tahara-Hanaoka S, Miyamoto A, et al. CD226 (DNAM-1) is involved in lymphocyte function-associated antigen 1 costimulatory signal for naive T cell differentiation and proliferation. The Journal of Experimental Medicine. 15 Dec 2003;**198**(12):1829-1839. DOI: 10.1084/jem.20030958. PMID: 14676297; PMCID: PMC2194159

[68] Chauvin J-M, Pagliano O, Fourcade J, Sun Z, Wang H, Sander C, et al. TIGIT and PD-1 impair tumor antigen-specific CD8⁺ T cells in melanoma patients. The Journal of Clinical Investigation. 2015;**125**(5):2046-2058

[69] Levin SD, Taft DW, Brandt CS, Bucher C, Howard ED, Chadwick EM, et al. Vstm3 is a member of the CD28 family and an important modulator of T-cell function. European Journal of Immunology. 2011;**41**(4):902-915

[70] Sanchez-Correa B, Valhondo I, Hassouneh F, Lopez-Sejas N, Pera A, Bergua JM, et al. DNAM-1 and the TIGIT/PVRIG/TACTILE Axis: Novel immune checkpoints for natural killer cell-based cancer immunotherapy. Cancers (Basel). 2019;**11**(6)

[71] Lupo KB, Matosevic S. CD155 immunoregulation as a target for natural killer cell immunotherapy in glioblastoma. Journal of Hematology & Oncology. 2020;**13**:76. DOI: 10.1186/s13045-020-00913-2

[72] Harjunpää H, Guillerey C. TIGIT as an emerging immune checkpoint. Clinical and Experimental Immunology. 2020;**200**(2):108-119

[73] Liu S, Zhang H, Li M, Hu D, Li C, Ge B, et al. Recruitment of Grb2 and SHIP1 by the ITT-like motif of TIGIT suppresses granule polarization and cytotoxicity of NK cells. Cell Death and Differentiation. 2013;**20**(3):456-464

[74] Li M, Xia P, Du Y, Liu S, Huang G, Chen J, et al. T-cell immunoglobulin and ITIM domain (TIGIT) receptor/poliovirus receptor (PVR) ligand engagement suppresses interferon-γ production of natural killer cells via β-arrestin 2-mediated negative signaling. The Journal of Biological Chemistry. 2014;**289**(25):17647-17657

[75] Zeng T, Cao Y, Jin T, et al. The CD112R/CD112 axis: A breakthrough in cancer immunotherapy. Journal of Experimental & Clinical Cancer Research. 2021;**40**:285. DOI: 10.1186/s13046-021-02053-y

Section 2

# Immune Checkpoints and Cancers

**Chapter 3**

# Immune Checkpoint Inhibitors Programmed Cell Death-1/ Programmed Cell Death-Ligand1 (PD-1/PD-L1) for Cancer Therapy

*Shaimaa M.M. Bebars*

## Abstract

Monoclonal antibodies that inhibit "immune checkpoint" through programmed cell death-1 and its ligand (PD-1/PD-L1) blockage have proven remarkable therapeutic action toward a range of cancer types. Hence, immunotherapy, binding the immune system to act against malignant tumors, has generated encouraging outcomes in clinical practice. Nevertheless, the robust advantage is not observed in a large number of patients. Recognizing patients that will probably respond and using therapies covering a larger number of patients necessitate an enhanced understanding of the biological action of PD-1 and cytotoxic T lymphocyte antigen (CTLA) at the cell level and reviewing the performed clinical studies and their outcomes to recognize the accumulating proof of its clinical significance. In this chapter, we will discuss and review the clinical and preclinical data regarding Immune Checkpoint Inhibitors PD-1/PD-L1 to recognize the advances and challenges of their implication in clinical practice.

**Keywords:** immune checkpoint, PD-1, PD-L1, target therapy, immunotherapy, resistance

## 1. Introduction

Twenty-two years ago, Freeman et al. were the first to introduce programmed cell death-1 and its ligand (PD-1/PD-L1) as an immune checkpoint that later on was the immune inhibitor target in cancer therapy. Generally, checkpoints play a role as a brake to slow down the immune function, and it was proposed that inhibition of these checkpoints may stimulate T cells and eradicate malignant cells more effectively [1, 2].

In immune regulation, CD4+ regulatory T cell's role is well recognized; they suppress autoimmunity and allergic reactions, on the other side, they enable cancer growth by inhibiting immunity against neoplasms [3, 4].

Immune evasion by cancer cells is mediated through acquiring mechanisms of resistance and escape including creating an environment of immunosuppression using immunosuppressive components such as molecules, cytokines of immune suppression type, and cells including CD4+ regulatory T cells to constrain active immunity against the tumor, thus endorsing tumor growth [4]. There is a suggestion of more malleability of the CD4+ regulatory T cell compartment expression with various aspects such as suppression function deactivation, inflammatory cytokines expression, and transcription reprogramming. Even though it is uncertain which element is responsible for CD4+ regulatory T cell malleability, there is probability that precise microenvironments have the inscription on CD4+ regulatory T cell destiny [5].

Numerous checkpoints of immune reaction have been established to bound the hyper-activation of immune cells involved in self-tolerance. One of the significant checkpoints is PD-1 and its ligands, PD-L1 and PD-L2 expressed mainly on the surface and in the body of lymphocytes, in antigen-presenting cells (APCs), and cancer cells and regulate responses toward antigens. Managing PD-1/PD-L actions facilitates the regulation of numerous immune-related disorders including infection, autoimmune disorders, and malignancies [6]. PD-L1 expression is related to microenvironment of T cells, cytokines produced by T cells of helper type, chemical mediators, interferons, and precise characters of gene expression. Continuous stimulation with an elevated level of PD-1 is frequently established in cancer inflammatory infiltrates mainly lymphocytes, as an expression of PD-L1 is utilized by neoplastic cells to escape immune damage. Blocking of these immune checkpoints is exploited to release the prospective of antagonistic therapy against cancer immune response as cancer treatment strategy [7].

Although there is a significant benefit in the outcome of patients attained with PD-L1/PD-1 blocking therapies, resistances are also commonly observed [8].

## 2. PD-1/PD-L1 immune checkpoint

Programmed cell death-1(PD-1/CD279) has two identified ligands, PD-L1 and 2 (CD274 and CD273 respectively), each with distinct expression patterns and regulations, of which PD-L1 is expressed in numerous cancers [9]. PD-1 is a transmembrane glycoprotein type 1 of the immunoglobulin superfamily, out of its total 288 amino acids, a 20% amino acid shows distinctiveness to cytotoxic T lymphocyte antigen 4 (CTLA4) and it is encoded by the PDCD1 gene on chromosome 2. PD-1 is formed of an extracellular domain of IgV-like and a transmembrane section. Its tyrosine-based switch motif (ITSM) and inhibitory motif tyrosine base are forming the tail which is located intracellularly. It was considered a CD28 receptor family member of T cells accessory molecules. Although PD-1 has similarities to the CD28 family, it shows distinctive properties distinguishing it from members of such family [10, 11].

PD-1 expression on effector T cells is mediated due to stimulation of the T cell receptor (TCR) and it plays a role as a receptor of immune inhibition. It binds the PD-L1 B7 homologs (B7-H1) and PD-L2 (B7-DC), existing mainly on APCs, and can be prompted in other tissues by cytokines of inflammation [1, 6]. PD-1 has a tendency concerning moderate local activation of T cells in tissues of the periphery. PD-1 may have delayed actions in the T cell activation and decay. Generally, PD-1/PD-L plays a significant role in sustaining T cell self-tolerance with the prevention of autoimmunity, and it reduces some anti-apoptotic molecules expression such as B-cell lymphoma-extra-large (BCL-XL) in addition to pro-inflammatory cytokines secretion [12, 13]. The inhibitory function of PD-1/PD-L1 is mediated primarily on effector T cells but also it acts on regulatory T cells by affecting phosphatidyl-inositol 3 kinase (PI3K) to control T cell autoimmunity and tolerance. In general, tolerance is the failure of T cells that may be manifested as ignorance (failure of activation), or "anergic" status (responding cells are persistent in a refractory status), or deletion (apoptosis of T cell) [3, 14].

PDCDL1 gene on chromosome 9 is responsible for PD-L1 coding in humans, PD-L1 a transmembrane protein type 1 was documented as a member of the family B7 protein. The length of PD-L1 is 290 amino acids of 40 kDa protein. PD-L1 consists of extracellular domains (IgV-like & IgC-like), a transmembrane domain (hydrophobic), and a 30 amino acids cytoplasmic tail. The PD-L1 constitutive expression can be detected at low levels, on inactive lymphocytes, APCs, and in syncytiotrophoblasts, corneal, endothelial, keratinocytes, and Langerhans' islet cells of the pancreas as it plays a role in inflammatory response tissue homeostasis and giving a state of "immune privileged", as the introduction of external antigens is tolerated with no immune or inflammatory response. PD-L1 is prompted as an inhibitory signal in inflammation acting upon immune, epithelial, and endothelial cells [15, 16].

Toll-like receptors (TLRs) in APCs affect PD-L1 expression through MEK/ERK (extracellular signal-regulated kinase) kinases activation, in addition to receptors of Interferon-gamma (IFN-γ) 1 & 2 via Jak (Janus kinase)/STAT (Signal transducer and activator of transcription)-mediated activation that can also influence MEK/ERK and PI3K/AKT pathway [17]. PD-1/PDL-1 ligation leads to SHP-1/SHP-2 recruitment to the ITSM with dephosphorylation of kinases e.g. CD3ζ, PKCθ, and ZAP70 leading to a general inhibition of T cell spreading out which results from PI3K-Akt and Ras-MEK-ERK cascade inhibition mostly through direct inactivation effect of PD-1of Ras &dephosphorylation of phospholipase Cγ [15, 18]. Dephosphorylation of Casein kinase 2 (CK-2), which is an SHP-2 target, causes uncontrolled activation of PTEN (PI3K-Akt signaling antagonist) [16, 17]. It was also suggested that CD28 receptor co-stimulation, maybe the main dephosphorylation target by SHP2 phosphatase [19]. PD-1/PD-L1 engagement modifies variable T cell activities including T cell proliferation deactivation, cytokine induction, survival, and other functions [20], the reaction between PI3K signaling and BCL-XL is a significant point of control where PD-1 inhibition of P13K decreases BCL-XL and endorses apoptosis [21] (**Figure 1**).

The PD-1/PD-L1 interaction is critical for immune tolerance development, whether central or peripheral in primary or secondary lymphoid tissue respectively [22]. PD-1/PD-L1 knock-out in animal experiments causes autoimmunity with glomerulonephritis lupus-like arthritis and diabetes. While in humans, using antibodies against PD-1/PD-L1 leads to immune-related disorders such as endocrinopathy, colitis, and dermatoses [23–25]. A principal feature of T cell exhaustion, which is a marked weakening of effector T cell function, embraces the generation of several co-inhibitory pathways such as PD-1/PD-L1. Such impairment could be detected through apoptosis or inhibition of T cell development or production of regulatory T cells [26, 27]. The role of PD-1/PD-L1 is manifested in cases of T cell exhaustion, not only in chronic infection but also in cancer state [28, 29].

The greatest documented evidence of this inhibitory role in human immunity is derived from the usage of mediators to block the PD-1/PD-L1 pathway, an important target for immunotherapy in malignancy. Nevertheless, PD-1–PD-L1 interaction inhibition in patients suffering from malignancy causes anticancer immunity activation and autoimmune symptoms known as immune-associated opposing incidents [30].

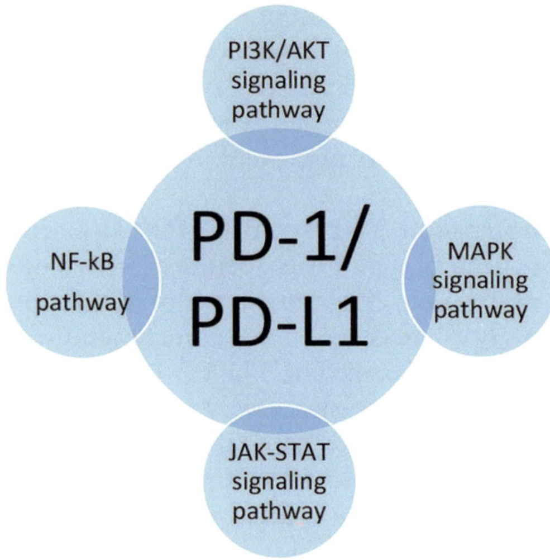


**Figure 1.**
*Activation pathways of PD-1/PD-L1 expression.*

## 3. PD-1/PD-L1 and cancer

### 3.1 PD-1/PD-L1 role in cancer

As PD-1/PD-L1 cardinal role is known in avoiding autoimmunity and preservation of normal peripheral tolerance, it is utilized by cancer cells in immune evasion eventually facilitating tumor growth, proliferation, and metastasis [6, 24].

Signaling of PD-1 in the tumor microenvironment, generated through interaction between cancer cells and non-transformed cells is an important player in the development and persistence of cancer through evasion of immune surveillance. PD-1 is markedly expressed in lymphocytes infiltrating a large number of cancers, also myeloid cells. While, PD-L1 is mainly conveyed on variable types of neoplastic cells such as melanoma, lung, renal and ovarian types. Moreover, PD-L1 expression can be up-regulated in different types of malignancy through carcinogenic signaling via aberrant PI3K-AKT activation or chromosomal amplifications and alterations, unrelated to inflammatory signaling in the microenvironment of malignancy [31–33].

Sometimes, PD-L1 expression is induced as a reaction to inflammation as an antitumor immune response via variable cytokines with IFN-γ being the most potent. IFN-γ causes PD-L1 activation and progression of ovarian neoplastic cells, while inhibition of IFN-γ receptor 1 can decrease PD-L1 expression in acute myeloid leukemia via the MEK/ERK and MYD88/TRAF6 pathways. Furthermore, IFN-γ prompts PKD2 (protein kinase D isoform 2), one of the PD-L1 regulator proteins. PD-L1 is also frequently expressed in cells of the microenvironment of tumors such as macrophages, dendritic cells, endothelial cells, and fibroblasts. PD-1/PD-L1 in tumor microenvironment endorses dysfunction and exhaustion of T cell, apoptosis, neutralization, and IL-10 secretion in a neoplastic mass generating resistance status against cancer cell destruction by a cytotoxic T cell (CD8+). Further infiltration by CD4+ regulatory T cells helps more suppression of effector immune response in tumors [31, 32].

The signaling of PD-L1 occurs via stimulation of PD-1which lead to pro-survival neoplastic signals induction helping anti-apoptotic effect via the cytoplasmic domain.

In addition, PD-L1 protects neoplastic cells from the IFNs (I & II) cytotoxicity and CTL cytolysis. Furthermore, targeting PD-L1 decreases the activity of mTOR and neoplastic cell glycolytic metabolism without T cells [31, 34, 35].

PD-L1 positivity or negativity in tumor cells can be achieved via variable biological processes. T cells infiltrating the malignant tumor may produce surface expression of PDL-1 which can be lost in absence of T cells. Also, genetic proceedings inside the neoplastic cells could prevent PD-L1 expression. Thus, the neoplastic cell surface expression or absence of PD-L1 may implicate diverse functional significances and treatment allegations according to the causal expression mechanism [36].

Immunohistochemical expression of PD-L1 in neoplastic tissues shows that PD-L1 positive immune reaction may appear membranous or cytoplasmic. Trans membranous structure of PD-L1 suggests that the positive immune reaction may be related to the binding of PD-L1 antibody to a specific domain. While the cytoplasmic reaction may be related to the translocation of receptors onto the surface as a part of the immune response [37–40].

Immunohistochemical expression of PD-L1 is still considered the merely broadly accessible, applicable, and cost-effective method for reviewing PD-L1 expression in cancer. Moreover, this method aids in recognizing patients who probably benefit from immunotherapy targeting PD-1/PD-L1. The FDA approval of such targeting therapy used trials depending on variable immunohistochemical platforms with different antibodies to evaluate PD-L1 expression on neoplastic cells, microenvironment immune cells, or both using specific scoring methods. These trials utilized particular PD-L1 inhibitors with particular assays and specific antibody reagents, thresholds, and protocols which should be standardized and validated. PD-L1 immunohistochemical procedure should be reproducible, both the staining technique and interpretation by pathologists which should be quality controlled starting from the tissue fixation and processing steps. Evolving applicable and reproducible scoring systems for PD-L1 is clinically important to identify patients who will probably benefit from targeted therapy. PD-L1 expression on both neoplastic and microenvironment immune cells has a greater association with clinical consequences in some neoplasms [41].

A recent systemic review and data analysis revealed the prognostic value of PD-L1. It shows high expression in solid malignancies which represents a bad prognostic feature regarding overall survival and progression-free survival [42]. The cytoplasmic expression and circulating tumor cells of PD-L1 were linked to better survival in thyroid carcinoma [43].

Blocking of PD-1 leads to suppression of transplanted myeloma cells growth in mice model while overexpressing PD-L1 in transplanted cells of mice model leads to the neoplastic establishment, load, and invasiveness which were reversed by using antibodies against PD-1/PD-L1. Thus, down-regulation of PD-1 and/or PD-L1 enriches T-cell activation against malignant cells which is the base for immunotherapy [33, 44].

### 3.2 PD-1/PD-L1 as a targeted therapy

Enhanced cancer suppression can be perceived when engaging different methodologies of PD-1/PD-L1 signaling disturbance, such as blocking using an antibody against PD-L1, DNA vaccination of PD-1 extracellular region, and injection of neoplasm-specific clones of T cells. The use of several immunotherapy approaches in combination may increase the therapeutic outcome [43–45].

The regulation of neoplastic cells' expression of PD-L1 includes signaling pathways (MAPK, PI3K/Akt), transcription factors (e.g., Hypoxia-Inducible Factor 1, STAT3, Nuclear Factor kappa B, Transforming Growth Factor beta, GATA-3, and T-bet), and epigenetic and micro RNAs regulation [11].

In clinical practice, blocking of PD-1/PD-L1 causes inhibition of immune checkpoints which provides long-term responses, and as such the blocking antibodies are approved to treat solid and hematologic neoplasms. As well, the cytoplasmic PD-L1 knockdown using particular RNAs could benefit tumor immunotherapy [46].

The PD-L1/PD-1 blocking antibodies are the mainstay of immunotherapy due to improved survival and their clinical effectiveness in various malignancies such as non-small cell lung carcinoma (NSCLC) [47, 48]. Neoplasms showing an increased capacity for mutation and antigenicity, e.g., high microsatellite instability (MSI) and mismatch repair deficiencies (dMMR) are good targets for PD-1 blocking therapies. Numerous elements play significant roles as a determinant of clinical response to blocking PD-L1/PD-1 pathway such as neoplasm mutation load densities of immune cells and tumor microenvironment types of cells, PD-1/PD-L1 level of expression, and cytokines [49, 50].

Immunotherapy is considered a safe treatment compared with other strategies such as chemotherapy, irradiation, and surgery, as the mechanism involves augmentation of self-immunity against malignancy. Moreover, as a checkpoint inhibitor, it is extremely precise to a targeted cell with fewer side effects and keeps antigenic memory of neoplasm. However, it has been observed that associated toxicities with PD-1 blocking antibodies is lower than the associated toxicity with other immunotherapies, e.g., CTLA-4 blocking agents [45, 47, 51–53].

PD-1/PD-L1-induced opposing events related to immunity are one of the disadvantages of this type of therapy. It can induce side effects related to immunity in different organs such as the endocrine, pancreas, skin, gastrointestinal tract, liver, and renal system. Furthermore, such antibodies induced lethal xenogeneic hypersensitivity reactions in an experimental model of breast cancer after repeated administration. It is worth mentioning that PD-1 blocking-related pneumonitis is a significant side event mostly observed in NSCLC patients. Other systemic side effects, e.g., cardiac arrhythmia and even heart failure due to myocarditis have also been reported [30, 54, 55]. Clinically, subcutaneous or intravenous route of administration in this type of therapy is considered as one of the drawbacks, especially with humble penetration of neoplastic tissue [56].

PD-1 blocking mediators are associated with increased rates of recurrence and progression of the disease, nevertheless, local therapy can produce long-term survival without progression in some of these patients [57]. PD-L1 expression is used as an authenticated and main biomarker for the prediction of therapy; still, this biomarker alone, due to tumor heterogeneity is considered insufficient for defining patients who can benefit from PD-1/PD-L1 blocking therapy. Then again, PDL-1 single nucleotide polymorphisms (genetic copy number gains) have been suggested to help predict treatment responders, [52, 58, 59], especially in lymphoma [60, 61]. This is because de-glycosylation of the natural heavily glycosylated surface PD-1 molecules by enzymes during immunohistochemistry increases antibody binding ability of anti-PD-L1, thus increasing the intensity of signals leading to better outcome prediction [62].

The prediction of patient response is an important issue in PD-1/PD-L1 blocking therapy as only one to two-thirds of patients show resistance to treatment due to heterogeneity [52, 63]. The absence of neoplastic antigens, neoantigens or gene mutations, dysfunction of T cell, expression of PD-L1 and tumor microenvironment, noncoding RNA, and gut microbiome are also underlying factors serving as mechanisms of resistance to PD-1/PD-L1 blocking treatment [64].

Furthermore, PD-1 blocking therapy is largely costing more than other immunotherapy treatments and original lines of treatment, especially in old patients with low income and there is a debate regarding the cost-benefit relationship in combined therapy [65]. Using such an immunotherapy line of treatment in patients with immune disease whether hyperactive or autoimmune or hypoactive or even deficient immunity is considered a challenge, particularly with the toxicity effect of such therapy [53, 66].

### 3.3 Improving the PD-1/PD-L1 blocking efficacy

The regulatory mechanisms and pathways of PD-L1 expression have been widely investigated to understand side effects and deficient responses in some patients. The combination approaches were introduced to concurrently enhance several cancer-immunity processes, eliminate brakes of immunosuppression, and coordinate an immune-enhanced neoplastic microenvironment [53, 67].

Combination lines of treatment, such as combining anti-PD-1/PD-L1 with radiotherapy, chemotherapy, other immune checkpoint inhibitors or targeted therapy, interferon genes agonists stimulator, transplantation/manipulation of microbiome, epigenetic or metabolic modulators may produce better treatment response. Furthermore, agents containing both PD-1 and PD-L1 targeting antibodies may also provoke a potent effect. Regulation of PD-L1 expression in the tumor microenvironment through medical treatment or regulation of genes expands the -PD-1/PD-L1 therapy effect [68–70].

Possible small-molecule mediators were suggested to be used for targeting PD-L1 which may help overcome the restrictions of monoclonal antibodies used in blocking PD-1/PD-L1. Preclinical investigations suggest that the combination of these small-molecule mediators with other immune checkpoints targeting agents may cause augmented antineoplastic action or use such small molecules to up-regulate PD-L1 and elevate the blocking efficacy [55, 71]. Moreover, prodrug nanoparticles conjugated with anti-PD-L1 peptide were suggested to be used to help inhibit neoplastic growth with minimum side events [72].

Other effective antineoplastic agents, e.g., antiangiogenic mediators, and immunogenic cell death inducers combined with immune checkpoint inhibitors may help as a preventive therapeutic method in improving blocking agents' efficacy [73, 74].

## 4. Conclusion

Taking into account the various potential strategies for successful PD-1/PD-L1 checkpoint inhibition such as blocking using antibodies against PD-L1, DNA vaccination of PD-1 extracellular region, injection of neoplasm-specific clones of T cell, with understanding mechanisms of action is important in clinical practice. A deep consideration of the mechanisms of resistance, whether cellular or molecular will benefit patients and improve therapeutic approaches. The combination approaches of immunotherapy or with other lines and strategies of therapy were introduced, also, small-molecule mediators and prodrug nanoparticle conjugation were suggested to be helpful in cases of anticipated resistance. The future perspective of combination therapy and investigation of predictive biomarkers will provide an important pathway for cancer patient care in cases treated with PD-1/PD-L1 checkpoint inhibition.

## Author details

Shaimaa M.M. Bebars
Faculty of Medicine Aswan University, Aswan, Egypt

*Address all correspondence to: bebars34@gmail.com; shaimaa_monir@aswu.edu.eg

## References

[1] Freeman GJ, Long AJ, Iwai Y, Bourque K, Chernova T, Nishimura H, et al. Engagement of the PD-1 immunoinhibitory receptor by a novel B7 family member leads to negative regulation of lymphocyte activation. The Journal of Experimental Medicine. 2000;**192**(7):1027-1034. DOI: 10.1084/jem.192.7.1027

[2] Ljunggren HG, Jonsson R, Hoglund P. Seminal immunologic discoveries with direct clinical implications: The 2018 nobel prize in physiology or medicine honours discoveries in cancer immunotherapy. Scandinavian Journal of Immunology. 2018;**88**:e12731. DOI: 10.1111/sji.12731

[3] Wing K, Sakaguchi S. Regulatory T cells exert checks and balances on self tolerance and autoimmunity. Nature Immunology. 2010;**11**(1):7-13. DOI: 10.1038/ni.1818

[4] Takeuchi Y, Nishikawa H. Roles of regulatory T cells in cancer immunity. International Immunology. 2016;**28**(8):401-409. DOI: 10.1093%2Fintimm%2Fdxw025

[5] Hatzioannou A, Boumpas A, Papadopoulou M, Papafragkos I, Varveri A, Alissafi T, et al. Regulatory T cells in autoimmunity and cancer: A duplicitous lifestyle. Frontiers in Immunology. 2021;**12**:731947. DOI: 10.3389/fimmu.2021.731947

[6] Nishikawa H, Sakaguchi S. Regulatory T cells in cancer immunotherapy. Current Opinion in Immunology. 2014;**27**:1-7. DOI: 10.1016/j.coi.2013.12.005

[7] Chamoto K, Al-Habsi M, Honjo T. Role of PD-1 in immunity and diseases. In: Akihiko Y, editor. Emerging Concepts Targeting Immune Checkpoints in Cancer and Autoimmunity. 2017. pp. 75-97. DOI: 10.1007/978-3-319-68929-6

[8] Pardoll D. The blockade of immune checkpoints in cancer immunotherapy. Nature Reviews. Cancer. 2012;**12**:252-264. DOI: 10.1038/nrc3239

[9] Hudson K, Cross N, Jordan-Mahy N, Leyland R. The extrinsic and intrinsic roles of PD-L1 and its receptor PD-1: Implications for immunotherapy treatment. Frontiers in Immunology. 2020;**2362**:568931. DOI: 10.3389/fimmu.2020.568931

[10] Dong H, Strome SE, Salomao DR, Tamura H, Hirano F, Flies DB, et al. Tumor-associated B7-H1 promotes T-cell apoptosis: a potential mechanism of immune evasion. Nature Medicine. 2002;**8**:793-800. DOI: 10.1038/nm730

[11] Carreno BM, Collins M. The B7 family of ligands and its receptors: New pathways of costimulation and inhibition of immune responses. Annual Review of Immunology. 2002;**20**:29. DOI: 10.1146/annurev.immunol.20.091101.091806

[12] Dermani FK, Samadi P, Rahmani G, Kohlan AK, Najafi R. PD-1/PD-L1 immune checkpoint: Potential target for cancer therapy. Journal of Cellular Physiology. 2019;**234**(2):1313-1325. DOI: 10.1002/jcp.27172

[13] Fife BT, Bluestone JA. Control of peripheral T-cell tolerance and autoimmunity via the CTLA-4 and PD-1 pathways. Immunological Reviews. 2008;**224**(1):166-182. DOI: 10.1111/j.1600-065X.2008.00662.x

[14] Tan CL, Kuchroo JR, Sage PT, Liang D, Francisco LM, Buck J, et al.

PD-1 restraint of regulatory T cell suppressive activity is critical for immune tolerance. Journal of Experimental Medicine. 2021;**218**(1):e20182232. DOI: 10.1084/jem.20182232

[15] Waldman AD, Fritz JM, Lenardo MJ. A guide to cancer immunotherapy: From T cell basic science to clinical practice. Nature Reviews Immunology. 2020;**20**(11):651-668. DOI: 10.1038/s41577-020-0306-5

[16] Kythreotou A, Siddique A, Mauri FA, Bower M, Pinato DJ. PD-L1. Journal of Clinical Pathology. 2018;**71**(3):189-194. DOI: 10.1136/jclinpath-2017-204853

[17] Boussiotis VA. Molecular and biochemical aspects of the PD-1 checkpoint pathway. New England Journal of Medicine. 2016;**375**(18):1767-1778. DOI: 10.1056/nejmra1514296

[18] Jiang X, Wang J, Deng X, Xiong F, Ge J, Xiang B, et al. Role of the tumor microenvironment in PD-L1/PD-1-mediated tumor immune escape. Molecular Cancer. 2019;**18**(1):1-7. DOI: 10.1186/s12943-018-0928-4

[19] Yokosuka T, Takamatsu M, Kobayashi-Imanishi W, et al. Programmed cell death 1 forms negative costimulatory microclusters that directly inhibit T cell receptor signaling by recruiting phosphatase SHP2. The Journal of Experimental Medicine. 2012;**209**:1201-1217. DOI: 10.1084/jem.20112741

[20] Hui E, Cheung J, Zhu J, Su X, Taylor MJ, Wallweber HA, et al. T cell costimulatory receptor CD28 is a primary target for PD-1-mediated inhibition. Science. 2017;**355**:1428-1433

[21] Butte MJ, Keir ME, Phamduy TB, Sharpe AH, Freeman GJ. Programmed death-1 ligand 1 interacts specifically with the B7-1 costimulatory molecule to inhibit T cell responses. Immunity. 2007;**27**:111-122

[22] Intlekofer AM, Thompson CB. At the bench: Preclinical rationale for CTLA-4 and PD-1 blockade as cancer immunotherapy. Journal of Leukocyte Biology. 2013;**94**(1):25-39. DOI: 10.1189%2Fjlb.1212621

[23] Xing Y, Hogquist KA. T-cell tolerance: Central and peripheral. Cold Spring Harbor Perspectives in Biology. 2012;**4**(6):a006957

[24] Nishimura H, Nose M, Hiai H, et al. Development of lupus-like autoimmune diseases by disruption of the PD-1 gene encoding an ITIM motif-carrying immunoreceptor. Immunity. 1999;**11**:141-151

[25] Keir ME, Liang SC, Guleria I, et al. Tissue expression of PD-L1 mediates peripheral T cell tolerance. The Journal of Experimental Medicine. 2006;**203**:883-895

[26] Kumar V, Chaudhary N, Garg M, et al. Current diagnosis and management of immune related adverse events (irAEs) induced by immune checkpoint inhibitor therapy. Frontiers in Pharmacology. 2017;**8**:49

[27] Wherry EJ, Kurachi M. Molecular and cellular insights into T cell exhaustion. Nature Reviews. Immunology. 2015;**15**:486-499

[28] Wherry EJ. T cell exhaustion. Nature Immunology. 2011;**131**:492-499

[29] Barber DL, Wherry EJ, Masopust D, Zhu B, Allison JP, Sharpe AH, et al. Restoring function in exhausted CD8 T cells during chronic viral infection. Nature. 2006;**439**:682-687

[30] Hofmann L, Forschner A, Loquai C, Goldinger SM, Zimmer L, Ugurel S, et al. Cutaneous, gastrointestinal, hepatic, endocrine, and renal side-effects of anti-PD-1 therapy. European Journal of Cancer. 2016;**60**:190-209. DOI: 10.1016/j.ejca.2016.02.025

[31] Hirano F, Kaneko K, Tamura H, Dong H, Wang S, Ichikawa M, et al. Blockade of B7-H1 and PD-1 by monoclonal antibodies potentiates cancer therapeutic immunity. Cancer Research. 2005;**65**:1089-1096

[32] Akinleye A, Rasool Z. Immune checkpoint inhibitors of PD-L1 as cancer therapeutics. Journal of Hematology & Oncology. 2019;**12**(1):1-3. DOI: 10.1186/s13045-019-0779-5

[33] Ai L, Xu A, Xu J. Roles of PD-1/PD-L1 pathway: Signaling, cancer, and beyond. Regulation of Cancer Immune Checkpoints. 2020;**1248**:33-59. DOI: 10.1007/978-981-15-3266-5_3

[34] Azuma T, Yao S, Zhu G, Flies AS, Flies SJ, Chen L. B7-H1 is a ubiquitous antiapoptotic receptor on cancer cells. Blood. 2008;**111**:3635-3643

[35] Chang CH, Qiu J, O'Sullivan D, Buck MD, Noguchi T, Curtis JD, et al. Metabolic competition in the tumor microenvironment is a driver of cancer progression. Cell. 2015;**162**:1229-1241

[36] Ribas A, Hu-Lieskovan S. What does PD-L1 positive or negative mean? The Journal of Experimental Medicine. 2016;**213**(13):2835-2840. DOI: 10.1084/jem.20161462

[37] Gato-Cañas M, Zuazo M, Arasanz H, Ibañez-Vea M, Lorenzo L, Fernandez-Hinojal G, et al. PDL1 signals through conserved sequence motifs to overcome interferon-mediated cytotoxicity. Cell Reports. 2017;**20**: 1818-1829

[38] Chen J, Jiang CC, Jin L, Zhang XD. Regulation of PD-L1: A novel role of pro-survival signalling in cancer. Annals of Oncology. 2016;**27**(3):409-416. DOI: 10.1093/annonc/mdv615

[39] Mahoney KM, Sun H, Liao X, Hua P, Callea M, Greenfield EA, et al. PD-L1 antibodies to its cytoplasmic domain most clearly delineate cell membranes in immunohistochemical staining of tumor cells immunohistochemical detection of membrane PD-L1. Cancer Immunology Research. 2015;**3**(12):1308-1315. DOI: 10.1158/2326-6066.CIR-15-0116

[40] Akhtar M, Rashid S, Al-Bozom IA. PD– L1 immunostaining: What pathologists need to know. Diagnostic Pathology. 2021;**16**(1):1-2

[41] Chowdhury S, Veyhl J, Jessa F, Polyakova O, Alenzi A, MacMillan C, et al. Programmed death-ligand 1 overexpression is a prognostic marker for aggressive papillary thyroid cancer and its variants. Oncotarget. 2016;7(22):32318

[42] D'Andréa G, Lassalle S, Guevara N, Mograbi B, Hofman P. From biomarkers to therapeutic targets: The promise of PD-L1 in thyroid autoimmunity and cancer. Theranostics. 2021;**11**(3):1310. DOI: 10.7150/thno.50333

[43] Wang Q, Liu F, Liu L. Prognostic significance of PD-L1 in solid tumor: An updated meta-analysis. Medicine. 2017;**96**(18):e6369 DOI: 10.1097/md.0000000000006369

[44] Iwai Y, Ishida M, Tanaka Y, Okazaki T, Honjo T, Minato N. Involvement of PD-L1 on tumor cells in the escape from host immune system and tumor immunotherapy

by PD-L1 blockade. Proceedings of the National Academy of Sciences. 2002;**99**(19):12293-12297. DOI: 10.1073/pnas.192461099

[45] Curiel TJ, Wei S, Dong H, Alvarez X, Cheng P, Mottram P, et al. Blockade of B7-H1 improves myeloid dendritic cell–mediated antitumor immunity. Nature Medicine. 2003;**9**(5):562-567. DOI: 10.1038/nm863

[46] He YF, Zhang GM, Wang XH, Zhang H, Yuan Y, Li D, et al. Blocking programmed death-1 ligand-PD-1 interactions by local gene therapy results in enhancement of antitumor effect of secondary lymphoid tissue chemokine. The Journal of Immunology. 2004;**173**(8):4919-4928. DOI: 10.4049/jimmunol.173.8.4919

[47] Blank C, Brown I, Peterson AC, Spiotto M, Iwai Y, Honjo T, et al. PD-L1/B7H-1 inhibits the effector phase of tumor rejection by T cell receptor (TCR) transgenic CD8+ T cells. Cancer Research. 2004;**64**(3):1140-1145. DOI: 10.1158/0008-5472.can-03-3259

[48] Wu X, Gu Z, Chen Y, Chen B, Chen W, Weng L, et al. Application of PD-1 blockade in cancer immunotherapy. Computational and Structural Biotechnology Journal. 2019;**17**:661-674. DOI: 10.1016%2Fj.csbj.2019.03.006

[49] Cui G. The mechanisms leading to distinct responses to PD-1/PD-L1 blockades in colorectal cancers with different MSI statuses. Frontiers in Oncology. 2021;**11**:573547. DOI: 10.3389/fonc.2021.573547

[50] Robert C, Ribas A, Schachter J, Arance A, Grob JJ, Mortier L, et al. Pembrolizumab versus ipilimumab in advanced melanoma (KEYNOTE-006): Post-hoc 5-year results from an open-label, multicentre, randomised, controlled, phase 3 study. The Lancet Oncology. 2019;**20**(9):1239-1251. DOI: 10.1016/S1470-2045(19)30388-2

[51] Khan M, Lin J, Liao G, Tian Y, Liang Y, Li R, et al. Comparative analysis of immune checkpoint inhibitors and chemotherapy in the treatment of advanced non-small cell lung cancer: A meta-analysis of randomized controlled trials. Medicine. 2018;**97**(33):e11936 DOI: 10.1097%2FMD.0000000000011936

[52] Kopetz S, Lonardi S, McDermott RS, Aglietta M, Hendlisz A, Morse M, et al. Concordance of DNA mismatch repair deficient (dMMR)/microsatellite instability (MSI) assessment by local and central testing in patients with metastatic CRC (mCRC) receiving nivolumab (nivo) in CheckMate 142 study. DOI: 10.1200/JCO.2017.35.15_suppl.3548

[53] Wu K, Yi M, Qin S, Chu Q, Zheng X, Wu K. The efficacy and safety of the combination of PD-1 and CTLA-4 inhibitors: A meta-analysis. Experimental Hematology & Oncology. 2019;**8**(1):1-2. DOI: 10.1186/s40164-019-0150-0

[54] Constantinidou A, Alifieris C, Trafalis DT. Targeting programmed cell death-1 (PD-1) and ligand (PD-L1): A new era in cancer active immunotherapy. Pharmacology & Therapeutics. 2019;**194**:84-106. DOI: 10.1016/j.pharmthera.2018.09.008

[55] Makuku R, Khalili N, Razi S, Keshavarz-Fathi M, Rezaei N. Current and future perspectives of PD-1/PDL-1 blockade in cancer immunotherapy. Journal of Immunology Research. 2021;**2021**:6661406. DOI: 10.1155/2021/6661406

[56] Naidoo J, Wang X, Woo KM, Iyriboz T, Halpenny D, Cunningham J,

et al. Pneumonitis in patients treated with anti-programmed death-1/ programmed death ligand 1 therapy. Journal of Clinical Oncology. 2017;**35**(7):709. DOI: 10.1200/ JCO.2016.68.2005

[57] Läubli H, Balmelli C, Bossard M, Pfister O, Glatz K, Zippelius A. Acute heart failure due to autoimmune myocarditis under pembrolizumab treatment for metastatic melanoma. Journal for Immunotherapy of Cancer. 2015;**3**(1):1-6. Available from: https://link.gale.com/apps/doc/A541676778/AONE?u=anon~af3806cf&sid=googleScholar&xid=e07d2490

[58] Yamaguchi H, Hsu JM, Yang WH, Hung MC. Mechanisms regulating PD-L1 expression in cancers and associated opportunities for novel small-molecule therapeutics. Nature Reviews Clinical Oncology. 2022;**19**(5):287-305. DOI: 10.1038/s41571-022-00601-9

[59] Klemen ND, Wang M, Feingold PL, Cooper K, Pavri SN, Han D, et al. Patterns of failure after immunotherapy with checkpoint inhibitors predict durable progression-free survival after local therapy for metastatic melanoma. Journal for Immunotherapy of Cancer. 2019;**7**(1):1-9. DOI: 10.1186/ s40425-019-0672-3

[60] Chen Q, Li T, Yue W. Drug response to PD-1/PD-L1 blockade: Based on biomarkers. OncoTargets and Therapy. 2018;**11**:4673. DOI: 10.2147/OTT.S168313

[61] Udall M, Rizzo M, Kenny J, Doherty J, Dahm S, Robbins P, et al. PD-L1 diagnostic tests: A systematic literature review of scoring algorithms and test-validation metrics. Diagnostic Pathology. 2018;**13**(1):1-1. DOI: 10.1186/ s13000-018-0689-9

[62] Budczies J, Denkert C, Győrffy B, Schirmacher P, Stenzinger A. Chromosome 9p copy number gains involving PD-L1 are associated with a specific proliferation and immune-modulating gene expression program active across major cancer types. BMC Medical Genomics. 2017;**10**(1):1-8. DOI: 10.1186/s12920-017-0308-8

[63] Nayak L, Iwamoto FM, LaCasce A, Mukundan S, Roemer MG, Chapuy B, et al. PD-1 blockade with nivolumab in relapsed/refractory primary central nervous system and testicular lymphoma. Blood, The Journal of the American Society of Hematology. 2017;**129**(23):3071-3073. DOI: 10.1182/ blood-2017-01-764209

[64] Xu J, Yang X, Mao Y, Mei J, Wang H, Ding J, et al. Removal of N-linked glycosylation enhances PD-L1 detection in colon cancer: Validation research based on immunohistochemistry analysis. Technology in Cancer Research & Treatment. 2021;**20**:15330338211019442

[65] LaFleur MW, Muroyama Y, Drake CG, Sharpe AH. Inhibitors of the PD-1 pathway in tumor therapy. The Journal of Immunology. 2018;**200**(2):375-383. DOI: 10.4049/ jimmunol.1701044

[66] Sun JY, Zhang D, Wu S, Xu M, Zhou X, Lu XJ, Ji J. Resistance to PD-1/ PD-L1 blockade cancer immunotherapy: Mechanisms, predictive factors, and future perspectives. Biomarker Research 2020;**8**(1):1-0. DOI: 10.1186/ s40364-020-00212-5

[67] Pike E, Hamidi V, Saeterdal I, Odgaard-Jensen J, Klemp M. Multiple treatment comparison of seven new drugs for patients with advanced malignant melanoma: A systematic review and health economic decision model in a Norwegian setting. BMJ

Open. 2017;**7**(8):e014880. DOI: 10.1136/bmjopen-2016-014880

[68] Alexander S, Swami U, Kaur A, Gao Y, Fatima M, Ginn MM, et al. Safety of immune checkpoint inhibitors in patients with cancer and pre-existing autoimmune disease. Annals of Translational Medicine. 2021;**9**(12):1033. DOI: 10.21037/atm-20-8124

[69] Guerrouahen BS, Maccalli C, Cugno C, Rutella S, Akporiaye ET. Reverting immune suppression to enhance cancer immunotherapy. Frontiers in Oncology. 2020;**9**:1554. DOI: 10.3389/fonc.2019.01554

[70] Yi M, Zheng X, Niu M, Zhu S, Ge H, Wu K. Combination strategies with PD-1/PD-L1 blockade: Current advances and future directions. Molecular Cancer. 2022;**21**(1):1-27. DOI: 10.1186/s12943-021-01489-2

[71] Dai X, Bu X, Gao Y, Guo J, Hu J, Jiang C, et al. Energy status dictates PD-L1 protein abundance and anti-tumor immunity to enable checkpoint blockade. Molecular Cell. 2021;**81**(11):2317-2331. DOI: 10.1016/j.molcel.2021.03.037

[72] Moon Y, Shim MK, Choi J, Yang S, Kim J, Yun WS, et al. Anti-PD-L1 peptide-conjugated prodrug nanoparticles for targeted cancer immunotherapy combining PD-L1 blockade with immunogenic cell death. Theranostics. 2022;**12**(5):1999. DOI: 10.7150/thno.69119

[73] Song Y, Fu Y, Xie Q, Zhu B, Wang J, Zhang B. Anti-angiogenic agents in combination with immune checkpoint inhibitors: A promising strategy for cancer treatment. Frontiers in Immunology. 2020;**11**:1956. DOI: 10.3389/fimmu.2020.01956

[74] Pandey P, Khan F, Qari HA, Upadhyay TK, Alkhateeb AF, Oves M. Revolutionization in cancer therapeutics via targeting major immune checkpoints PD-1, PD-L1 and CTLA-4. Pharmaceuticals. 2022;**15**(3):335. DOI: 10.3390/ph15030335

**Chapter 4**

# Immune Checkpoint and Tumor Therapy

*Pei Huang and Hongzhang Deng*

## Abstract

Cancer immunotherapy employing immune checkpoint inhibitors (ICI) has revolutionized the tumor therapy far beyond their impressing clinical effects. Immune checkpoint therapy (ICT), which is directly involved in different immunosuppressive mechanisms at tumor sites, has been thoroughly studied. Nevertheless, the "off-target" effects of ICIs following systemic administration is still challenging. In addition, the clinical response rate of ICT is still unsatisfactory in that only a few patients hold lasting benefits. In this chapter, the mechanism of most widely used ICIs, including those based on CTLA-4 and PD-1/PD-L1, has been introduced. The approaches to enhancing the efficacy of ICT have been highlighted, namely improving targeted delivery of ICI by employing nanotechnology, modulating the immunosuppressive tumor microenvironment (TME), and combining ICT with other therapies. We hope advanced strategies summarized in this chapter would further inspire the development of ICT to boost their effectiveness while minimize unwanted side effects.

**Keywords:** cancer immunotherapy, immune checkpoint, targeted delivery, immunomodulation, combined therapy

## 1. Introduction

Cancer immunotherapy is a promising strategy to combat cancer by leveraging host immune system, involving lymphocyte-promoting cytokines, cancer vaccines, immune checkpoint therapy (ICT), and engineered T cells [1, 2]. Among the diverse immunotherapeutic approaches, ICT is the most thoroughly investigated approach with broad impact. It can enhance antitumor immunity by inhibiting negative regulatory pathways. To date, several monoclonal antibodies against the cytotoxic T lymphocyte antigen 4 (CTLA-4) and programmed cell death 1 (PD1)–PD1 ligand 1 (PD-L1) axis have been clinically approved for various cancers, including melanoma, lung, and renal cancers (**Figure 1**) [3]. Some other checkpoint inhibitors are also in preclinical or earlier phases of clinical development, such as LAG3, TIGIT, TIM3, B7H3, CD39, CD73 and adenosine A2A receptors [4, 5].

Despite substantial progress of immune checkpoint inhibitors (ICIs) in the cancer treatment, there are still several key limitations. Firstly, systemically delivery of checkpoint inhibitors may cause serious side effects in several major organs.

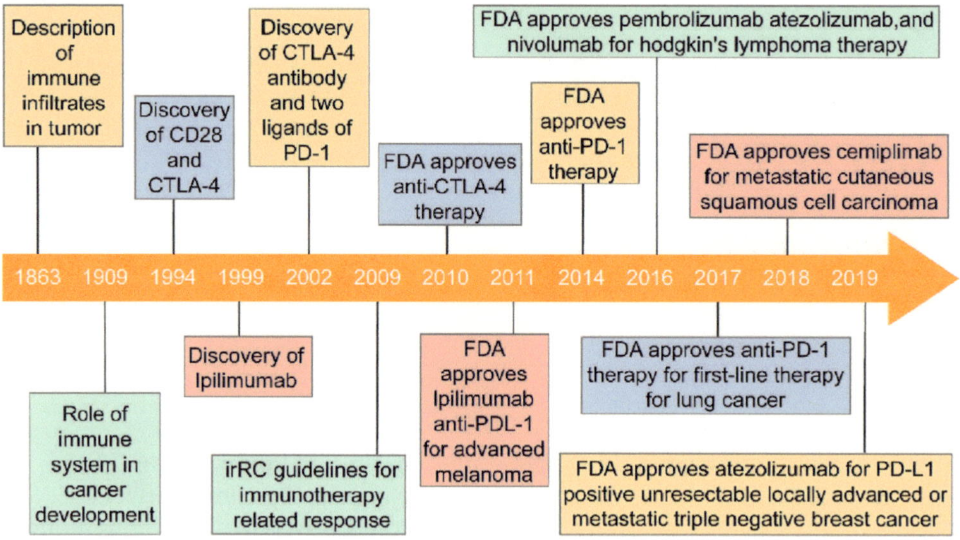


**Figure 1.**
*Timeline of significant milestones in the development of cancer immune checkpoint inhibitors. CD28: cluster of differentiation 28; CTLA-4: cytotoxic T lymphocyte-associated protein 4; FDA: US Food and Drug Administration; irRC: immune-related response criteria; PD-1: programmed cell death protein 1; and Tregs: regulatory T cells.*

In addition, many patients with nonimmunogenic tumor microenvironments (TMEs) showed therapeutic resistance to checkpoint inhibitors and do not respond to the treatment. The mechanism of the non-responsiveness to checkpoint inhibitors are still in investigation and may involve poor tumor-infiltration of T cells, checkpoints dysregulation in tumor cells and T cells, and adaptive resistance to checkpoint inhibition [6–8]. These drawbacks need to be overcome to achieve more satisfactory therapeutic outcomes against various cancer. In this chapter, we will introduce immunological mechanism of immune checkpoint blockade and highlight emerging approaches to enhancing ICT efficiency. It is foreseeable that ICT will lead to next-generation promising techniques and continuously contribute to the future cancer treatment.

## 2. Mechanisms of immune checkpoint therapy (ICT)

T cells enable to distinguish tumor cells from normal cells and launch attack accordingly, which plays a critical role in maintaining appropriate immune responses. However, such immunologic effects may be prevented in the TME. The prevention of T cells activation in the presence of antigen is related with the T cells dysfunction and inhibiting the receptors expression, such as those of CTLA-4 and PD-1 [9] ICP aim to block such inhibition and reverse the immunosuppressive TME, thus achieving functions mainly by activating normal immune system to eradicate cancer cells. Despite a few overlaps in inhibitory roles, each checkpoint inhibitor also performs some unique functions.

### 2.1 CTLA-4

The normal T cell activation requires the binding of CD28 on T cells with co-stimulatory B7 molecules (CD80 and CD86) on DC surface, also known as

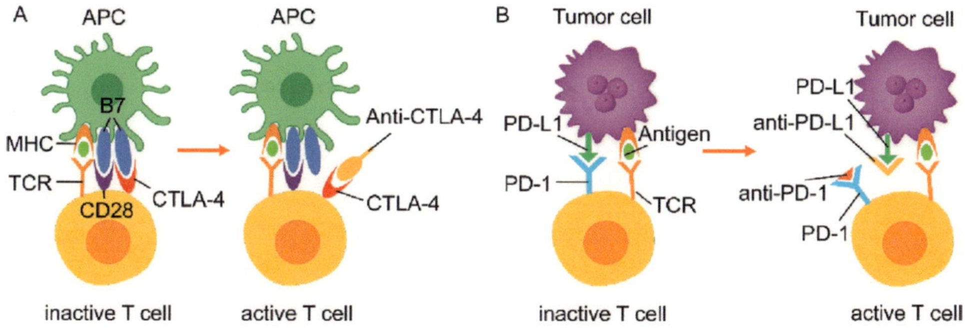


**Figure 2.**
*Scheme illustration showing the mechanism of (A) CTLA-4 blockade; and (B) PD-1 Blockade.*

signal 2 of T-cell receptors (TCR) activation [10]. However, CTLA-4 which is expressed on the surface of late-stage T cells can competitively bind with CD80/CD86 to prevent T-cell activation [5]. Regarding this, blockade with monoclonal antibody against CTLA-4 enables to proceed CD28/B7 pathway and restore T-cells activity. CTLA-4 is also constitutively overexpressed on regulatory T cells (Tregs), which can mediate dendritic cell (DC) function inhibition and suppress the T cell response against tumors [11]. Additionally, CTLA-4 was reported to be expressed in some other cells such as activated B cells, placental fibroblasts and monocytes, and may playing roles in immune regulation of other cells. For instance, it is associated with decreased circulating B cell amounts and antibody expression levels [12]. Of note, the exact cellular mechanisms underlying CTLA-4 blockade remains to be investigated and different anti-CTLA-4 antibody has distinct properties (**Figure 2**) [13].

### 2.2 PD-1/PD-L1

In normal physiological conditions, ICIs can modulate T cell activity and protect healthy tissues from immune attack. T cell activity can be suspended by the binding of PD-1 on T-cells with its ligands programmed death ligand 1 (PD-L1) and programmed death ligand 2 (PD-L2) which are largely distributed on tumor cells and DCs. Regarding this, PD1 PD-L1/2 blockade by using monoclonal antibody can lead to restoration of T cell activity. PD-L2 shows higher affinity to PD-1 but with more limited expression profile and is mainly expressed on activated DCs, macrophages, and some B cells [14]. PD-L1 is more widely expressed on DCs, macrophages, T and B cells, as well as some cell types in non-hematologic tissues, such as epithelia, endothelial cells, astrocytes and neurons.

### 2.3 Other immune checkpoints

Some other ICI molecules under investigation include positive regulators such as tumor necrosis factor receptor superfamily membrane 9 (4-1BB) and tumor necrosis factor receptor superfamily member 4 (OX-40), and negative regulators such as T-cell immunoglobulin and mucin domain (TIM-3) and lymphocyte activation gene-3 (LAG-3) [5]. These immune checkpoints also have been recognized for their roles in regulating tumor immunity and elicits antitumor response.

## 3. Approaches to enhancing ICB therapy efficiency

### 3.1 Improve targeted delivery of ICIs by employing nanotechnology

The ICP therapeutic effects depends on successful interaction of ICIs with the protein of interest. Nevertheless, the "off-target" effects of ICT therapeutics following systemic administration brings some side effects and limits the maximum allowable doses. Thus, it is significant to achieve targeted delivery and controlled release of ICIs in the desired cell types. To this end, several nanoparticle (NP) systems, such as liposome, polymeric NPs and inorganic NPs, have been used to achieve targeted delivery of ICIs to maximize the therapeutic effects while minimizing the unwanted side effects [15]. The nanotechnology-mediated ICT showed several advantages over traditional method and can improve therapeutic efficacy of ICT, as described below.

#### *3.1.1 Passive targeting*

Employing nanotechnology can improve the tumor accumulation of therapeutic ICIs via enhanced permeability and retention (EPR) effect, which refers to the higher permeability of tumor vessels to NPs than normal vessels and the increased retention of NPs in tumors due to the poor lymphatic clearance. For example, Nikpoor et al. developed PEGylated liposomes for the delivery of αCTLA-4 monoclonal antibodies [16]. They found that tumor accumulation of PEGylated liposomes encapsulated with anti-CTLA-4 antibodies was significantly greater than that of free antibodies in the CT26 colorectal tumor-bearing mice 18 h post-injection. Accordingly, the tumor-bearing mice receiving treatment of PEGylated liposomes loaded with antibody showed obviously extended survival time compared with free antibody group, suggesting that improved tumor accumulation led to greater therapeutic efficacy. It should be noted that the tumor accumulation effects of NPs via EPR effect are closely related with tumor type, heterogeneity, and perfusion.

The size and charges of NPs playing critical roles in passive targeting pattern by affecting the half-life and biodistribution. Such structure–activity relationships guide the rational design of targeted delivery nanoplatform. The size of the NPs should not be too small or too large. The NPs smaller than 7 nm tend to be cleared by renal filtration and urinary excretion [17, 18], while those larger than 200 nm are more likely to be cleared by the reticuloendothelial system (RES) [19]. As for the surface charge, the positively charged NPs show higher cellular uptake efficiency, while those slightly negatively charged and neutral NPs exhibit longer persistence during circulation. Besides, strongly positively or negatively charged NPs tend to be cleared by RES [17].

The surface properties of NPs also have impact on *in vivo* fate and performance by affecting their interaction with endogenous macromolecules. Poly(ethylene)glycol (PEG) is the most widely applied coatings to adjust the NPs surface properties. In a study, PEGylated and non-PEGylated liposomes in similar diameter of 140 nm were both applied to deliver anti-CTLA-4 mAb into C26 colon tumor-bearing mice to study antitumor therapeutic effects. PEGylated CTLA-4-liposomes were shown to prolong blood half-lives and induce higher intratumoral accumulation than free antibodies and non-PEGylated groups [16].

### *3.1.2 Active targeting*

In addition to passive targeting via EPR effects, achieving active targeting by introducing targeting moieties into NPs also can facilitate target site accumulation. Active targeting approaches can promote targeted delivery by directing NPs to action sites, either a specific location or a specific cellular type, and reduce off-target side effects. This strategy often leads to better therapeutic effects compared with those without targeting moieties through passive targeting. For example, LinTT1 is an active targeting peptide which can promote cellular uptake and tumor tissue penetration by intervening low-affinity binding with p32 cell surface receptors on tumor cells, and tumor-associated macrophages [20]. Li et al. incorporated an active targeting peptide LinTT1 into self-assembled micelles for the co-delivery of siRNA for PD-L1 and an IDO inhibitor [21]. The results showed that intravenous administration of LinTT-1-targeted NPs significantly enhanced tumor delivery of the therapeutic cargos than free therapeutics.

Moreover, introducing multiple targeting molecules into one nanoplatform can further enhance the active targeting ability. For instance, Chiang et al. fabricated anti-CD3 antibodies modified magnetic NPs for anti-PD-1 mAb delivery [22]. In addition to facilitating T cells delivery mediated by anti-CD3 antibodies bounding to the CD3 T-cell surface marker, ferromagnetic properties also facilitated tumor targeting under an external magnetic field. This dual-targeting strategy improved tumor accumulation of anti-PD-1 mAb drugs and antitumor therapeutic effects compared with the anti-CD3 single targeting group. Multivalent active targeting strategies not only can promote the NPs transportation to targeting sites, but also enable to attract specific immune cells to the site of interest. For example, Au et al. established a PEG-PLGA based trispecific NK cell engager platform for combining targeted chemoimmunotherapy and co-stimulatory 4-1BB molecule-based ICT [23]. The NPs were functionalized with tumor targeting anti-epidermal growth factor receptor (α-EGFR) antibody and two NK-activating components, anti-CD16 (α-CD16) and anti–4-1BB (α-4-1BB) antibodies, and encapsulated chemotherapeutics epirubicin (EPI). This trispecific α-EGFR/α-CD16/α-4-1BB NPs not only can achieve targeted delivery of EPI to EGFR-overexpressed tumor cells and NK cells, but also can recruit and activate circulating NK cells to the TME following systemic delivery. This multifunctional and multivalent active targeting strategy led to the greatest therapeutic efficacy and extended survival in EGFR-overexpressing murine tumor model compared with other treatment groups. These finding demonstrated that multiple targeting strategy can be applied to improve targeting specificity or drive two different targets together into spatial proximity to improve treatment outcomes.

### *3.1.3 Controlled release*

In addition to passive and active targeting strategy, the NPs also can be engineered to achieve selective and controlled release of ICI cargos at the action sites so as to maximize the therapeutic effects. Several NPs have been reported to utilize the characteristics of TME as triggers to realize controlled release of ICT drugs, such as acidic pH and matrix metalloproteinases (MMPs) in TME [24, 25]. For instance, Lang et al. encapsulated chemotherapeutic drug paclitaxel (PTX), anti- cancer stem cells (CSC) agent thioridazine (THZ), and the PD-1/PD-L1 inhibitor HY19991 (HY) into an

MMPs enzymes as well as pH dual-responsive double-layer structured NPs [25]. The MMPs in TME triggered outer layer degradation and achieved release of HY, THZ, and PTX-loaded. Subsequently, the micelles internalized into cells and disrupted under endosomes/lysosomes acidic, leading to the PTX release and cancer cell death. This controlled release strategy controlled spatial and temporal delivery to showed powerful synergy among different therapeutic effects.

#### *3.1.4 Codelivery of different therapeutics*

Utilizing nanotechnology enable co-delivery of different therapeutics simultaneously. Mi et al. explored the dual immunotherapy nanoparticles (DINP) for the co-delivery of αPD-1 monoclonal antibodies and agonistic antibodies for the co-stimulatory receptor αOX40, to prevent T-cell inhibition and elicit T-cell activation simultaneously [26]. They proved that using DINP induced higher levels of T-cell activation compared with free immunotherapeutic antibodies or single therapeutic NPs. This NP-based co-delivery strategy enabled to increase T-cell activation, improve therapeutic efficacy and enhance immunological memory. Cheng et al. developed amphiphilic peptides containing NPs for the codelivery of PD-1/PD-L1 peptide ICI, DPPA-1, and an IDO inhibitor, NLG919 [27]. At neutral conditions, the hydrophobic segments of amphiphilic peptides formed a tight shell to protect hydrophobic cargos. At the weak acidic pH at TME, the NP swelled and MMPs diffusing into the internal hydrophobic domain, leading to the disassembly of NP and release of DPPA-1 and NLG919. This co-delivery of DPPA-1 and NLG919 enhanced tumor inhibition effects and survival in tumor-bearing mice compared to the delivery of either therapeutic alone. These finding confirmed the superiorities of nanotechnology in terms of integrating different therapeutic into a single platform.

#### *3.1.5 Other superiorities of nanotechnology*

The application of nanotechnology allows for real-time delivery monitoring. For instance, Meir et al. developed an integrated diagnostic and therapeutic nanoplatform by conjugating α-PD-L1 antibodies to gold nanoparticles (αPDL1-GNPs) to stratify patient response to ICIs [28]. αPDL1-GNPs were intravenously injected into subcutaneous MC38 colon tumors bearing mice and accumulated in tumor, which generated CT signal contrast and could be used to predict response to ICT. A strong correlation was observed between αPD-L1-GNPs related CT signal and tumor growth, leading to the facile precise prediction of the ICT response via CT signal levels. Although more validation in other tumor models is required, this proof-of-concept study suggested that nanotechnology may promote non-invasive monitoring of ICT response.

Additionally, the combination of nanotechnology can promote development of novel delivery approaches. As an example, Wang et al. established a microneedle patch coated with pH-sensitive dextran nanoparticles for the sustained delivery of αPD1 [28]. The αPD1 was encapsulated into the NPs, which can dissociate at acidic pH and achieve controlled and sustained released αPD-1 antibodies over 3 days. This sustained release of αPD-1 antibodies improved tumor retention of antibodies and prolonged the survival time of subcutaneous B16F10 melanomas bearing mice. Nevertheless, this delivery approach seems be limited to superficial tumors, such as melanomas, and need more investigation to confirm strategies.

### 3.2 Modulate the immunosuppressive tumor microenvironment (TME)

ICT have showed great potential in increasing survival rate in various cancers. However, the low response rate of patients to ICT, which is related to immunosuppressive tumor microenvironments, remains a challenge to be addressed. Several studies have aimed to target and reverse the immunosuppressive TME, so as to increase the therapeutic effects and decrease side effects of ICT (**Figure 3**) [29].

#### *3.2.1 Modulate or eradicate the fibrotic stroma*

Fibroblastic stroma can reduce the efficacy of ICT by promoting tumor development and employing immunosuppressive immune cells. Several strategies have been applied to modulate or eradicate the fibrotic stroma to improve the effectiveness of ICT. For instance, Xu et al. constructed a puerarin loaded nano emulsion (nanoPue) for the targeted delivery of puerarin to the sigma receptor over-expressing cancer-associated fibroblasts (CAFs) and cancer cells [30]. Reactive oxygen species (ROS) play critical roles in activation of CAFs and puerarin was applied to decrease ROS production in the activated myofibroblast. In the desmoplastic triple-negative breast cancer (TNBC) model, nanoPue greatly reduced CAFs in mice and deactivated the stromal microenvironment, leading to enhanced chemotherapy effect of encapsulated paclitaxel. Importantly, combination therapy of nanoPue and α-PD-L1-based ICT induced more apoptosis and exhibited a significantly robust antitumor effect in 4 T1 tumor model compared to α-PD-L1 or nanoPue monotherapy. This suggests that CAFs deactivation is a promising approach to regulate tumor stroma and improve

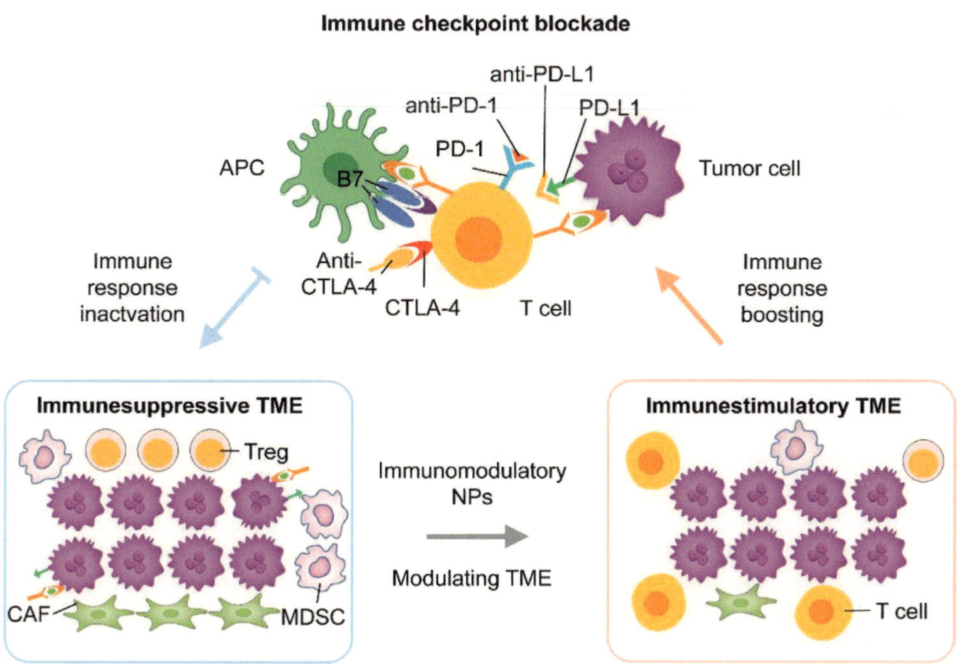


**Figure 3.**
*Modulate the immunosuppressive tumor microenvironment (TME) to boost the efficacy of immune checkpoint therapy (ICT). Treg: regulatory T cell; CAF: cancer-associated fibroblast; and MDSC: myeloid treated suppressor cell.*

the efficacy of ICT. In another study, Zhao et al. established cyclopamine (CPA) and paclitaxel (PTX) co-encapsulated polymeric micelles (M-CPA/PTX) to modulate desmoplastic stroma in pancreatic ductal adenocarcinoma (PDAC) and improve the efficacy of ICT [31]. The (M-CPA/PTX) plarform could regulated the tumor stroma to enhance intratumoral vasculature density, leading to increased tumor-infiltrating CTLs and decreased hypoxia. In a Kras model, the combination treatment of M-CPA/PTX with α-PD-1-based ICT upregulated $CD8^+$ T cells and IFN-γ levels in tumor tissues and prolonged the survival of mice compared to monotherapy of M-CPA/PTX or and α-PD-1 alone. These findings demonstrated the potential of fibrotic stroma modulation in enhancing the therapeutic efficacy of ICT.

#### *3.2.2 Targeted modulation of T cells*

Kosmides et al. fabricated an "immunoswitch" iron-dextran nanoparticle coated with two different antibodies which can simultaneously block the PD-L1 inhibitory signal and activate T cells through 4-1BB co-stimulatory pathway [32]. The intratumoral treatment with immunoswitch NPs suppressed tumor growth and prolonged survival time compared with direct co-injection of free antibodies in various tumor models-bearing mice. In addition, regulatory T (Treg) cells can induce immunosuppressive TME which is a major obstacle for cancer immunotherapy. In an exemplified study, Ou et al. constructed imatinib (IMT)-loaded, tLyp1 peptide-decorated hybrid NPs (IMT-loaded tLyp1-hNP) which exhibited good stability and effective targeting ability to neuropilin-1 (Nrp1) overexpressing Tregs in TME [33]. IMT was applied to reduce the proportion of Treg cells by blocking STAT3 and STAT5 signaling. The IMT-loaded tLyp1-hNP showed higher cellular uptake efficiency for Treg cells and boost the effect of imatinib in inhibiting Tregs-mediated suppression. The combination treatment of α-CTLA-4-based ICT and IMT-loaded tLyp-hNPs increased tumor-infiltrating CD8+ T cells and extended survival of B16BL/6 tumor-bearing mice, suggesting that reducing Tregs mediated by targeted IMT-loaded tLyp-hNPs enabled a synergistic effect with ICT.

#### *3.2.3 Targeted modulation of tumor-associated myeloid cells (TAMCs)*

To enhance the therapeutic effects of ICT and modulate the immunosuppressive TME, various approaches have been adopted for TAMCs targeting. As is known, polarization of macrophages in TME into M2 tumor-associated macrophages (TAMs) can facilitate tumor progression and inhibit antitumor efficacy of ICT by releasing anti-inflammatory cytokines and angiogenic factors. Based on this, Choo et al. exploited M1 macrophages derived nanovesicles (M1NVs) to repolarize M2 TAMs to M1 macrophages which can release pro-inflammatory cytokines and elicit antitumor immunity [34]. The results showed combination treatment of M1NVs and aPD-L1 significantly decreased the tumor volume compared to the treatment of M1NVs or aPD-L1 alone, proving that M1NV can repolarize M2 TAMs to M1 macrophages and potentiate the antitumor efficacy of ICT. Shae et al. constructed stimulator of interferon gene NPs (STING-NPs) based on endosomolytic polymersome possessing pH-responsive membrane [35]. The STING-NPs can enhance cytosolic delivery of 2′3' cyclic guanosine monophosphate–adenosine monophosphate (cGAMP), which is an endogenous ligand for cyclic dinucleotide (CDN) agonists of stimulator of interferon genes (STING). They demonstrated that STING-NPs treatment could remodel the TME and repolarize macrophages to block immunosuppressive characteristics in melanoma bearing mice. Importantly, the combination of STING-NPs enhanced response to α-PD-1 and α-CTLA-4, prolonged the survival and inhibit tumor growth compared with ICT or free cGAMP-ICT treatment. These results confirmed that STING-NPs can activate STING pathways in myeloid cell populations in TME and increases the therapeutic efficacy of ICT.

#### *3.2.4 Other approaches to regulating immune-suppressive TME*

There are plenty of other immune suppressive mechanisms related with the reduced effectiveness of ICT. In view of this, several therapeutic agents have been applied to regulate various immune suppressive mechanisms and increase the efficacy of ICT, such as pro-stromal signaling modulators [36], exosome release inhibitors [37], tumor-associated myeloid cells (TAMCs) eliminators [38], TAMC recruitment inhibitors [39], and TAMC reprogrammers [40]. For instance, inhibiting C-X-C motif chemokine ligand 12 (CXCL12), which is secreted by CAFs and promotes cancer cell migration and proliferation, is another approach to regulate the fibrotic stroma. Shen et al. downregulated the CXCL12 expression by employing small trap proteins targeting IL-10 and CXCL12, leading to elevated tumor-infiltrating DCs, NK cells, and tumor-infiltrated T cells [36]. TLR7 and TLR8 are highly expressed in leukocytes and myeloid cells. Lee et al. revealed the treatment of TLR agonist resiquimod which binds to TLR7 and TLR8 can promote the differentiation of myeloid derived suppressor cells (MDSCs) into macrophages and dendritic cells [40]. MDSCs were shown to lost immunosuppressive ability in T cells and result in increased proliferation of T cells.

### 3.3 Combine ICT with other therapies

ICT can combine with other immunotherapies, such as cancer vaccines, to augment antitumor immunity. Moreover, conventional therapeutic approaches, including chemotherapy, phototherapy, radiotherapy, not only can kill cancer cells but also show immunomodulation effects. ICT can combine with these different treatments to boost the antitumor immunotherapeutic effects.

#### *3.3.1 ICT combines with cancer vaccine*

Combined immunotherapies of ICT and cancer vaccine can potentiate antitumor immune response. Kuai et al. developed a nanodisc to co-deliver anti-PD-1 and anti-CTLA-4, in combination with the sHDL-Ag/CpG mediated cancer vaccine, for the MC-38 colon tumors and B16F10 melanomas treatment [41]. The combination of ICT with neoantigen vaccination markedly inhibit tumor growth and eradicate established tumors, suggesting the superiority of combined immunotherapeutic strategy. Zhu et al. further explored this strategy by constructing endogenously self-assembled albumin/AlbiVax nanocomplexes [42]. The AlbiVax nanovaccines are composed of antigens and adjuvants conjugated with maleimide-functionalized Evans Blue (MEB), namely MEB-Ag and MEB-CpG. MEB can bind with endogenous albumin which can work as a natural carrier and enable to direct the nanovaccine trafficking to the lymph nodes. The anti-PD-1 based ICT could prevent exhaustion of CTL responses, in combination with AlbiVax nanovaccine which can efficiently traffic to lymph nodes, leading to induction of robust antitumor immune response. The found that vaccination with AlbiVax led to 12.5% tumors regression, while combination treatment of AlbiVax + anti-PD-1 increased tumor regression to 60% in mice.

### *3.3.2 ICT combines with chemotherapy*

It has been realized that cytotoxic chemotherapy exerts therapeutic effects not only through direct tumor cells killing, but also may be related with immunoregulatory properties of chemotherapeutic agents. The chemotherapy achieve antitumor effects by facilitating tumor cell killing or inhibiting tumor cell division via multiple mechanism, such as causing DNA damage, disrupting DNA replication, preventing mitosis, cellular metabolism and microtubule assembly [43]. Although the precise mechanism remains further investigation, it is believed that chemotherapy can modulate T cell activity by promoting immunogenic cell death (ICD), increasing effector T-cell response, enhancing tumor antigenicity, or blocking immune suppressive pathways [44, 45]. Chemotherapy can induce ICD by releasing damage-associated molecular patterns (DAMP), which can be recognized by pattern-recognition receptors such as Toll-like receptors (TLRs) expressed on antigen-presenting cells (APCs). These DAMPs and tumor-associated antigens collectively elicit APCs maturation and induce a robust antitumor immunity. For instance, anthracycline-based chemotherapy has been shown to induce immunogenic cell death (ICD) which favors the DCs maturation and block immunosuppressive pathways in the TME [44]. In a genetically engineered mouse lung adenocarcinoma model, combined therapy of oxaliplatin and cyclophosphamide drive the T cell infiltration-lacking tumors sensitive to ICT based on PD1 and CTLA4 antibodies (**Figure 4**) [46].

### *3.3.3 ICT combines with radiotherapy*

When ICT combines with radiotherapy, abscopal effect can occur to facilitate regression of distant tumors or metastases. Specifically, APCs uptake tumor-associated antigens (TAAs) released by the dying tumor cells upon irradiation, accumulate to the lymph nodes and activate $CD8^+$ T-cells to eradicate the tumor cells in primary and distant tumors. It has been recognized that the abscopal effect can be augmented by combining radiotherapy with ICT. Ni et al. established a radiosensitizer (Hf12-DBA) for radiotherapy in combination with anti-PD-L1 based ICT, resulting antitumor response both in primary and distant tumors [47]. In dual subcutaneous colorectal CT26 tumors bearing mice, monotherapies of ICT and radiotherapy just lead to delayed primary and distant tumors growth, while combination of ICT and radiotherapy elicit complete regression of primary, treated tumor and shrinkage of

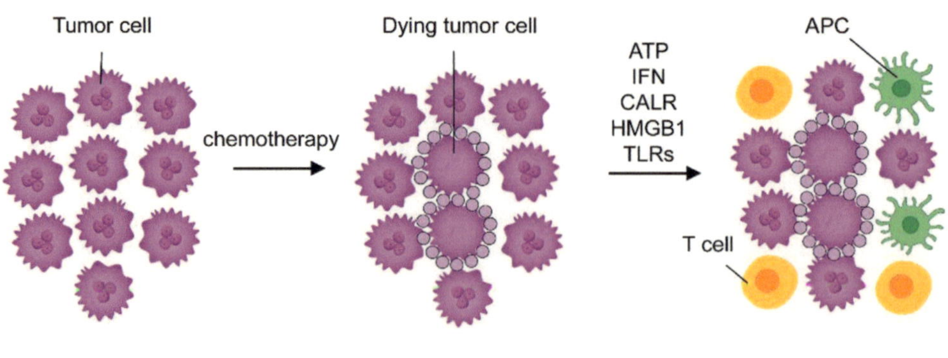


**Figure 4.**
*Scheme illustration showing the cancer treatment with chemotherapy which can elicit immune stimulation including: Secretion of ATP; expression of type 1 interferon (IFN); exposure of calreticulin (CALR) on the outer membrane; and release of high mobility group box 1 (HMGB1).*

distant, non-irradiated tumors. Accordingly, the abscopal effect was boosted and the antitumor immune responses was potentiated by the combination of ICT and radiotherapy. Min et al. developed a new strategy to improve abscopal effect by constructing antigen-capturing NPs mediated combination therapy of anti-PD-1-based ICT and radiotherapy [48]. In bilateral B16F10 melanomas bearing mice, ICT and radiotherapy combination therapy mediated by antigen-capturing NPs induced a 20% complete response rate and tumor re-challenge resistant 3 months later. By contrast, mice receiving the combination treatment without antigen-capturing succumbed to disease within 40 days, suggesting that antigen-capturing strategy play a critical role in improving the abscopal effect and enhance therapeutic effects.

#### *3.3.4 ICT combines with phototherapy*

Combination of phototherapy can induce abscopal effect, reduce tumor burden, and boost antitumor responses in various tumor models. Phototherapy relies on photosensitizers which can generate reactive oxygen species for photodynamic therapy (PDT) or heat for photothermal therapy (PTT) upon laser irradiation to eradicate tumor cells. Chen et al. combined PLGA-ICG-R837-based PTT with anti-CTLA-4-based ICT to induce robust anti-tumor immune responses for cancer immunotherapy [49]. In a 4 T1 breast tumor model with lung metastases, the combination treatment of PTT and ICT could protect treated mice against tumor rechallenging 40 days post ablation, while surgery + anti-CTLA-4 treatment or PLGA-ICG-R837-based-PTT alone can lead to metastases.

#### *3.3.5 Challenges for combination therapies*

Combination therapy is crucial for increasing sensitivity of ICT and enhancing antitumor efficacy. However, there are still some challenges need to be addressed. First, careful consideration needs to be given to for which therapies to combine. Preclinically determining whether there is an additive or synergistic therapeutic effect and determining the optimal combination can help identify and drive combinations that produce synergistic therapeutic effects into clinical trials. Second, strong rationale is needed for the spatiotemporal factors of combination therapy administration. The half-life, tumor accumulation and kinetics for each monotherapy should be examined. Nanotechnology exhibit superiorities in this aspect by integrating multiple therapies into a single platform to promote accumulation and co-localization at the target sites. Additionally, optimizing the dose and scheduling of combination therapy is also needed when considering spatiotemporal factors. Of note, nanotechnology shows the potential to solve the challenges related to combination therapy in a number of ways: through integrating multiple therapies into a single nanoplatform, or optimizing dosage and therapeutic schedule, or exploring the potential therapeutic mechanisms.

## 4. Conclusion

ICT-mediated immunotherapy has attracted extensive research interest and pioneered a new paradigm for cancer treatment over the past decades. The final goal of ICT is to induce a robust antitumor response by interfering immunosuppressive TMEs while alleviating side effects. Various strategies have been investigated for enhancing efficacy of ICT, including nanotechnology-mediated targeted delivery of ICIs, regulation of the immunosuppressive TME, and combination therapies. Despite substantial progress, the issues of immune-related adverse events (irAEs) and therapeutic resistance may lead to the failure of therapy and even patient mortality in some cases. Biomarkers can be employed to predict the efficacy of ICI treatment and irAEs by distinguishing responders and non-responders, which would promote patient selection and decision-making. Abundant opportunities remain in ICT for maximizing therapeutic effects, improving safety profiles, and reducing recurrence. We believe that expanding the understanding of immune checkpoint biology and nanotechnology will improve the efficacy of current ICT and continuously contribute to the next generation of novel immunotherapy for clinical translation.

## Acknowledgements

This research was supported by National Natural Science Foundation of China (NSFC) projects (Nos 32171320 and 81371667), Xi'an Association for Science and Technology young Talent Promotion Plan (Nos. 095920211324 and 095920221341), Qinchuangyuan cited the high-level innovation and entrepreneurship talent program (QCYRCXM-2022-27), State Key Laboratory of Veterinary Biotechnology Foundation (SKLVBF202207), the Fundamental Research Funds for the Central Universities (No. QTZX22067), the Opening Project of the State Key Laboratory of Microbial Resources (SKLMR-20220703).

## Conflict of interest

The authors declare no conflict of interest.

## Author details

Pei Huang[1,2] and Hongzhang Deng[1,2,3*]

1 Engineering Research Center of Molecular and Neuro-Imaging, Ministry of Education, School of Life Science and Technology, Xidian University, Xi'an, Shaanxi, P.R. China

2 Academy of Advanced Interdisciplinary Research, Xidian University, Xi'an, Shaanxi, P.R. China

3 National Institutes of Health, Tianjin University, Tianjin, China

*Address all correspondence to: dhz1989@163.com

## References

[1] Sanmamed MF, Chen L. A paradigm shift in cancer immunotherapy: From enhancement to normalization. Cell. 2018;**175**:313-326. DOI: 10.1016/j.cell.2018.09.035

[2] Finck A, Gill SI, June CH. Cancer immunotherapy comes of age and looks for maturity. Nature Communications. 2020;**11**:3325. DOI: 10.1038/s41467-020-17140-5

[3] Lou J, Zhang L, Zheng G. Advancing cancer immunotherapies with nanotechnology. Advanced Therapeutics. 2019;**2**:1800128. DOI: 10.1002/adtp.201800128

[4] Granier C, De Guillebon E, Blanc C, Roussel H, Badoual C, Colin E, et al. Mechanisms of action and rationale for the use of checkpoint inhibitors in cancer. ESMO Open. 2017;**2**:e000213. DOI: 10.1136/esmoopen-2017-000213

[5] Pardoll DM. The blockade of immune checkpoints in cancer immunotherapy. Nature Reviews. Cancer. 2012;**12**:252-264. DOI: 10.1038/nrc3239

[6] Restifo NP, Smyth MJ, Snyder A. Acquired resistance to immunotherapy and future challenges. Nature Reviews. Cancer. 2016;**16**:121-126. DOI: 10.1038/nrc.2016.2

[7] Garg AD, Coulie PG, Van den Eynde BJ, Agostinis P. Integrating next-generation dendritic cell vaccines into the current cancer immunotherapy landscape. Trends in Immunology. 2017;**38**:577-593. DOI: 10.1016/j.it.2017.05.006

[8] Dillman RO. Is there a role for therapeutic cancer vaccines in the age of checkpoint inhibitors? Human Vaccines & Immunotherapeutics. 2017;**13**:528-532. DOI: 10.1080/21645515.2016.1244149

[9] Singh S, Hassan D, Aldawsari HM, Molugulu N, Shukla R, Kesharwani P. Immune checkpoint inhibitors: A promising anticancer therapy. Drug Discovery Today. 2020;**25**:223-229. DOI: 10.1016/j.drudis.2019.11.003

[10] Chen DS, Mellman I. Elements of cancer immunity and the cancer-immune set point. Nature. 2017;**541**:321-330. DOI: 10.1038/nature21349

[11] Grosso JF, Jure-Kunkel MN. CTLA-4 blockade in tumor models: An overview of preclinical and translational research. Cancer Immunity. 2013;**13**:5. DOI: 10.1158/1424-9634.DCL-5.13.1

[12] Cremolini C, Vitale E, Rastaldo R, Giachino C. Advanced nanotechnology for enhancing immune checkpoint blockade therapy. Nanomaterials (Basel). 2021;**11**:661. DOI: 10.3390/nano11030661

[13] Arce Vargas F, Furness AJS, Litchfield K, Joshi K, Rosenthal R, Ghorani E, et al. Fc effector function contributes to the activity of human anti-CTLA-4 antibodies. Cancer Cell. 2018;**33**:649-663. DOI: 10.1016/j.ccell.2018.02.010

[14] Rotte A, Jin J, Lemaire V. Mechanistic overview of immune checkpoints to support the rational design of their combinations in cancer immunotherapy. Annals of Oncology. 2018;**29**:71-83. DOI: 10.1093/annonc/mdx686

[15] Shao K, Singha S, Clemente-Casares X, Tsai S, Yang Y, Santamaria P. Nanoparticle-based immunotherapy for cancer. ACS Nano. 2015;**9**:16-30. DOI: 10.1021/nn5062029

[16] Nikpoor AR, Tavakkol-Afshari J, Sadri K, Jalali SA, Jaafari MR. Improved tumor accumulation and therapeutic efficacy of CTLA-4-blocking antibody using liposome-encapsulated antibody: In vitro and in vivo studies. Nanomedicine: Nanotechnology, Biology and Medicine. 2017;**13**:2671-2682. DOI: 10.1016/j.nano.2017.08.010

[17] Wilhelm S, Tavares AJ, Dai Q, Ohta S, Audet J, Dvorak HF, et al. Analysis of nanoparticle delivery to tumours. Nature Reviews Materials. 2016;**1**:1-12. DOI: 10.1038/natrevmats.2016.14

[18] Soo Choi H, Liu W, Misra P, Tanaka E, Zimmer JP, Itty Ipe B, et al. Renal clearance of quantum dots. Nature Biotechnology. 2007;**25**:1165-1170. DOI: 10.1038/nbt1340

[19] Blanco E, Shen H, Ferrari M. Principles of nanoparticle design for overcoming biological barriers to drug delivery. Nature Biotechnology. 2015;**33**:941-951. DOI: 10.1038/nbt.3330

[20] Boone CE, Wang L, Gautam A, Newton IG, Steinmetz NF. Combining nanomedicine and immune checkpoint therapy for cancer immunotherapy. Wiley Interdisciplinary Reviews. Nanomedicine and Nanobiotechnology. 2022;**14**:e1739. DOI: 10.1002/wnan.1739

[21] Li G, Gao Y, Gong C, Han Z, Qiang L, Tai Z, et al. Dual-blockade immune checkpoint for beast cancer treatment based on a tumor-penetrating peptide assembling nanoparticle. ACS Applied Materials & Interfaces. 2019;**11**:39513-39524. DOI: 10.1021/acsami.9b13354

[22] Chiang CS, Lin YJ, Lee R, Lai YH, Cheng HW, Hsieh CH, et al. Combination of fucoidan-based magnetic nanoparticles and immunomodulators enhances tumour-localized immunotherapy. Nature Nanotechnology. 2018;**13**:746-754. DOI: 10.1038/s41565-018-0146-7

[23] Au KM, Park SI, Wang AZ. Trispecific natural killer cell nanoengagers for targeted chemoimmunotherapy. Science Advances. 2020;**6**:eaba8564. DOI: 10.1126/sciadv.aba8564

[24] Lang T, Liu Y, Zheng Z, Ran W, Zhai Y, Yin Q, et al. Cocktail strategy based on spatio-temporally controlled nano device improves therapy of breast cancer. Advanced Materials. 2019;**31**:1806202. DOI: 10.1002/adma.201806202

[25] Feng B, Zhou F, Hou B, Wang D, Wang T, Fu Y, et al. Binary cooperative prodrug nanoparticles improve immunotherapy by synergistically modulating immune tumor microenvironment. Advanced Materials. 2018;**30**:e1803001. DOI: 10.1002/adma.201803001

[26] Mi Y, Smith CC, Yang F, Qi Y, Roche KC, Serody JS, et al. A dual immunotherapy nanoparticle improves T-cell activation and cancer immunotherapy. Advanced Materials. 2018;**30**:e1706098. DOI: 10.1002/adma.201706098

[27] Cheng K, Ding Y, Zhao Y, Ye S, Zhao X, Zhang Y, et al. Sequentially responsive therapeutic peptide assembling nanoparticles for dual-targeted cancer immunotherapy. Nano Letters. 2018;**18**:3250-3258. DOI: 10.1021/acs.nanolett.8b01071

[28] Meir R, Shamalov K, Sadan T, Motiei M, Yaari G, Cohen CJ, et al. Fast image-guided stratification using anti-programmed death ligand 1 gold nanoparticles for cancer immunotherapy. ACS Nano. 2017;**11**:11127-11134. DOI: 10.1021/acsnano.7b05299

[29] Kim J, Hong J, Lee J, Fakhraei Lahiji S, Kim YH. Recent advances in tumor microenvironment-targeted nanomedicine delivery approaches to overcome limitations of immune checkpoint blockade-based immunotherapy. Journal of Controlled Release. 2021;**332**:109-126. DOI: 10.1016/j.jconrel.2021.02.002

[30] Xu H, Hu M, Liu M, An S, Guan K, Wang M, et al. Nano-puerarin regulates tumor microenvironment and facilitates chemo- and immunotherapy in murine triple negative breast cancer model. Biomaterials. 2020;**235**:119769. DOI: 10.1016/j.biomaterials.2020.119769

[31] Zhao J, Xiao Z, Li T, Chen H, Yuan Y, Wang YA, et al. Stromal modulation reverses primary resistance to immune checkpoint blockade in pancreatic cancer. ACS Nano. 2018;**12**:9881-9893. DOI: 10.1021/acsnano.8b02481

[32] Kosmides AK, Sidhom JW, Fraser A, Bessell CA, Schneck JP. Dual targeting nanoparticle stimulates the immune system to inhibit tumor growth. ACS Nano. 2017;**11**:5417-5429. DOI: 10.1021/acsnano.6b08152

[33] Ou W, Thapa RK, Jiang L, Soe ZC, Gautam M, Chang JH, et al. Regulatory T cell-targeted hybrid nanoparticles combined with immuno-checkpoint blockage for cancer immunotherapy. Journal of Controlled Release. 2018;**281**:84-96. DOI: 10.1016/j.jconrel.2018.05.018

[34] Choo YW, Kang M, Kim HY, Han J, Kang S, Lee JR, et al. M1 macrophage-derived nanovesicles potentiate the anticancer efficacy of immune checkpoint inhibitors. ACS Nano. 2018;**12**:8977-8993. DOI: 10.1021/acsnano.8b02446

[35] Shae D, Becker KW, Christov P, Yun DS, Lytton-Jean AKR, Sevimli S, et al. Endosomolytic polymersomes increase the activity of cyclic dinucleotide STING agonists to enhance cancer immunotherapy. Nature Nanotechnology. 2019;**14**:269-278. DOI: 10.1038/s41565-018-0342-5

[36] Shen L, Li J, Liu Q, Song W, Zhang X, Tiruthani K, et al. Local blockade of interleukin 10 and CXC motif chemokine ligand 12 with nano-delivery promotes antitumor response in murine cancers. ACS Nano. 2018;**12**:9830-9841. DOI: 10.1021/acsnano.8b00967

[37] Poggio M, Hu T, Pai C-C, Chu B, Belair CD, Chang A, et al. Suppression of exosomal PD-L1 induces systemic anti-tumor immunity and memory. Cell. 2019;**177**:414-427. DOI: 10.1016/j.cell.2019.02.016

[38] Grauers Wiktorin H, Nilsson MS, Kiffin R, Sander FE, Lenox B, Rydström A, et al. Histamine targets myeloid-derived suppressor cells and improves the anti-tumor efficacy of PD-1/PD-L1 checkpoint blockade. Cancer Immunology, Immunotherapy. 2019;**68**:163-174. DOI: 10.1007/s00262-018-2253-6

[39] Nywening TM, Belt BA, Cullinan DR, Panni RZ, Han BJ, Sanford DE, et al. Targeting both tumour-associated CXCR2+ neutrophils and CCR2+ macrophages disrupts myeloid recruitment and improves chemotherapeutic responses in pancreatic ductal adenocarcinoma. Gut. 2018;**67**:1112-1123. DOI: 10.1136/gutjnl-2017-315443

[40] Lee M, Park C-S, Lee Y-R, Im S-A, Song S, Lee C-K. Resiquimod, a TLR7/8 agonist, promotes differentiation of myeloid-derived suppressor cells into macrophages and dendritic cells.

Archives of Pharmacal Research. 2014;**37**:1234-1240. DOI: 10.1007/s12272-014-0379-4

[41] Kuai R, Ochyl LJ, Bahjat KS, Schwendeman A, Moon JJ. Designer vaccine nanodiscs for personalized cancer immunotherapy. Nature Materials. 2017;**16**:489-496. DOI: 10.1038/nmat4822

[42] Zhu G, Lynn GM, Jacobson O, Chen K, Liu Y, Zhang H, et al. Albumin/vaccine nanocomplexes that assemble in vivo for combination cancer immunotherapy. Nature Communications. 2017;**8**:1-15. DOI: 10.1038/s41467-017-02191-y

[43] DeVita VT Jr, Chu E. A history of cancer chemotherapy. Cancer Research. 2008;**68**:8643-8653. DOI: 10.1158/0008-5472.CAN-07-6611

[44] Galluzzi L, Buque A, Kepp O, Zitvogel L, Kroemer G. Immunological effects of conventional chemotherapy and targeted anticancer agents. Cancer Cell. 2015;**28**:690-714. DOI: 10.1016/j.ccell.2015.10.012

[45] Gotwals P, Cameron S, Cipolletta D, Cremasco V, Crystal A, Hewes B, et al. Prospects for combining targeted and conventional cancer therapy with immunotherapy. Nature Reviews. Cancer. 2017;**17**:286-301. DOI: 10.1038/nrc.2017.17

[46] Pfirschke C, Engblom C, Rickelt S, Cortez-Retamozo V, Garris C, Pucci F, et al. Immunogenic chemotherapy sensitizes tumors to checkpoint blockade therapy. Immunity. 2016;**44**:343-354. DOI: 10.1016/j.immuni.2015.11.024

[47] Ni K, Lan G, Chan C, Quigley B, Lu K, Aung T, et al. Nanoscale metal-organic frameworks enhance radiotherapy to potentiate checkpoint blockade immunotherapy. Nature Communications. 2018;**9**:2351. DOI: 10.1038/s41467-018-04703-w

[48] Min Y, Roche KC, Tian S, Eblan MJ, McKinnon KP, Caster JM, et al. Antigen-capturing nanoparticles improve the abscopal effect and cancer immunotherapy. Nature Nanotechnology. 2017;**12**:877-882. DOI: 10.1038/nnano.2017.113

[49] Chen Q, Xu L, Liang C, Wang C, Peng R, Liu Z. Photothermal therapy with immune-adjuvant nanoparticles together with checkpoint blockade for effective cancer immunotherapy. Nature Communications. 2016;7:13193. DOI: 10.1038/ncomms13193

Chapter 5

# Immune Checkpoint Inhibitors in Hodgkin Lymphoma and Non-Hodgkin Lymphoma

*Jiawen Huang and Juan Huang*

## Abstract

Lymphoma, which mainly includes Hodgkin lymphoma (HL) and Non-Hodgkin lymphoma (NHL), is the most common hematological malignance of the lymphoid tissues with significantly heterogeneous characteristics. Tumor immune disequilibrium is involved in tumor development and progression, evading tumor immunosurveillance and suppressing anti-tumor immune responses. The tumor microenvironment (TME) is a complex network that comprises stromal cells and extracellular matrix, playing important roles in the pathogenesis, progression, and drug resistance of lymphoma. Therefore, a promising therapeutic strategy for lymphoma is by targeting the TME to stimulate anticancer immunity either by enhancing the release of immunostimulatory molecules or by mediating immune cell populations. Notably, immune checkpoint therapy (ICT) can provide durable clinical responses and improve overall survival in HL and NHL. However, different subsets of patients with lymphoma have different responses to ICT. Thus, significant challenges remain, including understanding pathways of resistance, optimizing patient selection, improving the management of immune-related adverse events, and identifying rational therapeutic combinations. This will allow a better understanding of the potential applications of ICT in lymphoma, guiding decisions to develop novel combination strategies with maximum efficacy and minimal toxicities for patients.

**Keywords:** tumor microenvironment (TME), immune checkpoint therapy (ICT), lymphoma, Hodgkin lymphoma (HL) and non-Hodgkin lymphoma (NHL)

## 1. Introduction

### 1.1 Biology of immune checkpoints inhibitors (ICIs)

T-cell activation is central to the immune response [1]. However, uncontrolled T cell activation leads to T cell exhaustion and autoimmune diseases [2, 3]. Therefore, it is crucial to maintain immune homeostasis and the balance of both co-stimulatory and co-inhibitory signals. These signals are thus referred as immune checkpoints. The major co-inhibitory receptors expressed on activated T cells are programmed cell death 1 (PD-1) and cytotoxic T-lymphocyte-associated protein 4 (CTLA-4). Here, we will briefly discuss their mechanisms of action.

 IntechOpen

### *1.1.1 Programmed cell death 1*

PD-1 is mainly expressed on mature effector T cells within the peripheral and tumor microenvironment [4], responsible for immune tolerance. Besides T cells, PD-1 expression is also found on B cells, natural killer (NK) cells, dendritic cells (DCs), macrophages, and monocytes [5]. Therefore, it is an inhibitor of both innate and adaptive immunity. In cancers, numerous pathways are responsible for the upregulation of PD-1/PD-L1 signaling; and these major pathways include phosphoinositide 3-kinase (PI3K)/protein kinase B (Akt) pathway, mitogen-activated protein kinase (MAPK) pathway, Jak-Stat pathway, Wnt pathway, NF-κB pathway, and Hedgehog (Hh) pathway [6]. Upon interaction with its ligands, programmed **cell death-ligand 1** or 2 (PD-L1 or PD-L2) expressed on cancer cells or antigen-presenting cells (APCs) of the tumor microenvironments [7–9], PD-1 signaling leads to T cell dysfunction, reduced cytokine production and anergy, thus protecting cancer cells from immune attack [10].

However, the detailed underlying mechanism of PD-1 signaling requires further elucidation. The inhibitory signal transduction of PD-1 needs both the interaction of PD-1/PD-L1 and peptide/MHC class I complex (MHC-I) from the same cells [11]. Src homology region 2 domain-containing phosphatase-2 (SHP-2) is a major downstream mediator of PD-1 and is capable of inhibiting key molecules and pathways such as ZAP70, PI3K/Akt pathway, and Ras pathway. Ultimately, PD-1 signaling counters the T-cell receptor (TCR) cascade and co-stimulatory receptor CD28 signaling in T cells, leading to reduced T cell activation and proliferation [11, 12]. Moreover, PD-1 can

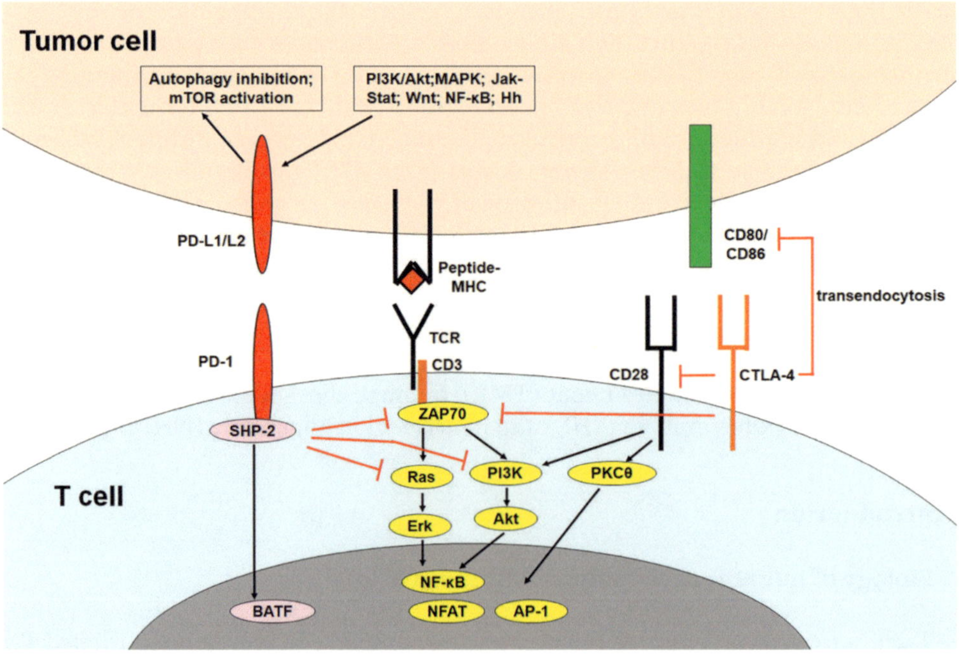


**Figure 1.**
*Major immune checkpoints on T cells. PD-1 and CTLA-4 are the major co-inhibitory receptors expressed on activated T cells. Through ZAP70, PD-1 signaling is able to inhibit ZAP70, PI3K/Akt pathway, and Ras pathway, resulting in reduced T-cell activation. PD-1 can also directly induce T cell exhaustion by upregulating BATF. Furthermore, PD-L1 protects cancer cells in a PD-1-independent manner. CTLA-4 is a competitive inhibitor of co-stimulatory receptor CD28. It also inhibits T cell function via inhibition of ZAP70, PI3K/Akt pathway, cell-cycle progression, and trans-endocytosis of CD80/CD86.*

directly exhaust T cells by upregulating the basic leucine transcription factor, ATF-like (BATF) [13]. Interestingly, PD-L1 may protect cancer cells in a PD-1 independent manner, leading to inhibition of autophagy and activation of mammalian target of rapamycin (mTOR; **Figure 1**) [14]. In addition, PD-1 is also highly expressed on regulatory T cells (Treg), enhancing its proliferation and immunosuppressive effects [12].

#### *1.1.2 Cytotoxic T-lymphocyte-associated protein 4*

In contrast to PD-1, CTLA-4 is mainly expressed in the endocytic vesicles of naïve T cells, and it translocates to the cell surface upon TCR activation. CTLA-4 shares the same ligands (CD80 and CD86) with co-stimulatory receptor CD28 (as competitive binding with higher affinity). Therefore, it can suppress T-cell activation [15, 16]. In addition, like PD-1, CTLA-4 is also able to directly inhibit ZAP70 to suppress TCR signaling and reverse T cell activation [17, 18]. Moreover, CTLA-4 exerts its immunosuppressive function via inhibition of PI3K/Akt pathway, cell-cycle progression, and removal of CD80/CD86 from the APCs via trans-endocytosis (**Figure 1**) [19–22]. Similar to PD-1, CTLA-4 is constitutively expressed in Tregs for immunosuppression and ligand (CD80/CD86) masking [4].

#### *1.1.3 Blockade of immune checkpoints for cancer therapy*

In cancers, the suppressive immune checkpoints introduced above are likely dysregulated, allowing them to escape from immune surveillance [23]. Therefore, blocking such immune checkpoints by antibodies is able to reverse the immune suppression for the treatment of cancers [24]. Preclinical studies have indicated that inhibition of immune checkpoints is able to enhance anti-tumor immunity. In the 1990s, initial research already indicated that the blockade of CTLA-4 by antibodies is able to reduce tumor burden in murine models [25, 26]. Since then, enormous advancements have been achieved in the use of immune checkpoint inhibition in cancer treatment, and the monoclonal antibodies targeting CTLA-4 and PD-1 have been approved by US Food and Drug Administration (FDA) for different cancers [27, 28]. In the following part of the chapter, we will summarize the current applications of immune checkpoint inhibitors (ICIs) for Hodgkin lymphomas (HLs) and non-Hodgkin lymphomas (NHLs).

## 2. Immune checkpoint inhibitors in Hodgkin lymphoma

### 2.1 Anti-PD-1 checkpoint inhibitors

In classical HL (cHL), malignant Reed-Sternberg cells harbor a recurrent chromosome 9p24.1 amplification. Such genetic abnormality encodes *PD-L1* and *PD-L2*, as well as *JAK2*, which further upregulates PD-1 ligand via the JAK-STAT pathway [29]. This upregulated PD-1 signaling allows cHL to suppress surrounding immune cells and survive from immune surveillance. Therefore, blocking PD-1 is likely to restore anti-tumor immunity and eradicate HL cells.

#### *2.1.1 Nivolumab and pembrolizumab*

Nivolumab and pembrolizumab are among the first fully human anti-PD-1 IgG4 monoclonal antibodies approved by the US FDA (May 2016 for nivolumab and March

2017 for pembrolizumab) for the treatment of relapsed or progressed cHL after autologous hematopoietic stem cell transplantation (auto-HSCT) and brentuximab vedotin (therefore referred as relapsed/refractory, r/r) [30, 31]. Since then, numerous clinical trials and real-world experiences have demonstrated the efficacy and safety profiles of nivolumab and pembrolizumab against HL, which is mainly (but not limited to) r/r cHL. Nivolumab and pembrolizumab are the most common ICIs used for r/r cHL patients, and many groups use both drugs in the same clinical trials (refers to them both as PD-1 ICIs). The clinical data of pembrolizumab are summarized in **Table 1** together with nivolumab.

As shown in **Table 1**, the objective response rate (ORR) for PD-1 ICIs is generally high (usually over 70%). However, the CR is rarely achieved, with a CR rate of around 30%–40%. Notably, some preconditions or previous treatments the patients experienced significantly enhance the outcomes of anti-PD-1 therapy. For example, 5 of 5 r/r cHL patients who have been given hypomethylating agents 5-azacitidine all achieved CR after ICI treatment [37]. This may suggest some potential combination therapies and numerous groups are assessing the efficacy of different treatment combinations.

#### *2.1.1.1 Combination of PD-1 inhibitors and HSCT*

The poor CR rate of anti-PD-1 antibodies suggests that monotherapy of PD-1 blockade alone may be not sufficient to cure r/r HL. Therefore, combined therapy of PD-1 blockade with other additional canonical treatments is necessary. It has been demonstrated that administration of PD-1 inhibitors before/after allogenic (allo-) or autologous (auto-) HSCT significantly enhances response rate and prolongs patient survival. Manson et al. [54] reported that none of the 13 r/r HL patients who underwent consolidation treatment of allo-HSCT together with nivolumab suffered from disease relapse. On contrary, 62.2% of those ($n$ = 37) who did not undergo subsequent allo-HSCT relapsed. In another similar study, Merryman et al. [55] studied the 209 cHL patients who underwent subsequent allo-HSCT after PD-1 inhibition. With a median follow-up of 24 months, they reported that the 2-year progression-free survival (PFS) and overall survival (OS) were 69% and 82%, respectively. Merryman et al. also suggested that a shorter interval between PD-1 inhibition and allo-HSCT can significantly boost the graft-versus-lymphoma (GVL) effect of allo-HSCT. The real-life experience of 74 patients who underwent allo-HSCT after nivolumab treatment in Spain provided a similar conclusion (i.e., improved PFS and OS) as well [56].

Similarly, consolidation after auto-HSCT by PD-1 blockade also improves the treatment outcomes [57]. In this clinical trial (NCT02362997), the expected PFS after auto-HSCT increased from 60 to 82% upon pembrolizumab administration. Casadei et al. [58] also reported that auto-HSCT after PD-1 blockade further improved patient survival, with an estimated 5-year PFS of 73.4% and 4.8-year OS of 92.3%.

Although the combination of PD-1 inhibition and allo-HSCT seems to be a promising strategy against HL, increased graft-versus-host disease (GVHD) upon anti-PD-1 administration is a major concern of this treatment option [55, 56, 59]. Such GVHD can be severe and may cause multi-organ failure and even death [55, 56, 59–64]. Therefore, multiple studies indicated that post-transplant cyclophosphamide (PTCy)-based GVHD prophylaxis is required for improved PFS and therefore strongly suggested [55, 59].

| Groups | Study status | | | | Responses | | | Survival | | AEs | |
|---|---|---|---|---|---|---|---|---|---|---|---|
| | Disease | Drug | Number | Follow-up | ORR | CR | PR | PFS | OS | Treatment-related AEs | >Grade 3 |
| Liput et al. [32] | cHL | Nivo | 10 | NA | 70% | 60% | 10% | — | — | 80% | 20% |
| Davis et al. [33] | r/r cHL (young patients) | Nivo | 10 | 30 d | 30% | 10% | 20% | — | — | Not reported for cHL separately | — |
| Kasamon et al. [34] | r/r cHL | Nivo | 95 | 6 mo | 65% | 7% | 58% | — | — | Lack overall summary | — |
| Bair et al. [35] | r/r cHL | Nivo, Pembro | 53 | 13 mo | 68% | 45% | 23% | 12 mo: 75% Median: 29 mo | 12 mo: 89% | Lack overall summary | — |
| Armand et al. [36] | r/r cHL after auto-HSCT | Nivo | 243 | 18 mo | 69% | 16% | 53% | Median: 14.7% | 12 mo: 92% | Lack overall summary | — |
| Falchi et al. [37] | r/r cHL | Nivo, Pembro | 9 | 9.9 mo | 89% | 78% | 11% | — | — | 100% | 67% |
| Armand et al. [38] | r/r cHL | Pembro | 31 | 17 mo | 65% | 16% | 48% | 24 wk.: 69% 52 wk.: 46% | 24 wk.: 100% | 97% | 16% |
| Ansell et al. [39] | r/r cHL | Nivo | 23 | 40 week | 87% | 17% | 70% | 24 wk.: 86% | — | 78% | 22% |
| Chen et al. [40] | r/r cHL | Pembro | 210 | 27.6 mo | 72% | 28% | 44% | Median: 13.7 mo | 24 mo: 100% | 73% | 12% |
| Younes et al. [41] | r/r cHL | Nivo | 80 | 8.9 mo | 66% | 9% | 57% | 6 mo: 76.9% | 6 mo: 98.7% | 99% | 40% |
| Bekoz et al. [42, 43] | r/r cHL | Nivo | 87 | 29 mo | 70% | 36% | 34% | 24 mo: 58.5% | 24 mo: 78.7% | 58% | 12% of AEs |
| Geoerger et al. [44] | r/r HL pediatric patients | Pembro | 15 | 8.6 mo | 60% | 13% | 47% | Median: 12.2 mo 6 mo: 72.7% 12 mo: 51.9% | 6 and 12 mo: 100% | Not reported for cHL separately | — |
| Maruyama et al. [45] | r/r cHL | Nivo | 16 | 38.8 mo | 87.5% | 31.3% | 56.3% | Median: 11.7 mo | 3 yr.: 80.4% | 100% | 50% |

| Groups | Study status | | | | Responses | | | Survival | | AEs | |
|---|---|---|---|---|---|---|---|---|---|---|---|
| | Disease | Drug | Number | Follow-up | ORR | CR | PR | PFS | OS | Treatment-related AEs | >Grade 3 |
| Ramchandren et al. [46] | untreated, advanced-stage cHL | Nivo | 51 | 9.4 mo | 84% | 67% | 17% | 9 mo: 92% | — | 96% | 59% |
| Chan et al. [47] | r/r cHL | Pembro (low dose) | 11 | — | 100% | 73% | 27% | Median: 35 mo | — | 27.2 | 0% |
| Chan et al. [47] | r/r cHL | Nivo (low dose) | 6 | — | 100% | 67% | 17% | Median: 33 mo | — | 67% | 0% |
| Dada et al. [48] | r/r cHL | Nivo | 10 | 12.3 mo | 80% | 70% | 10% | — | — | 40% | 0% |
| Kuruvilla et al. [49] | r/r cHL | Pembro | 151 | 25.7 mo | 65.6% | 25% | 41% | Median: 13.2 mo | — | 75% | 20% |
| Momotow et al. [50] | r/r HL | Nivo, Pembro | 60 | 20.4 mo | 65% | 18% | 47% | 2 yr.: 42.3% | 2 yr.: 78.4%<br>3 yr.: 65.8% | — | 32% |
| Hur et al. [51] | Pretreated cHL | Nivo, Pembro | 20 | 14 mo | 75% | 45% | 30% | Median: 18 mo | Median: 36 mo | Lack overall summary | — |
| Lepik et al. [52] | r/r cHL | Nivo | 99 | 21 mo | 64% | 31% | 33% | Median: 19.4 mo | — | 88% | 17% |
| Armand et al. [53] | cHL after BV failure | Pembro | 31 | 52.8 mo | 58% | 19% | 39% | Median: 11.4 mo<br>24 mo: 30% | 24 mo: 87%<br>36 mo: 81% | 71% | 19% |

*Numbers: number of patients; Follow-up: median or minimum follow-up; ORR: overall response rate; CR: complete response; PR: partial response; PFS: progression free survival; OS: overall survival; AEs: adverse events; r/r cHL: relapsed/refractory classical Hodgkin's lymphoma; d: days; mo: months; yr.: years; Nivo: nivolumab; Pembro: pembrolizumab; BV: brentuximab vedotin.*

**Table 1.**
*Overview of clinical efficiency and toxicity results of PD-1 inhibitors, nivolumab and pembrolizumab, in Hodgkin's lymphoma.*

#### *2.1.1.2 Other combined therapy*

The regimen AVD regimen (doxorubicin, vinblastine, and dacarbazine) is the backbone of the well-established chemotherapy regimen ABVD (doxorubicin, bleomycin, vinblastine, and dacarbazine) for HL [65]. Therefore, the efficacy of nivolumab and AVD combination in early-stage cHL was assessed [66]. In total, 109 patients were given two different treatment strategies (of dosing and sequencing), and both groups displayed promising outcomes, with over 90% CR and nearly 100% 12-month PFS. Another multicenter, single-arm, phase II trial proved that pembrolizumab followed by AVD was both effective and safe in patients with untreated early unfavorable and advanced-stage cHL, with all patients ($n$ = 30) achieving complete metabolic response (CMR) [67]. At the median follow-up of 22.5 months, the PFS and OS are 100%, indicating the superior efficacy of the strategy.

Brentuximab vedotin (BV) is a CD30-based antibody-drug conjugate. When used alone, it can lead to an ORR of 72% and CR rate of 33% in r/r HL patients [68]. Advani et al. [69] reported that BV combined with nivolumab can be the first salvage therapy in patients with r/r cHL, with an ORR of 85% and CR rate of 67%. In a median follow-up of 34.3 months, the estimated 3-year PFS and OS were 77% and 93%, respectively. Such combination treatment can be applied as a first-line option for older or chemotherapy-ineligible cHL patients, as demonstrated by Cheson et al. [70]. With a total of 46 patients and a median follow-up of 21.2 months, 48% of patients achieved CR and 13% achieved PR, with an ORR of 61%. Due to the high efficacy of this combination, it was considered as a salvage option after PD-1 blockade failure. In 21 r/r cHL patients who failed nivolumab monotherapy previously, BV combined with nivolumab resulted in an ORR of 57% [71]. Twenty-four-month PFS and OS were 31% and 80%, respectively. In total, 63% of patients suffered from adverse effects (AEs), but AEs of grade 3 or 4 were only observed in 10% of patients.

The potential synergistic effect of radiotherapy and ICIs has been proposed as well. In a cohort of 12 patients with r/r cHL, patients were given a combined treatment of radiotherapy and nivolumab/pembrolizumab, with an ORR of 100% and a CR rate of 58% [72]. With a median follow-up of 18 months, 92% of patients remained in CR (9 of 12 patients underwent HSCT consolidation). Forceville et al. [73] presented two case reports supporting that radiotherapy combined with nivolumab can lead to excellent outcomes.

Gemcitabine, vinorelbine, and liposomal doxorubicin (GVD) are traditional second-line treatment options for r/r cHL, with a CR rate of around 50% [74]. In comparison, the combination of GVD and pembrolizumab resulted in an ORR of 100% and a CR rate of 95%, with a total of 39 enrolled r/r cHL patients [75]. In total, 36 of these 39 patients underwent subsequent auto-HSCT, and they all remained in CR at a median post-transplant follow-up of 13.5 months. In a similar trial consisting of 103 patients (27 for GVD + PD-1 blockade, 76 for GVD), the combination group had a higher CR rate of 85.2% (65.8% for the GVD group) and an extended PFS (1-year PFS of 82.2% vs. 67.9% for GVD group) [76].

### *2.1.2 Camrelizumab*

Camrelizumab (SHR-1210), which was developed in China, is a humanized high-affinity anti-PD-1 IgG4 monoclonal antibody. It has shown promising efficacy against numerous advanced solid tumors including nasopharyngeal carcinoma, esophageal carcinoma, gastric and gastroesophageal junction cancer [77–81]. In a single-arm, multicenter, phase II study (NCT03155425), a total of 75 patients with r/r cHL were given Camrelizumab 200 mg every 2 weeks intravenously. In a median follow-up of 12.9 months, 21 (28.0%) and 36 (48.0%) patients achieved complete or partial remission, respectively (i.e., objective response rate is 76.0%). Treatment-related adverse events (AE) were observed in all patients enrolled, with 20 (26.7%) of them exhibiting grade 3 or 4 treatment-related AEs [82]. The group further extended the follow-up of this clinical trial till 2020, with a median follow-up duration of 36.2 months. The objective response rate remained almost unchanged. The median PFS was 22.5 months and 3-year OS was 82.7%.

#### *2.1.2.1 Combined therapy*

Like other checkpoint inhibitors, although camrelizumab exhibits a high objective response rate in patients with r/r cHL, the CR rate remains low (as shown above). It has been proven that inhibition of *de novo* DNA methylation can boost T-cell function upon PD-1 blockade [83, 84]. Decitabine is a DNA demethylating agent [85]; therefore, clinical trial combining a low dose of decitabine with camrelizumab against r/r cHL was conducted (NCT02961101, NCT03250962). Indeed, when compared with camrelizumab monotherapy, r/r cHL patients receiving decitabine plus camrelizumab exhibited a higher CR rate (79% vs. 32%) and longer median PFS (35.0 vs. 15.5 months) [86, 87]. In addition, the administration of decitabine plus camrelizumab showed promising efficacy against HL with resistance to anti-PD-1 [86, 87]. Similarly, combination treatment of anti-angiogenic agent apatinib and camrelizumab might be a salvage option for r/r cHL patients who failed PD-1/PD-L1 inhibitor therapy, as demonstrated in the case reports presented by Yan et al. [88]. Out of seven enrolled patients, two achieved CR, and four achieved PR. The median PFS was 10 months, and no unexpected side effects were observed.

### *2.1.3 Sintilimab*

Sintilimab is an anti-PD-1 antibody developed by Innovent Biologics, Suzhou, China. Shi et al. reported it exhibits comparable activity to nivolumab and pembrolizumab in patients with r/r cHL [89]. In their single-arm, multicenter, phase II trial (NCT03114683), 6-months PFS was 77.6%, and 74 of 92 fully analyzed patients (80.4%) achieved an objective response. Among those with objective responses, 31 (34%) had CR and 43 (47%) had PR. As for AE, 89 (93%) of 96 patients demonstrated treatment-related AE, including 17 (18%) with grade 3 or 4 and 11 (11%) with serious treatment-related AE (all expected).

### *2.1.4 Tislelizumab*

Tislelizumab is a specially engineered humanized anti-PD-1 IgG4 monoclonal antibody. In contrast to other conventional PD-1 inhibitors, the Fcγ receptor (FcγR) fragment of tislelizumab was modified to minimize the binding of macrophages and the subsequent antibody-dependent phagocytosis. The antibody-dependent phagocytosis by macrophages could potentially lead to T-cell clearance and greatly affect the efficacy of anti-PD-1 therapy [90]. Therefore, the FcγR modification allows tislelizumab to exhibit improved anti-tumor function. In the single-arm, multicenter, phase II trial of tislelizumab in patients with r/r cHL (NCT03209973) [91], 61 of 70

(87.1%) patients achieved an objective response, including a high CR rate of 62.9% (44 of 70). The estimated median 9-month PFS was 74.5%. AEs were observed in 65 of 70 (92.9%) patients, with 15 (21.4%) experiencing grade 3 or 4 AEs.

#### *2.1.4.1 Combined therapy.*

Similar to other anti-PD-1 antibodies, co-administration of low-dose decitabine and tislelizumab for the treatment of r/r cHL has been reported. A 27-year-old male r/r cHL patient who failed eight lines of therapy (including PD-1 inhibition) achieved partial remission upon receiving decitabine plus tislelizumab treatment. No disease progression was observed during the entire 11.5 months of follow-up [92].

### *2.1.5 Zimberelimab*

Zimberelimab (GLS-010) is the first fully human anti-PD-1 monoclonal antibody produced in a transgenic rat platform. While sharing the same heavy chain constant region as nivolumab and pembrolizumab, zimberelimab has two different modifications, namely S228P and N95S, in IgG4 core-hinge area and CDR3 area of the light chain, respectively. The S228P mutation prevents Fab-arm exchange, and the N95S mutation prevents the glycosylation of the antigen-binding domain [93]. Phase I studies for advanced solid tumors [94, 95] or preliminary studies for r/r cHL [96] have suggested high efficacy and acceptable safety. In a phase II trial for patients with r/r cHL (NCT03655483), 77 of 85 (90.6%) patients had objective responses, with a CR rate of 32.9% (28 patients). Twelve-month PFS and OS were 78% and 99%, respectively. Treatment-related AEs were found in 79 of 85 (92.9%) patients, with 24 (28.2%) of them demonstrated grade 3 or 4 and 1 exhibited grade 5 treatment-related AE (gastrointestinal infection) [93].

### *2.1.6 Penpulimab*

Penpulimab is a humanized anti-PD-1 monoclonal antibody co-developed by Akeso Biopharma and Chia Tai Tianqing for the treatment of solid tumors. Similar to tislelizumab, the FcγR fragment region of penpulimab is engineered, through which the FcγR bindings of effectors (such as macrophages) are eliminated. As the results, T cells are protected from antibody-dependent cell-mediated cytotoxicity (ADCC), and the efficacy of tislelizumab is expected to be enhanced. In the open-label, multicenter, single-arm, phase I/II study (NCT03722147), the objective response rate was 89.4% (76 of 85 patients), with 40 (47.1%) patients achieving CR. Twelve-month PFS was 72.1%. Treatment-related AEs were observed in 97.9% (92 of 94) patients, with 25 (26.6%) experienced grade 3 or above treatment-related AEs [97, 98].

## 2.2 Anti-PD-L1 checkpoint inhibitors

Besides PD-1 blockade, targeting PD-L1 is an alternative strategy to avoid PD-1/PD-L1 immune checkpoints. However, it should be noted that PD-L1 and PD-L2, the two ligands to PD-1, are differentially expressed in the tumor microenvironment of cHL [29, 99]. Therefore, anti-PD-L1 monotherapy may be not sufficient to completely inhibit the PD-1 pathway, its efficacy may be lower than PD-1 inhibition alone. The use of PD-L1 inhibitors in HL should be carefully evaluated.

#### *2.2.1 Avelumab*

Avelumab (MSB0010718C) is a human anti-PD-L1 IgG1 monoclonal antibody. Besides blocking PD-1/PD-L1 interactions, the binding of avelumab on tumor cells induces ADCC via the FcɣR binding [100, 101]. Unlike the ADCC induced by anti-PD-1 antibodies that impair T-cell function and dampen the efficacy of treatment, the ADCC induced by anti-PD-L1 antibodies provides another mechanism of tumor clearance and further enhances treatment efficacy. In a phase Ib trial of avelumab against r/r cHL [102], 13 of 31 (41.2%) patients showed an objective response, with six (19.4%) achieving CR and seven (22.6%) achieved PR. Twelve-month PFS was 18.2%, and the median PFS was 5.7 months. Treatment-related AEs were observed in 26 (86.7%) patients and 13 (43.3%) of them are grade 3 or 4.

#### *2.2.2 Sugemalimab*

Sugemalimab is a fully human, full-length, anti-PD-L1 IgG4 monoclonal antibody developed by CStone Pharmaceuticals for advanced solid tumors and lymphoma. In 2021, it has been approved in China for the first-line treatment of various forms of non-small-cell lung cancer in combination with different treatments. Phase Ia and Ib studies have been finished for sugemalimab against advanced malignancies (including 5 cHL patients in phase Ia study) [103]. They have demonstrated the safety and anti-tumor efficacy of sugemalimab. Currently, a single-arm, phase 2 trial of sugemalimab against r/r cHL (as monotherapy) is underway (NCT03505996) and has enrolled 80 patients [104].

#### *2.2.3 Durvalumab*

Durvalumab is another human anti-PD-L1 monoclonal antibody and has been approved by US FDA for urothelial carcinoma and stage III non-small-cell lung cancer [105]. Ogasawara et al. have conducted a pharmacokinetic analysis of durvalumab in 267 patients with hematological malignancies (including HL) [105]. They suggested the dosing regimen (1500 mg every 4 weeks) for hematologic malignancies can be the same as other solid tumors. This suggests a potential application of durvalumab against HL.

#### *2.2.4 Atezolizumab*

Atezolizumab is an inhibitor of PD-L1, and it has been approved by the US FDA and the European Medicines Agency for certain forms of solid tumors (such as triple-negative breast cancer or non-small-cell lung carcinoma, as monotherapy or used in combination) [106]. iMATRIX was a multicenter, open-label, phase I/II trial of young patients (<30 years old) with solid tumors or lymphomas (including nine HL patients, NCT02541604) [106]. Unfortunately, only two patients demonstrated objective response (PR). For the rest of the HL patients, two of them remained with stable disease, and five suffered from disease progression. Another phase II clinical trial of atezolizumab in r/r HL (NCT03120676) was also terminated due to lack of accrual.

### 2.3 Anti-CTLA-4 checkpoint inhibitors

#### *2.3.1 Ipilimumab*

In contrast to the wild application of anti-PD-1/PD-L1 inhibitor for the treatment of HL, very few studies have been conducted to assess the efficacy of anti-CTLA-4 inhibitor against HL. Ipilimumab is a fully humanized anti-CTLA-4 IgG1κ monoclonal antibody. Although several clinical trials of ipilimumab have been conducted for numerous solid tumors [107–110], and there are some ongoing clinical trials assessing the possibility of using ipilimumab in r/r cHL (like NCT04938232); currently very few reports have demonstrated the efficacy of ipilimumab as monotherapy in the treatment of HL. Bashey et al. reported that two out of 14 relapsed HL patients after allo-HSCT achieved CR upon ipilimumab treatment [111]. In comparison, the possibility of co-administrating ipilimumab with other agents against HL has been evaluated.

#### *2.3.1.1 Combined therapy*

In an open-label, multicenter, phase I trial assessing the efficacy of combination therapy in 61 patients with r/r HL (NCT01896999), patients were divided into three groups: combinations of brentuximab vedotin with ipilimumab (ipi-group) or nivolumab (nivo-group) or both (triplet-group) [112]. Although the overall response rates were similar for all three groups (76% for ipi-group, 89% for nivo-group, and 82% for triplet-group), triplet groups demonstrated a higher CR rate (73%), as compared with ipi- (57%) and nivo-groups (61%). These are also higher than the expected individual monotherapies. However, the inclusion of ipilimumab in the combination therapy significantly increased the chance of severe (grade 3 or 4) treatment-related AEs, with 43% in the ipi-group and 50% in the triplet-group. On contrary, this number is only 16% in the nivo-group. This may raise concerns for the possible higher toxicity of ipilimumab in treating Hodgkin lymphoma.

Lenalidomide is an FDA-approved drug for the treatment of multiple myeloma, with the ability of modulating cellular and humoral immunity and antiangiogenesis [113]. In a phase I dose-escalation study of ipilimumab and lenalidomide including seven refractory HL patients (NCT01750983) [114], PR was observed in one patient, and three patients experienced tumor shrinkage (less than PR).

### **2.4 Other potential immune checkpoint inhibitors**

Besides the well-known immune checkpoints PD-1 and CTLA-4, novel immune checkpoints may be used as therapeutic targets for the treatment of HL. Halabi et al. found that lymphocyte-activation gene 3 (LAG-3) and T-cell immunoglobulin and mucin-domain containing 3 (TIM-3) are almost constitutively expressed in cHL [115]. Therefore, clinical trials targeting LAG-3 (relatlimab, NCT02061761) or TIM-3 (BMS-986258, NCT03446040) alone or in combination with nivolumab in the treatment of r/r HL are completed, and results will be released soon. In addition, T-cell Ig and ITIM domains (TIGIT) are another immune checkpoint receptor that is found to be highly co-expressed with PD-1 in r/r cHL patients [116]. Therefore, co-inhibition of PD-1 and TIGIT could be a novel strategy for treating r/r cHL.

Immune checkpoints are expressed in immune cells other than T cells, which could be targeted as well. In a phase Ib study, Armand et al. evaluated the efficacy and safety of dual inhibition of PD-1 and CTLA-4 (65 patients) or killer immunoglobulin-like receptors (KIRs) (72 patients) for r/r cHL [117]. KIR is expressed on NK cells and inhibits their function by interacting with MHC I [118]. However, the authors reported that the combination failed to further improve the efficacy, as compared with nivolumab monotherapy.

## 3. Immune checkpoints inhibitors in non-Hodgkin lymphoma

Non-Hodgkin lymphoma (NHL) is a mostly common and heterogeneous group of lymphomas derived from B and T lymphocytes, natural killer (NK), cells or precursors of these cells. Its pathology remains largely unexplained. Recent studies identified that tumor microenvironment (TME) in NHL is now playing a significant role in immune suppression and propagating tumor growth [119, 120]. Therefore, immunotherapies have been widely used and investigated in NHL to enhance or manipulate host anti-tumor immunity. In recent years, interference of PD-1/PD-L1 signaling, the immune checkpoint (therefore also known as checkpoint blockade), has been used in these kinds of lymphomas for its clinical efficacy by enhancing anti-tumor immune response. More importantly, therapeutic interference of checkpoint blockade has enjoyed significant success in cHL, but clinical response greatly varied in NHLs [121].

PD-1 and its ligands (PD-Ls), PD-L1 (also known as CD274 or B7-H1) and PD-L2 (as known as CD273 or B7-DC), form a signaling network that serves as a checkpoint to limit T-cell immunity, causing T-cell exhaustion [6, 122, 123]. Targeting PD-1 signaling to block T-cell activity with immune inhibitory antibodies can promote the activation, maturation, and proliferation of T-cells, eventually regulating anti-tumor activity, which has been investigated in NHL. Recent studies suggested that ICIs have been considered a promising and effective treatment strategy for some types of NHLs. Thus, PD-1 antibodies have been approved by the US FDA including nivolumab and pembrolizumab. Now, let us review the effectiveness of ICIs in NHL.

### 3.1 Immune checkpoints inhibitors in B-non-Hodgkin lymphoma

#### *3.1.1 Diffuse large B-cell lymphoma (DLBCL)*

Diffuse large B-cell lymphoma (DLBCL) represents 30–40% of all non-Hodgkin lymphomas (NHL) with a 60–70% curable rate in Rituximab Era [120]. However, about one-third of these patients are refractory or resistant to standard treatment. In addition, there are several subtypes of DLBCL in the 2016 World Health Organization (WHO) classification of lymphoid malignancies according to unique clinical and pathological features, including primary DLBCL of the central nervous system (PCNSL), primary cutaneous DLBCL, leg type, T-cell/histiocyte-rich large cell lymphoma, and EBV positive DLBCL of the elderly [124]. Nevertheless, most cases of DLBCL fall into the "not otherwise specified" (NOS) category [125]. As we know, immune evasion plays an important pathogenetic mechanism in DLBCL evolution, and immune checkpoint blockade therapy was explored in all kinds of lymphomas. But the outcome of immunotherapy remained controversial.

PD-L1 expression in DLBCL, with an incidence of ~25%, is associated with inferior outcomes, involving in DLBCL pathogenesis, which is considered a potential target [126, 127]. Importantly, chromosome 9p24.1 copy number alteration observed in DLBCL, in addition to cHL, is also involved in negative T cell regulation and NF-κb signaling pathway, which is associated with responsiveness to ICIs in relapsed/refractory DLBCL (r/r DLBCL) [126]. However, the results of ICIs in r/r DLBCL are disappointing [128, 129]. A phase I study to evaluate the safety and efficacy of nivolumab enrolled 81 r/r lymphoma patients (11 DLBCL) and showed an ORR of 36% in DLBCL. A recent phase II study (NCT02038933) showed that nivolumab monotherapy had good safety profiles but low ORR in DLBCL patients [130]. However, clinical trials of nivolumab combined with other immunochemotherapies are still in progress.

Pembrolizumab (Keytruda), a humanized anti-PD-1 MoAb with excellent anti-tumor activity, was explored in DLBCL. This study including 30 DLBCL patients, evaluated the efficacy of pembrolizumab (200 mg) with R-CHOP, and showed a 90% ORR, 77% CR, and 83% 2y-PFS at a median follow-up of 25.5 months, suggesting that this combination may be a promising treatment strategy [131]. All in all, the results of anti-PD-1 antibody in DLBCL patients are not promising in the current clinical trials, and anti-PD-1 antibody combination therapy is also under investigation [126].

It is a worthy note that anti-PD-L1 antibody atezolizumab (MPDL-3280A) combined chemotherapy seems a promising approach in DLBCL. In a phase I/II study, atezolizumab-R-CHOP for DLBCL demonstrated high efficacy (ORR of 87.5%) and durable responses (24 months for 80% of patients) for the combinational group [132]. Fifty-eight DLBCL patients enrolled in the study to assess the anti-tumor activity of atezolizumab associated with Venetolax (a BCL-2 inhibitor) and Obinutuzumab with 23.6% ORR (NCT03276468). In another phase 1/2 study, atezolizumab in combination with rituximab and polatuzumab in 21 participants with r/r DLBCL showed 57.14% ORR and 33.33% CR. In additional, atezolizumab with mosunetuzumab (a bispecific CD20-CD3 monoclonal antibody) was evaluated (NCT02500407). Certainly, anti-PD-L1 antibodies have been extensively investigated in combination with new-generation CD20 antibodies (NCT03533283), Chimeric antigen receptor (CAR)-T (NCT02926833), and ASCT (NCT02362997).

Durvalumab, another humanized IgG1-kappa monoclonal antibody against PD-L1, showed markedly anti-tumor activity in vivo. Thus, like atezolizumab, numbers of clinical trials are ongoing to investigate the value of durvalumab as a single agent or in combination with other treatment approaches or CAR T-cells in B-NHL patients. Encouraging results were commonly seen in patients treated with durvalumab in combination therapy in early studies. Durvalumab with Ibrutinib in DLBCL has 25% ORR and 4.6 months PFS [133]. Also, durvalumab combined with R-CHOP showed 54.10% CR but 51% serious AEs [134]. More interesting, remarkable results were found when combined with durvalumab and CAR T-cells in B-NHL including 12 DLBCLs, 2 high-grade B-cell lymphomas, and 1 PMBL (NCT03310619 (PLATFORM) and NCT02706405), which reported an ORR of 91%, including 64% CR [135, 136]. From these clinical results, AEs were frequently seen in combination therapy, which needed to be noted [137, 138].

Another inhibitor signaling of CTLA-4 including ipilimumab was not explored for its efficacy and safety. Recently, the combination of ipilimumab and nivolumab in patients with high-risk DLBCL after Allo-SCT has been opened (NCT02681302) [139]. More results should be worthy of expectation.

#### *3.1.2 Primary mediastinal large B-cell lymphoma (PMBCL)*

Importantly, anti-PD-1 MoAb has promising results in some special DLBCL. Primary mediastinal large B-cell lymphoma (PMBCL) comprises approximately 10% of DLBCL with different clinicopathologic and molecular signature, which have a good prognosis with R-CHOP/R-DAEPOCH combined with radiotherapy, with a 5-year event-free survival rate of 93% and OS rate of 97% [140]. However, more than 10% of patients still suffered relapsed or refractory, and the outcomes in r/r PMBCL remain poor. Studies have elucidated that PMBCL shared many similar biological features with cHL, including the importance of JAK-STAT and NF-κB signaling pathways as well as immune evasion [141]. Aberration expressions of PD-L1 and PD-L2 were found in PMBCL tumors, and the efficacy of anti-PD-1 antibody (pembrolizumab) in r/r PMBCL was confirmed in phase 1 KEYNOTE-013 study [142]. Subsequently, a phase 2 study (KEYNOTE-170) has evaluated the efficacy of pembrolizumab in r/r PMBCL, and similar results were observed, with 45% ORR, and 13% CR, and median duration of response (DOR) not yet reached [143]. Thus, pembrolizumab has been approved in r/r PMBCL by FDA. After that, ICIs combined with other therapeutic agents for r/r PMBCL have been widely studied all over the world. Nivolumab combined with the anti-CD30 antibody-drug conjugate (ADC) brentuximab vedotin (BV) has been studied for r/r PMBCL in the CheckMate 436 study with an ORR was 73% and CR 37% [144]. These studies have identified the efficacy of PD-1 in PMBCL, especially combined with other agents. Numerous clinical trials assessing combination therapies with immune checkpoint inhibitors are ongoing [145].

#### *3.1.3 Epstein-Barr virus (EBV)+ diffuse large B-cell lymphoma (DLBCL) and primary DLBCL of the central nervous system (PCNSL)*

Epstein-Barr virus (EBV) is detected in a variety of B-cell lymphomas (BCLs) and lymphoproliferative disorders (B-LPD) with poor prognosis, associated with immunodeficiency, a key factor of lymphomagenesis. EBV+ DLBCL-NOS was first described as age-related EBV-associated LPD in 2003 with poor outcomes compared with EBV-negative DLBCL patients [146]. Unfortunately, the biology of EBV+ DLBCL-NOS remains unsure, and no standard approaches for these kinds of patients. Researchers have identified that 100% PD-L1 expression was seen in EBV+ DLBCL in a larger cohort study ($n$ = 1100), which was significantly associated with EBV+ status [147, 148]. Liu et al. have identified that anti-PD-1 antibodies can restore and active function of T cells in EBV+ DLBCL [149]. Thus, the PD-L1/PD-1 pathway may be a potential therapeutic target for EBV+ DLBCL. Many studies are ongoing to assess the application of ICIs combined with chemotherapies in EBV+ DLBCL (e.g., NCT03212807, NCT04181489, NCT04705129, and so on).

Also, primary central nervous lymphoma (PCNSL) is a rare extra-nodal lymphoma with a high refractory/relapse rate using high-dose MTX-based treatment [150, 151]. For relapsed/refractory PCNSL (r/r PCNSL), new strategies have been explored including immunotherapy. PD-1 antibodies in r/r PCNSL have been reported with good efficacy in some case reports [152, 153]. Thus, some retrospective and prospective studies discussed the efficacy of anti-PD-1 antibody as monotherapy and in combination with other drugs [153, 154]. Unluckily, the results of ICIs in r/r PCNSL varied. Especially, we have seen promising efficacy in PCNSL with Bruton's Tyrosine Kinase and Immune Modulatory Small Molecules. Some explorations of ICIs in primary and r/r PCNSL are under study, especially for those who have higher PD-L1 expression and no chance to do MTX-based chemotherapy (NCT04899427, NCT05425654, and NCT04831658).

In other B-NHL entities, the rates of PD-L1 expression on neoplastic B cells are low: ~5% in FL, ~10% in high-grade MZL, and 0% in MCL. Therefore, slightly rare studies have been explored in these types of B-NHL.

### 3.2 Immune checkpoints inhibitors in T-non-Hodgkin lymphoma

PD-1 or PD-L1 has been used in various kinds of NHLs, either alone or in combination with other agents, which have promising results in some Lymphoma. For T-cell lymphomas, this strategy has been challenging because these markers may be expressed on the tumor cells themselves resulting in inadvertent tumor growth.

Peripheral T-cell lymphoma (PTCL) is a group of lymphoproliferative disorders, originating from mature T/NK cells with highly heterogeneous, aggressive characteristics and poor prognosis. There are 27 subtypes of PTCL in the World Health Organization 2016 classification of lymphoid neoplasm, including extranodal NK/T-cell lymphoma, nasal-type (ENKTL), nonspecific (PTCL-NOS), angioimmunoblastic T-cell lymphoma (AITL), and anaplastic lymphoma kinase (ALK)+/− anaplastic large cell lymphoma (ALCL) [155, 156]. CHOP-based regimens are the first-line treatments for PTCL other than NK/T-cell lymphoma, but the efficacy is limited [157, 158]. Thus, effective treatments for relapsed or refractory (r/r) PTCL are urgently needed. PD-1 and PD-L1 expression is commonly observed in PTCL cells, and PD-1 or PD-L1 is considered a prognostic biomarker and target. A phase I study (five patients with r/r PTCL) and phase 2 study (12 patients with r/r PTCL) have identified the clinical value of Nivolumab in r/r PTCL patients with 33% ORR [159, 160]. Also, the promising results using pembrolizumab have been seen in seven relapsed ENKT lymphoma with 100% overall response rates after a median of 7 weeks of treatment, either EBV DNA-positive or negative. The remission has been maintained at a median follow-up of 6 months. Similar results were reported for nivolumab. Thus, several studies are ongoing to explore the efficacy of PD-1 inhibitors in the treatment of ENKL. Studies showed that the response is correlated with the level of PD-1 expression, especially in EBV DNA positive patients. Although, studies were halted early due to the short duration of response and concern for hyperprogression. Encouraging results were also seen with pembrolizumab in patients with r/r cutaneous T-cell lymphoma with 38% ORR in a phase 2 study [142]. There was an alarming report of hyperprogression in three patients with ATLL that were enrolled in the nivolumab trial. Clinical progression was also accompanied by an increase in the viral load [143]. In these cases, PD-1 tumor suppressor function may have been lifted by PD-1 blockade. The use of PD-1 and PD-L1 antibodies in ATLL has to be viewed with caution. Therefore, more clinical trials should be done to evaluate the efficacy and safety of ICIs in different subtypes of PTCL.

Ipilimumab, an inhibitor of CTLA-4 (also known as CD152), provides both positive and negative feedback for T-cell activation when combined with its costimulatory receptor CD28. But the effect of CTLA-4 inhibitors in PTCL is not well characterized. In general, immunotherapy for PTCL is promising. For other immune checkpoint proteins, such as TIGIT, TIM-3, and LAG-3, their evaluation in PTCL is still at the preclinical stage and needed to be further explored via relevant clinical trials. Some studies have shown that the combined blockade of the TIM-3 and PD-1 pathways has significant efficacy in hematological tumors [161]. More importantly, the combination of PD-1/PD-L1 inhibitors and CAR-T cell therapy are worthy of exploring [162]. These ICIs combined therapies may be the best strategy for tumor therapy and promote the prognosis in near future.

## 4. Immune checkpoints inhibitors toxicity

As reported by the current clinical trials, treatment-related AEs were very common in patients undergoing anti-PD-1 treatment (**Table 1**). However, grade 3 or above treatment-related AEs were generally only observed in less than 30% of patients. Here, we use the studies with most patients enrolled as examples (i.e., $n$ = 243 for Armand et al. [36] and $n$ = 210 for Chen et al. [40]). As reported by Armand et al. [36], the most common treatment-related AEs of any grade were fatigue (23%), diarrhea (15%), and infusion-related reactions (14%). However, none of them were severe (grade 3 or above). On contrary, the most common grade 3 or 4 treatment-related AEs were lipase increases (5%), neutropenia (3%), and ALT increases. The most common treatment-related AEs that led to treatment discontinuation were pneumonitis (2%) and autoimmune hepatitis (1%). Other serious treatment-relate AEs included infusion-related reactions (2%), pneumonia (1%), pleural effusion (1%), and pyrexia (1%). For the study conducted by Chen et al. [40], the most common treatment-related AEs were hypothyroidism (14.3%), pyrexia (11.4%), rash (11.0%), and fatigue (11.0%). The most common grade 3 or 4 treatment-relate AEs were neutropenia (2.4%) and diarrhea (1.4%). Fourteen patients discontinued treatment due to treatment-related AEs, and the most common causes were pneumonitis in seven (3.3%) and infusion-related reactions in two (1.0%). Here, we will briefly discuss some cases that deserve special attention.

### 4.1 Thyroid dysfunction

Thyroid dysfunction is one of the most common AEs observed during PD-1 inhibition and is heterogeneous in nature. In a study of 73 patients who underwent nivolumab therapy, Peiro et al. [163] reported that 23.3% of patients developed thyroid dysfunction. Among them, seven patients showed thyrotoxicosis and 10 patients showed primary hypothyroidism (four required levothyroxine treatment). They concluded that thyrotoxicosis occurred earlier than hypothyroidism. Before the onset of hypothyroidism, 33% of patients exhibited transient thyroiditis and five patients had hyperthyroid, which became hypothyroid later. In cases of thyroiditis, patients can be treated with beta-blockers, and thyroid hormone replacement may be required for hypothyroidism. For hyperthyroidism, beta-blockers and corticosteroids are very effective [164].

### 4.2 Treatment-related pneumonitis

In a meta-analysis of 11 clinical trials in patients treated with ICI (PD-1 or CTLA-4 blockade), the use of ICIs led to an increased risk of pneumonitis of all grades [165]. Younger age (<60 years old) may be a major risk factor [166]. Corticosteroids can be used for the treatment of pneumonitis, and those refractory cases should be treated with steroid-free immunosuppressants. For cases of grade 3 or above pneumonitis, potential infections should be considered. In cases of severe pneumonitis, the use of ICI should be stopped [167].

### 4.3 Treatment-related colitis/diarrhea

Gastrointestinal AEs are another most common treatment-related AEs during ICI therapy. Physicians should carefully distinguish colitis from diarrhea; and when colitis symptoms emerge, hospitalization and discontinuation of ICIs should be considered. In cases of mild symptoms, administration of corticosteroids or antidiarrheals could be applied [168], and additional infliximab may be needed [169].

### 4.4 Treatment-related cardiovascular disease

The incidences of treatment-related cardiovascular diseases are frequently underestimated, as reported by Jain et al. [170]. They identified 16,574 patients who received ICIs from a total of 2,687,301 patients and 1:1 matched to 2875 patients who received chemotherapy or 4611 patients who received targeted agents. They observed the onsets of treatment-related cardiovascular diseases included stroke (4.6%), heart failure (3.5%), atrial fibrillation (2.1%), conduction disorders (1.5%), myocardial infarction (0.9%), myocarditis (0.05%), vasculitis (0.05%), and pericarditis (0.2%). In addition, anti-CTLA-4 therapy was more commonly related to treatment-related cardiovascular diseases. Moreover, another retrospective analysis indicated that inhibition of PD-1/PD-L1 was significantly associated with the risk of myocarditis, and males may have an increased risk of certain cardiovascular AEs [171]. In another meta-analysis including 2576 trials/studies and 20,244 patients, combined therapy of PD-1 blockade and chemotherapy may increase the risk of myocardial disease of all grades; although there was no significant increase in the risk of other cardiovascular diseases [172].

### 4.5 Other autoimmune diseases

As PD-1 blockade non-specifically activates the immune system, the induction of autoimmune-like diseases is the major concern of the toxicity incurred. Examples of symptoms during the treatment of HL include autoimmune type I diabetes [173–176], autoimmune encephalitis [177–179], autoimmune hepatitis [36], autoimmune nephritis [36, 38], and autoimmune hemolytic anemia [180, 181]. In cases of autoimmune diseases, the use of immunosuppressive treatment or delay of ICI therapy should be seriously considered.

### 4.6 Association between toxicity and efficacy

Although treatment-related AEs severely affect the treatment outcomes of ICIs, the onset of AEs that are immune-related may be directly associated with the efficacy of ICIs. In a study of 106 patients who underwent PD-1 blockade monotherapy, Rogado et al. [182] observed that patients with immune-related AEs have a higher ORR of 82.5% (vs 16.6%) and longer PFS of 10 months (vs 3 months), as compared with those without immune-related AEs. Although the detailed underlying mechanisms remain to be elucidated, concerns about the effect of corticosteroids and other immunosuppressants administration on ICI efficacy have been raised. However, some studies suggested that the use of corticosteroids and other immunosuppressants may not impair the anti-tumor activities of ICIs [183, 184].

## 5. Conclusions

ICIs therapies have demonstrated remarkable efficacy in several subtypes of HL and NHL, and some ICIs (e.g., pembrolizumab) have been approved to use in HL and PMBCL. Especially, anti-PD-1/PD-L1 antibodies in a combination with other therapies have acquired promising results, and AEs are common in these treatments. Thus, we need to do more clinical trials and real-world studies to further explore the effectiveness and safety of ICIs treatment in lymphoma.

## Funding

This work was financially supported by National Natural Science Foundation of China (NSFC 81500173).

## Author details

Jiawen Huang and Juan Huang*
Department of Hematology, Sichuan Academy of Medical Sciences and Sichuan Provincial People's Hospital, School of Medicine UESTC, Chengdu, Sichuan Province, China

*Address all correspondence to: huangjuanxy@med.uestc.edu.cn

## References

[1] Lenschow DJ, Bluestone JA. T cell co-stimulation and in vivo tolerance. Current Opinion in Immunology. 1993;**5**(5):747-752

[2] Wherry EJ, Kurachi M. Molecular and cellular insights into T cell exhaustion. Nature Reviews. Immunology. 2015;**15**(8):486-499

[3] Takeuchi Y, Hirota K, Sakaguchi S. Impaired T cell receptor signaling and development of T cell-mediated autoimmune arthritis. Immunological Reviews. 2020;**294**(1):164-176

[4] Pardoll DM. The blockade of immune checkpoints in cancer immunotherapy. Nature Reviews. Cancer. 2012;**12**(4):252-264

[5] Ahmadzadeh M, Johnson LA, Heemskerk B, Wunderlich JR, Dudley ME, White DE, et al. Tumor antigen-specific CD8 T cells infiltrating the tumor express high levels of PD-1 and are functionally impaired. Blood. 2009;**114**(8):1537-1544

[6] Han Y, Liu D, Li L. PD-1/PD-L1 pathway: Current researches in cancer. American Journal of Cancer Research. 2020;**10**(3):727-742

[7] Latchman Y, Wood CR, Chernova T, Chaudhary D, Borde M, Chernova I, et al. PD-L2 is a second ligand for PD-1 and inhibits T cell activation. Nature Immunology. 2001;**2**(3):261-268

[8] Dong H, Strome SE, Salomao DR, Tamura H, Hirano F, Flies DB, et al. Tumor-associated B7-H1 promotes T-cell apoptosis: A potential mechanism of immune evasion. Nature Medicine. 2002;**8**(8):793-800

[9] Curiel TJ, Wei S, Dong H, Alvarez X, Cheng P, Mottram P, et al. Blockade of B7-H1 improves myeloid dendritic cell-mediated antitumor immunity. Nature Medicine. 2003;**9**(5):562-567

[10] Dermani FK, Samadi P, Rahmani G, Kohlan AK, Najafi R. PD-1/PD-L1 immune checkpoint: Potential target for cancer therapy. Journal of Cellular Physiology. 2019;**234**(2):1313-1325

[11] Sharpe AH, Pauken KE. The diverse functions of the PD1 inhibitory pathway. Nature Reviews. Immunology. 2018;**18**(3):153-167

[12] Patsoukis N, Wang Q, Strauss L, Boussiotis VA. Revisiting the PD-1 pathway. Science Advances. 2020;**6**(38):eabd2712

[13] Quigley M, Pereyra F, Nilsson B, Porichis F, Fonseca C, Eichbaum Q, et al. Transcriptional analysis of HIV-specific CD8+ T cells shows that PD-1 inhibits T cell function by upregulating BATF. Nature Medicine. 2010;**16**(10):1147-1151

[14] Clark CA, Gupta HB, Sareddy G, Pandeswara S, Lao S, Yuan B, et al. Tumor-intrinsic PD-L1 signals regulate cell growth, pathogenesis, and autophagy in ovarian Cancer and melanoma. Cancer Research. 2016;**76**(23):6964-6974

[15] Linsley PS, Greene JL, Brady W, Bajorath J, Ledbetter JA, Peach R. Human B7-1 (CD80) and B7-2 (CD86) bind with similar avidities but distinct kinetics to CD28 and CTLA-4 receptors. Immunity. 1994;**1**(9):793-801

[16] Linsley PS, Bradshaw J, Greene J, Peach R, Bennett KL, Mittler RS. Intracellular trafficking of CTLA-4 and focal localization towards sites of TCR engagement. Immunity. 1996;**4**(6):535-543

[17] Schneider H, Smith X, Liu H, Bismuth G, Rudd CE. CTLA-4 disrupts

ZAP70 microcluster formation with reduced T cell/APC dwell times and calcium mobilization. European Journal of Immunology. 2008;**38**(1):40-47

[18] Guntermann C, Alexander DR. CTLA-4 suppresses proximal TCR signaling in resting human CD4(+) T cells by inhibiting ZAP-70 Tyr(319) phosphorylation: A potential role for tyrosine phosphatases. Journal of Immunology. 2002;**168**(9):4420-4429

[19] Qureshi OS, Zheng Y, Nakamura K, Attridge K, Manzotti C, Schmidt EM, et al. Trans-endocytosis of CD80 and CD86: A molecular basis for the cell-extrinsic function of CTLA-4. Science. 2011;**332**(6029):600-603

[20] Parry RV, Chemnitz JM, Frauwirth KA, Lanfranco AR, Braunstein I, Kobayashi SV, et al. CTLA-4 and PD-1 receptors inhibit T-cell activation by distinct mechanisms. Molecular and Cellular Biology. 2005;**25**(21):9543-9553

[21] Kubsch S, Graulich E, Knop J, Steinbrink K. Suppressor activity of anergic T cells induced by IL-10-treated human dendritic cells: Association with IL-2- and CTLA-4-dependent G1 arrest of the cell cycle regulated by p27Kip1. European Journal of Immunology. 2003;**33**(7):1988-1997

[22] Brunner MC, Chambers CA, Chan FK, Hanke J, Winoto A, Allison JP. CTLA-4-mediated inhibition of early events of T cell proliferation. Journal of Immunology. 1999;**162**(10):5813-5820

[23] Finn OJ. Immuno-oncology: Understanding the function and dysfunction of the immune system in cancer. Annals of Oncology. 2012;**23**(Suppl. 8):viii6-viii9

[24] Bagchi S, Yuan R, Engleman EG. Immune checkpoint inhibitors for the treatment of Cancer: Clinical impact and mechanisms of response and resistance. Annual Review of Pathology. 2021;**16**:223-249

[25] van Elsas A, Hurwitz AA, Allison JP. Combination immunotherapy of B16 melanoma using anti-cytotoxic T lymphocyte-associated antigen 4 (CTLA-4) and granulocyte/macrophage colony-stimulating factor (GM-CSF)-producing vaccines induces rejection of subcutaneous and metastatic tumors accompanied by autoimmune depigmentation. The Journal of Experimental Medicine. 1999;**190**(3):355-366

[26] Leach DR, Krummel MF, Allison JP. Enhancement of antitumor immunity by CTLA-4 blockade. Science. 1996;**271**(5256):1734-1736

[27] Peggs KS, Quezada SA, Korman AJ, Allison JP. Principles and use of anti-CTLA4 antibody in human cancer immunotherapy. Current Opinion in Immunology. 2006;**18**(2):206-213

[28] Hodi FS, O'Day SJ, McDermott DF, Weber RW, Sosman JA, Haanen JB, et al. Improved survival with ipilimumab in patients with metastatic melanoma. The New England Journal of Medicine. 2010;**363**(8):711-723

[29] Green MR, Monti S, Rodig SJ, Juszczynski P, Currie T, O'Donnell E, et al. Integrative analysis reveals selective 9p24.1 amplification, increased PD-1 ligand expression, and further induction via JAK2 in nodular sclerosing Hodgkin lymphoma and primary mediastinal large B-cell lymphoma. Blood. 2010;**116**(17):3268-3277

[30] U.S. Food and Drug Administration (FDA). Nivolumab (Opdivo) for Hodgkin Lymphoma. 2016. Available from: https://www.fda.gov/drugs/resources-information-approved-drugs/

nivolumab-opdivo-hodgkin-lymphoma [Accessed: Jun 17, 2022]

[31] U.S. Food and Drug Administration (FDA). Pembrolizumab (KEYTRUDA) for classical Hodgkin lymphoma. 2017. Available from: https://www.fda.gov/drugs/resources-information-approved-drugs/pembrolizumab-keytruda-classical-hodgkin-lymphoma [Accessed: Jun 17, 2022]

[32] Liput J, Guler E, Smith DA, Tirumani SH, Hoimes C, Caimi PF, et al. Clinical, imaging findings, responses, and outcomes of patients with classical Hodgkin lymphoma and non-Hodgkin lymphoma undergoing immune checkpoint inhibitor therapy: A single-institution experience. Journal of Computer Assisted Tomography. 2020;**44**:619-626. DOI: 10.1097/RCT.0000000000001043

[33] Davis KL, Fox E, Merchant MS, Reid JM, Kudgus RA, Liu X, et al. Nivolumab in children and young adults with relapsed or refractory solid tumours or lymphoma (ADVL1412): A multicentre, open-label, single-arm, phase 1-2 trial. The Lancet Oncology. 2020;**21**:541-550. DOI: 10.1016/S1470-2045(20)30023-1

[34] Kasamon YL, de Claro RA, Wang Y, Shen YL, Farrell AT, Pazdur R. FDA approval summary: Nivolumab for the treatment of relapsed or progressive classical Hodgkin lymphoma. The Oncologist. 2017;**22**:585-591. DOI: 10.1634/theoncologist.2017-0004

[35] Bair SM, Strelec LE, Feldman TA, Ahmed G, Armand P, Shah NN, et al. Outcomes and toxicities of programmed Death-1 (PD-1) inhibitors in Hodgkin lymphoma patients in the United States: A real-world, Multicenter retrospective analysis. The Oncologist. 2019;**24**:955-962. DOI: 10.1634/theoncologist.2018-0538

[36] Armand P, Engert A, Younes A, Fanale M, Santoro A, Zinzani PL, et al. Nivolumab for relapsed/refractory classic Hodgkin lymphoma after failure of autologous hematopoietic cell transplantation: Extended follow-up of the multicohort single-arm phase II CheckMate 205 trial. Journal of Clinical Oncology. 2018;**36**(14):1428-1439. DOI: 10.1200/JCO.2017.76.0793

[37] Falchi L, Sawas A, Deng C, Amengual JE, Colbourn DS, Lichtenstein EA, et al. High rate of complete responses to immune checkpoint inhibitors in patients with relapsed or refractory Hodgkin lymphoma previously exposed to epigenetic therapy. Journal of Hematology & Oncology. 2016;**9**(1):132. DOI: 10.1186/s13045-016-0363-1

[38] Armand P, Shipp MA, Ribrag V, Michot JM, Zinzani PL, Kuruvilla J, et al. Programmed Death-1 blockade with pembrolizumab in patients with classical Hodgkin lymphoma after brentuximab Vedotin failure. Journal of Clinical Oncology. 2016;**34**(31):3733-3739. DOI: 10.1200/JCO.2016.67.3467

[39] Ansell SM, Lesokhin AM, Borrello I, Halwani A, Scott EC, Gutierrez M, et al. PD-1 blockade with nivolumab in relapsed or refractory Hodgkin's lymphoma. The New England Journal of Medicine. 2015;**372**:311-319. DOI: 10.1056/NEJMoa1411087

[40] Chen R, Zinzani PL, Lee HJ, Armand P, Johnson NA, Brice P, et al. Pembrolizumab in relapsed or refractory Hodgkin lymphoma: 2-year follow-up of KEYNOTE-087. Blood. 2019;**134**(14):1144-1153. DOI: 10.1182/blood.2019000324

[41] Younes A, Santoro A, Shipp M, Zinzani PL, Timmerman JM, Ansell S, et al. Nivolumab for classical Hodgkin's lymphoma after failure of both

autologous stem-cell transplantation and brentuximab vedotin: A multicentre, multicohort, single-arm phase 2 trial. The Lancet Oncology. 2016;**17**:1283-1294. DOI: 10.1016/S1470-2045(16)30167-X

[42] Bekoz H, Ozbalak M, Karadurmus N, Paydas S, Turker A, Toptas T, et al. Nivolumab for relapsed or refractory Hodgkin lymphoma: Real-life experience. Annals of Hematology. 2020;**99**:2565-2576. DOI: 10.1007/s00277-020-04077-4

[43] Bekoz H, Karadurmus N, Paydas S, Turker A, Toptas T, Firatli Tuglular T, et al. Nivolumab for relapsed or refractory Hodgkin lymphoma: Real-life experience. Annals of Oncology. 2017;**28**:2496-2502. DOI: 10.1093/annonc/mdx341

[44] Geoerger B, Kang HJ, Yalon-Oren M, Marshall LV, Vezina C, Pappo A, et al. Pembrolizumab in paediatric patients with advanced melanoma or a PD-L1-positive, advanced, relapsed, or refractory solid tumour or lymphoma (KEYNOTE-051): Interim analysis of an open-label, single-arm, phase 1-2 trial. The Lancet Oncology. 2020;**21**:121-133. DOI: 10.1016/S1470-2045(19)30671-0

[45] Maruyama D, Terui Y, Yamamoto K, Fukuhara N, Choi I, Kuroda J, et al. Final results of a phase II study of nivolumab in Japanese patients with relapsed or refractory classical Hodgkin lymphoma. Japanese Journal of Clinical Oncology. 2020;**50**:1265-1273. DOI: 10.1093/jjco/hyaa117

[46] Ramchandren R, Domingo-Domenech E, Rueda A, Trneny M, Feldman TA, Lee HJ, et al. Nivolumab for newly diagnosed advanced-stage classic Hodgkin lymphoma: Safety and efficacy in the phase II CheckMate 205 study. Journal of Clinical Oncology. 2019;**37**:1997-2007. DOI: 10.1200/JCO.19.00315

[47] Chan TSY, Hwang YY, Khong PL, Leung AYH, Chim CS, Tse EWC, et al. Low-dose pembrolizumab and nivolumab were efficacious and safe in relapsed and refractory classical Hodgkin lymphoma: Experience in a resource-constrained setting. Hematological Oncology. 2020;**38**:726-736. DOI: 10.1002/hon.2787

[48] Dada R, Zabani Y. Nivolumab induces impressive responses in relapsed/refractory classic Hodgkin lymphoma: Single institutional experience. Journal of Oncology Pharmacy Practice. 2019;**25**:1586-1589. DOI: 10.1177/1078155218800150

[49] Kuruvilla J, Ramchandren R, Santoro A, Paszkiewicz-Kozik E, Gasiorowski R, Johnson NA, et al. Pembrolizumab versus brentuximab vedotin in relapsed or refractory classical Hodgkin lymphoma (KEYNOTE-204): An interim analysis of a multicentre, randomised, open-label, phase 3 study. The Lancet Oncology. 2021;**22**:512-524. DOI: 10.1016/S1470-2045(21)00005-X

[50] Momotow J, Buhnen I, Trautmann-Grill K, Kobbe G, Hahn D, Schroers R, et al. Outcomes of anti-programmed death 1 treatment for relapsed/refractory Hodgkin lymphoma: A German Hodgkin study group multicentre real-world analysis. British Journal of Haematology. 2022;**198**(2):401-404. DOI: 10.1111/bjh.18231

[51] Hur JY, Yoon SE, Kim SJ, Kim WS. Immune checkpoint inhibitors in patients with pretreated HodgkinEs lymphoma: A Korean single-center, retrospective study. Blood Res. 2020;**55**:85-90. DOI: 10.5045/br.2020.2020014

[52] Lepik KV, Mikhailova NB, Moiseev IS, Kondakova EV, Tsvetkova LA, Zalyalov YR, et al. Nivolumab for the treatment of relapsed and refractory

classical Hodgkin lymphoma after ASCT and in ASCT-naive patients. Leukemia & Lymphoma. 2019;**60**:2316-2319. DOI: 10.1080/10428194.2019.1573368

[53] Armand P, Kuruvilla J, Michot JM, Ribrag V, Zinzani PL, Zhu Y, et al. KEYNOTE-013 4-year follow-up of pembrolizumab in classical Hodgkin lymphoma after brentuximab vedotin failure. Blood Advances. 2020;**4**:2617-2622. DOI: 10.1182/bloodadvances.2019001367

[54] Manson G, Mear JB, Herbaux C, Schiano JM, Casasnovas O, Stamatoullas A, et al. Long-term efficacy of anti-PD1 therapy in Hodgkin lymphoma with and without allogenic stem cell transplantation. European Journal of Cancer. 2019;**115**:47-56

[55] Merryman RW, Castagna L, Giordano L, Ho VT, Corradini P, Guidetti A, et al. Allogeneic transplantation after PD-1 blockade for classic Hodgkin lymphoma. Leukemia. 2021;**35**(9):2672-2683

[56] Martinez C, Carpio C, Heras I, Rios-Herranz E, Buch J, Gutierrez A, et al. Potential survival benefit for patients receiving allogeneic hematopoietic stem cell transplantation after nivolumab therapy for relapse/refractory Hodgkin lymphoma: Real-life experience in Spain. Biology of Blood and Marrow Transplantation. 2020;**26**(8):1534-1542

[57] Armand P, Chen YB, Redd RA, Joyce RM, Bsat J, Jeter E, et al. PD-1 blockade with pembrolizumab for classical Hodgkin lymphoma after autologous stem cell transplantation. Blood. 2019;**134**(1):22-29

[58] Casadei B, Argnani L, Morigi A, Lolli G, Broccoli A, Pellegrini C, et al. Potential survival benefit for patients receiving autologous hematopoietic stem cell transplantation after checkpoint inhibitors for relapsed/refractory Hodgkin lymphoma: A real-life experience. Hematological Oncology. 2020;**38**(5):737-741

[59] Ito A, Kim SW, Matsuoka KI, Kawakita T, Tanaka T, Inamoto Y, et al. Safety and efficacy of anti-programmed cell death-1 monoclonal antibodies before and after allogeneic hematopoietic cell transplantation for relapsed or refractory Hodgkin lymphoma: A multicenter retrospective study. International Journal of Hematology. 2020;**112**(5):674-689

[60] Singh AK, Porrata LF, Aljitawi O, Lin T, Shune L, Ganguly S, et al. Fatal GvHD induced by PD-1 inhibitor pembrolizumab in a patient with Hodgkin's lymphoma. Bone Marrow Transplantation. 2016;**51**(9):1268-1270

[61] Charles J, Giovannini D, Terzi N, Schwebel C, Sturm N, Masson D, et al. Multi-organ failure induced by nivolumab in the context of Allo-stem cell transplantation. Experimental Hematology & Oncology. 2019;**8**:8

[62] Steinerova K, Jindra P, Lysak D, Karas M. Development of resistant GvHD in a patient treated with nivolumab for Hodgkins lymphoma relapse after allogeneic unrelated transplantation. Klinická Onkologie;**32**(1):66-69

[63] Minson A, Douglas G, Bilmon I, Grigg A. Low dose PD-1 inhibition in relapsed refractory Hodgkin lymphoma after allogeneic stem cell transplant with concomitant active GVHD. British Journal of Haematology. 2019;**184**(5):840-844

[64] Amerikanou R, Neill L, Shafat M, Roddy H, Hyare H, Hughes S, et al.

Multi-organ graft-versus-host disease after nivolumab for relapsed Hodgkin lymphoma: The role of plasma exchange. Lancet Haematol. 2021;**8**(11):e862

[65] Sasse S, Brockelmann PJ, Goergen H, Plutschow A, Muller H, Kreissl S, et al. Long-term follow-up of contemporary treatment in early-stage Hodgkin lymphoma: Updated analyses of the German Hodgkin study group HD7, HD8, HD10, and HD11 trials. Journal of Clinical Oncology. 2017;**35**(18):1999-2007

[66] Brockelmann PJ, Goergen H, Keller U, Meissner J, Ordemann R, Halbsguth TV, et al. Efficacy of nivolumab and AVD in early-stage Unfavorable classic Hodgkin lymphoma: The randomized phase 2 German Hodgkin study group NIVAHL trial. JAMA Oncology. 2020;**6**(6):872-880

[67] Allen PB, Savas H, Evens AM, Advani RH, Palmer B, Pro B, et al. Pembrolizumab followed by AVD in untreated early unfavorable and advanced-stage classical Hodgkin lymphoma. Blood. 2021;**137**(10):1318-1326

[68] Younes A, Gopal AK, Smith SE, Ansell SM, Rosenblatt JD, Savage KJ, et al. Results of a pivotal phase II study of brentuximab vedotin for patients with relapsed or refractory Hodgkin's lymphoma. Journal of Clinical Oncology. 2012;**30**(18):2183-2189

[69] Advani RH, Moskowitz AJ, Bartlett NL, Vose JM, Ramchandren R, Feldman TA, et al. Brentuximab vedotin in combination with nivolumab in relapsed or refractory Hodgkin lymphoma: 3-year study results. Blood. 2021;**138**(6):427-438

[70] Cheson BD, Bartlett NL, LaPlant B, Lee HJ, Advani RJ, Christian B, et al. Brentuximab vedotin plus nivolumab as first-line therapy in older or chemotherapy-ineligible patients with Hodgkin lymphoma (ACCRU): A multicentre, single-arm, phase 2 trial. Lancet Haematology. 2020;**7**(11):e808-e815

[71] Fedorova LV, Lepik KV, Volkov NP, Kotselyabina PV, Borzenkova ES, Popova MO, et al. Efficacy and safety of nivolumab combined with brentuximab vedotin after nivolumab monotherapy failure in patients with relapsed and refractory classic Hodgkin lymphoma. International Journal of Clinical Oncology. 2022;**27**(3):626-632

[72] Lucchini E, Rusconi C, Levis M, Ricci F, Santoro A, Ricardi U, et al. Immune checkpoint inhibitors in combination with radiotherapy as salvage treatment for relapsed/refractory classical Hodgkin lymphoma: A retrospective analysis in 12 patients. Hematology Reports. 2021;**13**(2):9080

[73] de Forceville L, Deau-Fischer B, Franchi P, Arsene-Henry A, Cassou Mounat T, Bouscary D, et al. Radiotherapy in combination with nivolumab for relapsed/refractory classical Hodgkin lymphoma: About two cases. Cancer Radiothérapie. 2019;**23**(3):232-239

[74] Bai B, Huang HQ, Cai QQ, Wang XX, Cai QC, Lin ZX, et al. Promising long-term outcome of gemcitabine, vinorelbine, liposomal doxorubicin (GVD) in 14-day schedule as salvage regimen for patients with previously heavily treated Hodgkin's lymphoma and aggressive non-Hodgkin's lymphoma. Medical Oncology. 2013;**30**(1):350

[75] Moskowitz AJ, Shah G, Schoder H, Ganesan N, Drill E, Hancock H, et al. Phase II trial of pembrolizumab plus gemcitabine, vinorelbine, and liposomal doxorubicin as second-line therapy for relapsed or refractory classical Hodgkin lymphoma. Journal of Clinical Oncology. 2021;**39**(28):3109-3117

[76] Zhang YC, Wang JN, Ma SY, Cai J, Su N, Huang HQ, et al. Combination of PD-1 inhibitor with GVD (gemcitabine, vinorelbine, liposomal doxorubicin) versus GVD regimen as second-line therapy for relapsed/refractory classical Hodgkin lymphoma. British Journal of Haematology. 2022;**196**(1):127-135

[77] Xu J, Zhang Y, Jia R, Yue C, Chang L, Liu R, et al. Anti-PD-1 antibody SHR-1210 combined with Apatinib for advanced hepatocellular carcinoma, gastric, or esophagogastric junction cancer: An open-label, dose escalation and expansion study. Clinical Cancer Research. 2019;**25**(2):515-523

[78] Huang J, Mo H, Zhang W, Chen X, Qu D, Wang X, et al. Promising efficacy of SHR-1210, a novel anti-programmed cell death 1 antibody, in patients with advanced gastric and gastroesophageal junction cancer in China. Cancer. 2019;**125**(5):742-749

[79] Huang J, Xu B, Mo H, Zhang W, Chen X, Wu D, et al. Safety, activity, and biomarkers of SHR-1210, an anti-PD-1 antibody, for patients with advanced Esophageal carcinoma. Clinical Cancer Research. 2018;**24**(6):1296-1304

[80] Mo H, Huang J, Xu J, Chen X, Wu D, Qu D, et al. Safety, anti-tumour activity, and pharmacokinetics of fixed-dose SHR-1210, an anti-PD-1 antibody in advanced solid tumours: A dose-escalation, phase 1 study. British Journal of Cancer. 2018;**119**(5):538-545

[81] Fang W, Yang Y, Ma Y, Hong S, Lin L, He X, et al. Camrelizumab (SHR-1210) alone or in combination with gemcitabine plus cisplatin for nasopharyngeal carcinoma: Results from two single-arm, phase 1 trials. The Lancet Oncology. 2018;**19**(10):1338-1350

[82] Song Y, Wu J, Chen X, Lin T, Cao J, Liu Y, et al. A single-arm, multicenter, phase II study of Camrelizumab in relapsed or refractory classical Hodgkin lymphoma. Clinical Cancer Research. 2019;**25**(24):7363-7369

[83] Pauken KE, Sammons MA, Odorizzi PM, Manne S, Godec J, Khan O, et al. Epigenetic stability of exhausted T cells limits durability of reinvigoration by PD-1 blockade. Science. 2016;**354**(6316):1160-1165

[84] Ghoneim HE, Fan Y, Moustaki A, Abdelsamed HA, Dash P, Dogra P, et al. De novo epigenetic programs inhibit PD-1 blockade-mediated T cell rejuvenation. Cell. 2017;**170**(1):142-157 e119

[85] Gore SD, Jones C, Kirkpatrick P. Decitabine. Nature Reviews. Drug Discovery. 2006;**5**(11):891-892

[86] Nie J, Wang C, Liu Y, Yang Q, Mei Q, Dong L, et al. Addition of low-dose decitabine to anti-PD-1 antibody Camrelizumab in relapsed/refractory classical Hodgkin lymphoma. Journal of Clinical Oncology. 2019;**37**(17):1479-1489

[87] Liu Y, Wang C, Li X, Dong L, Yang Q, Chen M, et al. Improved clinical outcome in a randomized phase II study of anti-PD-1 camrelizumab plus decitabine in relapsed/refractory Hodgkin lymphoma. Journal for Immunotherapy of Cancer. 2021;**9**(4):e002347

[88] Yan Z, Ma J, Yao S, Yao Z, Wang H, Chu J, et al. Anti-angiogenic agent combined with anti-PD-1 immunotherapy showed activity in patients with classical Hodgkin lymphoma who have failed immunotherapy: A retrospective case report study. Frontiers in Immunology. 2021;**12**:727464

[89] Shi Y, Su H, Song Y, Jiang W, Sun X, Qian W, et al. Safety and activity of

sintilimab in patients with relapsed or refractory classical Hodgkin lymphoma (ORIENT-1): A multicentre, single-arm, phase 2 trial. Lancet Haematology. 2019;**6**(1):e12-e19

[90] Dahan R, Sega E, Engelhardt J, Selby M, Korman AJ, Ravetch JV. FcgammaRs modulate the anti-tumor activity of antibodies targeting the PD-1/PD-L1 axis. Cancer Cell. 2015;**28**(3):285-295

[91] Song Y, Gao Q, Zhang H, Fan L, Zhou J, Zou D, et al. Treatment of relapsed or refractory classical Hodgkin lymphoma with the anti-PD-1, tislelizumab: Results of a phase 2, single-arm, multicenter study. Leukemia. 2020;**34**(2):533-542

[92] Ding XS, Mi L, Song YQ, Liu WP, Yu H, Lin NJ, et al. Relapsed/refractory classical Hodgkin lymphoma effectively treated with low-dose decitabine plus tislelizumab: A case report. World Journal of Clinical Cases. 2021;**9**(21):6041-6048

[93] Lin N, Zhang M, Bai H, Liu H, Cui J, Ke X, et al. Efficacy and safety of GLS-010 (zimberelimab) in patients with relapsed or refractory classical Hodgkin lymphoma: A multicenter, single-arm, phase II study. European Journal of Cancer. 2022;**164**:117-126

[94] Shen L, Gong J, Xu Y, Zhang X, Peng Z, Qi C, et al. A novel recombinant human anti-PD-1 monoclonal antibody GLS-010 in patients with advanced cancer: Result of a phase Ia clinical trial. Annals of Oncology. 2018;**29**:x22-x23

[95] Lin S, Gong J, Xu Y, Zhang X, Peng Z, Qi C, et al. Gls-010, a novel anti-PD-1 mAb in Chinese advanced gastrointestinal tumor: Result of a phase Ib clinical trial. Journal of Clinical Oncology. 2019;**37**(4_suppl):125-125

[96] Song Y, Zhu J, Lin N, Zhang C, Zhang M, Bai H, et al. GLS-010, a novel anti-PD-1 mAb in Chinese patients with relapsed or refractory classical Hodgkin's lymphoma: Preliminary result of a phase II clinical trial. Journal of Clinical Oncology. 2019;**37**(15_suppl):e14072-e14072

[97] Song Y, Zhou K, Jin C, Qian Z, Hou M, Fan L, et al. A phase II study of penpulimab, an anti-PD-1 antibody, in patients with relapsed or refractoryclassic Hodgkin lymphoma (cHL). Journal of Clinical Oncology. 2021;**39**(15_suppl):7529-7529

[98] Dhillon S. Penpulimab: First approval. Drugs. 2021;**81**(18): 2159-2166

[99] Chen X, Kong H, Luo L, Han S, Lei T, Yu H, et al. High efficacy of PD-1 inhibitor after initial failure of PD-L1 inhibitor in relapsed/refractory classical Hodgkin lymphoma. BMC Cancer. 2022;**22**(1):9

[100] Fujii R, Friedman ER, Richards J, Tsang KY, Heery CR, Schlom J, et al. Enhanced killing of chordoma cells by antibody-dependent cell-mediated cytotoxicity employing the novel anti-PD-L1 antibody avelumab. Oncotarget. 2016;**7**(23):33498-33511

[101] Boyerinas B, Jochems C, Fantini M, Heery CR, Gulley JL, Tsang KY, et al. Antibody-dependent cellular cytotoxicity activity of a novel anti-PD-L1 antibody avelumab (MSB0010718C) on human tumor cells. Cancer Immunology Research. 2015;**3**(10):1148-1157

[102] Herrera AF, Burton C, Radford J, Miall F, Townsend W, Santoro A, et al. Avelumab in relapsed/refractory classical Hodgkin lymphoma: Phase 1b results from the JAVELIN Hodgkins trial. Blood Advances. 2021;**5**(17):3387-3396

[103] Gong J, Cao J, Zhang Q, Xu N, Zhao Y, Xing B, et al. Safety, antitumor activity and biomarkers of sugemalimab in Chinese patients with advanced solid tumors or lymphomas: Results from the first-in-human phase 1 trial. Cancer Immunology, Immunotherapy. 2022;**71**(8):1897-1908

[104] Dhillon S, Duggan S. Sugemalimab: First Approval. Drugs. 2022;**82**(5): 593-599

[105] Ogasawara K, Newhall K, Maxwell SE, Dell'Aringa J, Komashko V, Kilavuz N, et al. Population pharmacokinetics of an anti-PD-L1 antibody, durvalumab in patients with hematologic malignancies. Clinical Pharmacokinetics. 2020;**59**(2):217-227

[106] Geoerger B, Zwaan CM, Marshall LV, Michon J, Bourdeaut F, Casanova M, et al. Atezolizumab for children and young adults with previously treated solid tumours, non-Hodgkin lymphoma, and Hodgkin lymphoma (iMATRIX): A multicentre phase 1-2 study. The Lancet Oncology. 2020;**21**(1):134-144

[107] Ansell SM, Hurvitz SA, Koenig PA, LaPlant BR, Kabat BF, Fernando D, et al. Phase I study of ipilimumab, an anti-CTLA-4 monoclonal antibody, in patients with relapsed and refractory B-cell non-Hodgkin lymphoma. Clinical Cancer Research. 2009;**15**(20):6446-6453

[108] Wolchok JD, Neyns B, Linette G, Negrier S, Lutzky J, Thomas L, et al. Ipilimumab monotherapy in patients with pretreated advanced melanoma: A randomised, double-blind, multicentre, phase 2, dose-ranging study. The Lancet Oncology. 2010;**11**(2):155-164

[109] Weber JS, O'Day S, Urba W, Powderly J, Nichol G, Yellin M, et al. Phase I/II study of ipilimumab for patients with metastatic melanoma. Journal of Clinical Oncology. 2008;**26**(36):5950-5956

[110] Phan GQ, Yang JC, Sherry RM, Hwu P, Topalian SL, Schwartzentruber DJ, et al. Cancer regression and autoimmunity induced by cytotoxic T lymphocyte-associated antigen 4 blockade in patients with metastatic melanoma. Proceedings of the National Academy of Sciences of the United States of America. 2003;**100**(14):8372-8377

[111] Bashey A, Medina B, Corringham S, Pasek M, Carrier E, Vrooman L, et al. CTLA4 blockade with ipilimumab to treat relapse of malignancy after allogeneic hematopoietic cell transplantation. Blood. 2009;**113**(7):1581-1588

[112] Diefenbach CS, Hong F, Ambinder RF, Cohen JB, Robertson MJ, David KA, et al. Ipilimumab, nivolumab, and brentuximab vedotin combination therapies in patients with relapsed or refractory Hodgkin lymphoma: Phase 1 results of an open-label, multicentre, phase 1/2 trial. Lancet Haematology. 2020;**7**(9):e660-e670

[113] Zeldis JB, Knight R, Hussein M, Chopra R, Muller G. A review of the history, properties, and use of the immunomodulatory compound lenalidomide. Annals of the New York Academy of Sciences. 2011;**1222**:76-82

[114] Sakamuri D, Glitza IC, Betancourt Cuellar SL, Subbiah V, Fu S, Tsimberidou AM, et al. Phase I dose-escalation study of anti-CTLA-4 antibody ipilimumab and lenalidomide in patients with advanced cancers. Molecular Cancer Therapeutics. 2018;**17**(3):671-676

[115] El Halabi L, Adam J, Gravelle P, Marty V, Danu A, Lazarovici J, et al.

Expression of the immune checkpoint regulators LAG-3 and TIM-3 in classical Hodgkin lymphoma. Clinical Lymphoma, Myeloma and Leukemia. 2021;**21**(4):257-266 e253

[116] Annibali O, Bianchi A, Grifoni A, Tomarchio V, Tafuri M, Verri M, et al. A novel scoring system for TIGIT expression in classic Hodgkin lymphoma. Scientific Reports. 2021;**11**(1):7059

[117] Armand P, Lesokhin A, Borrello I, Timmerman J, Gutierrez M, Zhu L, et al. A phase 1b study of dual PD-1 and CTLA-4 or KIR blockade in patients with relapsed/refractory lymphoid malignancies. Leukemia. 2021;**35**(3):777-786

[118] Cao Y, Wang X, Jin T, Tian Y, Dai C, Widarma C, et al. Immune checkpoint molecules in natural killer cells as potential targets for cancer immunotherapy. Signal Transduction and Targeted Therapy. 2020;**5**(1):250

[119] Tun AM, Ansell SM. Immunotherapy in Hodgkin and non-Hodgkin lymphoma: Innate, adaptive and targeted immunological strategies. Cancer Treatment Reviews. 2020;**88**:102042

[120] Alizadeh AA, Eisen MB, Davis RE, Ma C, Lossos IS, Rosenwald A, et al. Distinct types of diffuse large B-cell lymphoma identified by gene expression profiling. Nature. 2000;**403**(6769):503-511

[121] Modi D, Potugari B, Uberti J. Immunotherapy for diffuse large B-cell lymphoma: Current landscape and future directions. Cancers (Basel). 2021;**13**(22):5827

[122] Gu Q, Li J, Chen Z, Zhang J, Shen H, Miao X, et al. Expression and prognostic significance of PD-L2 in diffuse large B-cell lymphoma. Frontiers in Oncology. 2021;**11**:664032

[123] Dong H, Zhu G, Tamada K, Chen L. B7-H1, a third member of the B7 family, co-stimulates T-cell proliferation and interleukin-10 secretion. Nature Medicine. 1999;**5**(12):1365-1369

[124] Li S, Young KH, Medeiros LJ. Diffuse large B-cell lymphoma. Pathology. 2018;**50**(1):74-87

[125] Grimm KE, O'Malley DP. Aggressive B cell lymphomas in the 2017 revised WHO classification of tumors of hematopoietic and lymphoid tissues. Annals of Diagnostic Pathology. 2019;**38**:6-10

[126] Godfrey J, Tumuluru S, Bao R, Leukam M, Venkataraman G, Phillip J, et al. PD-L1 gene alterations identify a subset of diffuse large B-cell lymphoma harboring a T-cell-inflamed phenotype. Blood. 2019;**133**(21):2279-2290

[127] Kiyasu J, Miyoshi H, Hirata A, Arakawa F, Ichikawa A, Niino D, et al. Expression of programmed cell death ligand 1 is associated with poor overall survival in patients with diffuse large B-cell lymphoma. Blood. 2015;**126**(19):2193-2201

[128] Wang Y, Farooq U, Link BK, Larson MC, King RL, Maurer MJ, et al. Late relapses in patients with diffuse large B-cell lymphoma treated with immunochemotherapy. Journal of Clinical Oncology. 2019;**37**(21):1819-1827

[129] Ansell SM, Minnema MC, Johnson P, Timmerman JM, Armand P, Shipp MA, et al. Nivolumab for relapsed/refractory diffuse large B-cell lymphoma in patients ineligible for or having failed autologous transplantation: A single-arm, phase II study. Journal of Clinical Oncology. 2019;**37**(6):481-489

[130] Zheng Y, Si J, Yuan T, Ding S, Tian C. Immune targeted therapy for diffuse large B cell lymphoma. Blood Science. 2021;**3**(4):136-148

[131] Smith SD, Till BG, Shadman MS, Lynch RC, Cowan AJ, Wu QV, et al. Pembrolizumab with R-CHOP in previously untreated diffuse large B-cell lymphoma: Potential for biomarker driven therapy. British Journal of Haematology. 2020;**189**(6):1119-1126

[132] Younes A, Burke JM, Cheson BD, Diefenbach C, Ferrari S, Hahn UH, et al. Safety and efficacy of atezolizumab in combination with rituximab plus CHOP in previously untreated patients with diffuse large B-cell lymphoma (DLBCL): Updated analysis of a phase I/II study. Blood. 2019;**134**(Supplement_1):2874-2874

[133] Herrera AF, Goy A, Mehta A, Ramchandren R, Pagel JM, Svoboda J, et al. Safety and activity of ibrutinib in combination with durvalumab in patients with relapsed or refractory follicular lymphoma or diffuse large B-cell lymphoma. American Journal of Hematology. 2020;**95**(1):18-27

[134] Younes A, Burke JM, Cheson B, Diefenbach C, Ferrari S, Hahn U, et al. Safety and efficacy of atezolizumab in combination with rituximab plus CHOP in previously untreated patients with diffuse large B-cell lymphoma (DLBCL): Primary analysis of a phase I/II study. Blood. 2018;**132**(Supplement 1):2969-2969

[135] Schuster SJ, Bartlett NL, Assouline S, Yoon S-S, Bosch F, Sehn LH, et al. Mosunetuzumab induces complete remissions in poor prognosis non-Hodgkin lymphoma patients, including those who are resistant to or relapsing after chimeric antigen receptor T-cell (CAR-T) therapies, and is active in treatment through multiple lines. Blood. 2019;**134**(Supplement_1):6-6

[136] Hutchings M, Gritti G, Sureda A, Terol MJ, Dyer MJ, Iacoboni G, et al. CD20-TCB, a novel T-cell-engaging bispecific antibody, can be safely combined with the anti-PD-L1 antibody atezolizumab in relapsed or refractory B-cell non-Hodgkin lymphoma. Blood. 2019;**134**(Supplement_1): 2871-2871

[137] Hirayama AV, Gauthier J, Hay KA, Sheih A, Cherian S, Chen X, et al. Efficacy and toxicity of JCAR014 in combination with durvalumab for the treatment of patients with relapsed/refractory aggressive B-cell non-Hodgkin lymphoma. Blood. 2018;**132**(Supplement 1):1680-1680

[138] Argnani L, Casadei B, Pelusi C, Lo Preiato V, Pagotto U, Bertoni F, et al. Immune-related adverse events in the treatment of non-Hodgkin lymphoma with immune checkpoint inhibitors. Scientific Reports. 2022;**12**(1):1753

[139] Ansell S, Gutierrez ME, Shipp MA, Gladstone D, Moskowitz A, Borello I, et al. A phase 1 study of nivolumab in combination with ipilimumab for relapsed or refractory hematologic malignancies (CheckMate 039). Blood. 2016;**128**(22):183-183

[140] Savage KJ. Primary mediastinal large B-cell lymphoma. Blood. 2021;**140**(9):955-970

[141] Chen H, Pan T, He Y, Zeng R, Li Y, Yi L, et al. Primary mediastinal B-cell lymphoma: Novel precision therapies and future directions. Frontiers in Oncology. 2021;**11**:654854

[142] Al Hadidi SA, Lee HJ. Pembrolizumab for the treatment of Hodgkin lymphoma. Expert Opinion on Biological Therapy. 2020;**20**(11):1275-1282

[143] Armand P, Rodig S, Melnichenko V, Thieblemont C, Bouabdallah K, Tumyan G, et al. Pembrolizumab in relapsed or refractory primary mediastinal large

B-cell lymphoma. Journal of Clinical Oncology. 2019;**37**(34):3291-3299

[144] Zinzani PL, Santoro A, Gritti G, Brice P, Barr PM, Kuruvilla J, et al. Nivolumab combined with brentuximab Vedotin for relapsed/refractory primary mediastinal large B-cell lymphoma: Efficacy and safety from the phase II CheckMate 436 study. Journal of Clinical Oncology. 2019;**37**(33):3081-3089

[145] Fakhri B, Ai W. Current and emerging treatment options in primary mediastinal B-cell lymphoma. Therapeutic Advances in Hematology. 2021;**12**:20406207211048959

[146] Beltran BE, Castro D, Paredes S, Miranda RN, Castillo JJ. EBV-positive diffuse large B-cell lymphoma, not otherwise specified: 2020 update on diagnosis, risk-stratification and management. American Journal of Hematology. 2020;**95**(4):435-445

[147] Chen BJ, Chapuy B, Ouyang J, Sun HH, Roemer MG, Xu ML, et al. PD-L1 expression is characteristic of a subset of aggressive B-cell lymphomas and virus-associated malignancies. Clinical Cancer Research. 2013;**19**(13):3462-3473

[148] Satou A, Nakamura S. EBV-positive B-cell lymphomas and lymphoproliferative disorders: Review from the perspective of immune escape and immunodeficiency. Cancer Medicine. 2021;**10**(19):6777-6785

[149] Quan L, Chen X, Liu A, Zhang Y, Guo X, Yan S, et al. PD-1 blockade can restore functions of T-cells in Epstein-Barr virus-positive diffuse large B-cell lymphoma In vitro. PLoS One. 2015;**10**(9):e0136476

[150] Soussain C, Malaise D, Cassoux N. Primary vitreoretinal lymphoma: A diagnostic and management challenge. Blood. 2021;**138**(17):1519-1534

[151] Ferreri AJM, Cwynarski K, Pulczynski E, Fox CP, Schorb E, La Rosee P, et al. Whole-brain radiotherapy or autologous stem-cell transplantation as consolidation strategies after high-dose methotrexate-based chemoimmunotherapy in patients with primary CNS lymphoma: Results of the second randomisation of the international Extranodal lymphoma study Group-32 phase 2 trial. Lancet Haematology. 2017;**4**(11):e510-e523

[152] Yamanaka R, Morii K, Shinbo Y, Sano M, Homma J, Tsuchiya N, et al. Late relapse of primary central nervous system lymphoma. Leukemia & Lymphoma. 2017;**58**(2):475-477

[153] Schaff LR, Grommes C. Update on novel therapeutics for primary CNS lymphoma. Cancers (Basel). 2021;**13**(21):5372

[154] Nayak L, Iwamoto FM, LaCasce A, Mukundan S, Roemer MGM, Chapuy B, et al. PD-1 blockade with nivolumab in relapsed/refractory primary central nervous system and testicular lymphoma. Blood. 2017;**129**(23):3071-3073

[155] Zain JM, Hanona P. Aggressive T-cell lymphomas: 2021 updates on diagnosis, risk stratification and management. American Journal of Hematology. 2021;**96**(8):1027-1046

[156] Hathuc V, Kreisel F. Genetic landscape of peripheral T-cell lymphoma. Life (Basel). 2022;**12**(3):410

[157] Kim J, Cho J, Byeon S, Kim WS, Kim SJ. Comparison of first-line treatments of peripheral T-cell lymphoma according to regimen: A systematic review and meta-analysis. Hematological Oncology. 2021;**39**(5):664-673

[158] Liu X, Yang M, Wu M, Zheng W, Xie Y, Zhu J, et al. A retrospective study

of the CHOP, CHOPE, and CHOPE/G regimens as the first-line treatment of peripheral T-cell lymphomas. Cancer Chemotherapy and Pharmacology. 2019;**83**(3):443-449

[159] Boku N, Ryu MH, Kato K, Chung HC, Minashi K, Lee KW, et al. Safety and efficacy of nivolumab in combination with S-1/capecitabine plus oxaliplatin in patients with previously untreated, unresectable, advanced, or recurrent gastric/gastroesophageal junction cancer: Interim results of a randomized, phase II trial (ATTRACTION-4). Annals of Oncology. 2019;**30**(2):250-258

[160] Lesokhin AM, Ansell SM, Armand P, Scott EC, Halwani A, Gutierrez M, et al. Nivolumab in patients with relapsed or refractory hematologic malignancy: Preliminary results of a phase Ib study. Journal of Clinical Oncology. 2016;**34**(23):2698-2704

[161] Yang R, Sun L, Li CF, Wang YH, Yao J, Li H, et al. Galectin-9 interacts with PD-1 and TIM-3 to regulate T cell death and is a target for cancer immunotherapy. Nature Communications. 2021;**12**(1):832

[162] Wang H, Kaur G, Sankin AI, Chen F, Guan F, Zang X. Immune checkpoint blockade and CAR-T cell therapy in hematologic malignancies. Journal of Hematology & Oncology. 2019;**12**(1):59

[163] Peiro I, Palmero R, Iglesias P, Diez JJ, Simo-Servat A, Marin JA, et al. Thyroid dysfunction induced by nivolumab: Searching for disease patterns and outcomes. Endocrine. 2019;**64**(3):605-613

[164] Naidoo J, Page DB, Li BT, Connell LC, Schindler K, Lacouture ME, et al. Toxicities of the anti-PD-1 and anti-PD-L1 immune checkpoint antibodies. Annals of Oncology. 2015;**26**(12):2375-2391

[165] Abdel-Rahman O, Fouad M. Risk of pneumonitis in cancer patients treated with immune checkpoint inhibitors: A meta-analysis. Therapeutic Advances in Respiratory Disease. 2016;**10**(3):183-193

[166] Asada M, Mikami T, Niimura T, Zamami Y, Uesawa Y, Chuma M, et al. The risk factors associated with immune checkpoint inhibitor-related pneumonitis. Oncology. 2021;**99**(4):256-259

[167] Vardhana S, Cicero K, Velez MJ, Moskowitz CH. Strategies for recognizing and managing immune-mediated adverse events in the treatment of Hodgkin lymphoma with checkpoint inhibitors. The Oncologist. 2019;**24**(1):86-95

[168] Brahmer JR, Lacchetti C, Schneider BJ, Atkins MB, Brassil KJ, Caterino JM, et al. Management of Immune-related adverse events in patients treated with immune checkpoint inhibitor therapy: American Society of Clinical Oncology clinical practice guideline. Journal of Clinical Oncology. 2018;**36**(17):1714-1768

[169] Miyahara K, Noda T, Ito Y, Hidaka H, Fujimoto S, Takedomi H, et al. An investigation of nine patients with gastrointestinal immune-related adverse events caused by immune checkpoint inhibitors. Digestion. 2020;**101**(1):60-65

[170] Jain P, Gutierrez Bugarin J, Guha A, Jain C, Patil N, Shen T, et al. Cardiovascular adverse events are associated with usage of immune checkpoint inhibitors in real-world clinical data across the United States. ESMO Open. 2021;**6**(5):100252

[171] Lal JC, Brown SA, Collier P, Cheng F. A retrospective analysis of cardiovascular adverse events associated with immune checkpoint inhibitors. Cardiooncology. 2021;**7**(1):19

[172] Hu J, Tian R, Ma Y, Zhen H, Ma X, Su Q, et al. Risk of cardiac adverse events in patients treated with immune checkpoint inhibitor regimens: A systematic review and Meta-analysis. Frontiers in Oncology. 2021;**11**:645245

[173] Wen L, Zou X, Chen Y, Bai X, Liang T. Sintilimab-induced autoimmune diabetes in a patient with the anti-tumor effect of partial regression. Frontiers in Immunology. 2020;**11**:2076

[174] Samoa RA, Lee HS, Kil SH, Roep BO. Anti-PD-1 therapy-associated type 1 diabetes in a Pediatric patient with relapsed classical Hodgkin lymphoma. Diabetes Care. 2020;**43**(9):2293-2295

[175] Munakata W, Ohashi K, Yamauchi N, Tobinai K. Fulminant type I diabetes mellitus associated with nivolumab in a patient with relapsed classical Hodgkin lymphoma. International Journal of Hematology. 2017;**105**(3):383-386

[176] Hughes MS, Pietropaolo M, Vasudevan MM, Marcelli M, Nguyen H. Checking the checkpoint inhibitors: A case of autoimmune diabetes after PD-1 inhibition in a patient with HIV. Journal of the Endocrine Society. 2020;**4**(12):bvaa150

[177] Nalbantoglu M, Altunrende B, Tuncer OG, Akman G. Autoimmune encephalitis after treatment of Hodgkin's lymphoma with the immune checkpoint inhibitor nivolumab. Noro Psikiyatri Arsivi. 2021;**58**(2):163-165

[178] Erol-Yildiz R, Kizilay T, Tuzun E, Misirli H, Turkoglu R. Nivolumab-induced autoantibody negative limbic encephalitis in a patient with Hodgkin lymphoma. Leukemia & Lymphoma. 2020;**61**(6):1519-1521

[179] De la Hoz A, Foolad F, Gallegos C, Kornblau S, Kontoyiannis DP. Nivolumab-induced encephalitis post allogeneic stem cell transplant in a patient with Hodgkin's disease. Bone Marrow Transplantation. 2019;**54**(5):749-751

[180] Tardy MP, Gastaud L, Boscagli A, Peyrade F, Gallamini A, Thyss A. Autoimmune hemolytic anemia after nivolumab treatment in Hodgkin lymphoma responsive to immunosuppressive treatment. A case report. Hematological Oncology. 2017;**35**(4):875-877

[181] Palla AR, Kennedy D, Mosharraf H, Doll D. Autoimmune Hemolytic Anemia as a complication of nivolumab therapy. Case Reports in Oncology. 2016;**9**(3):691-697

[182] Rogado J, Sanchez-Torres JM, Romero-Laorden N, Ballesteros AI, Pacheco-Barcia V, Ramos-Levi A, et al. Immune-related adverse events predict the therapeutic efficacy of anti-PD-1 antibodies in cancer patients. European Journal of Cancer. 2019;**109**:21-27

[183] Weber JS, Hodi FS, Wolchok JD, Topalian SL, Schadendorf D, Larkin J, et al. Safety profile of nivolumab monotherapy: A pooled analysis of patients with advanced melanoma. Journal of Clinical Oncology. 2017;**35**(7):785-792

[184] Eggermont AMM, Kicinski M, Blank CU, Mandala M, Long GV, Atkinson V, et al. Association between immune-related adverse events and recurrence-free survival among patients with stage III melanoma randomized to receive pembrolizumab or placebo: A secondary analysis of a randomized clinical trial. JAMA Oncology. 2020;**6**(4):519-527

**Chapter 6**

# Immunotherapy and Hepatocellular Carcinoma

*Jacob Zaemes, Muneeb Rehman, Coleman Smith and Ruth He*

## Abstract

The management of hepatocellular carcinoma (HCC) has been transformed by the incorporation of immune checkpoint inhibitor therapy. Compared to traditional chemotherapy, these regimens have markedly improved outcomes in patients with HCC. Additionally, they are generally well-tolerated in patients with impaired hepatic function. This chapter will review the landmark trials which have paved the way for the use of ICIs in the treatment of HCC and summarize current consensus on best practices regarding their use in this setting. It will also discuss other prospective uses of immunotherapy for the treatment of HCC currently being investigated, including further incorporation of both checkpoint inhibitor and non-checkpoint inhibitor agents into treatment strategies. Furthermore, it will summarize the existing safety and efficacy data regarding the use of checkpoint inhibitors in patients who have previously undergone liver transplant.

**Keywords:** hepatocellular carcinoma, checkpoint inhibitor therapy, nivolumab, pembrolizumab, sorafenib, Lenvatinib, liver transplant, liver rejection

## 1. Introduction

Hepatocellular carcinoma (HCC) is estimated to be the sixth most prevalent cancer worldwide and the fourth leading cause of cancer-related death [1]. HCC typically develops in the background of chronic liver disease often in the setting of either chronic infection with hepatitis B or C, alcohol abuse, or metabolic syndrome [2].

The immune system plays a vital role in controlling cancer development and progression [2]. Dysfunction of the tumor and immune system interaction leads to immune evasion through impaired antigen recognition or by tumor creating an immunosuppressive microenvironment [3]. Immune checkpoints are inhibitor molecules expressed by lymphocytes that prevent their overaction. Tumor cells exploit this normal physiological mechanism by expressing these ligands in the tumor microenvironment [4]. The recent emergence of immune checkpoint inhibitors has significantly changed the cancer treatment landscape. These monoclonal antibodies block the interaction of checkpoint proteins with their ligands, preventing the inactivation of T cells [5]. The ligands that are targeted include cytotoxic T lymphocyte-associated antigen (CTLA4), programmed death 1 (PD-1), programmed death-ligand 1 (PD-L1), lymphocyte-activation gene 3 (LAG3), etc. [6].

Immune checkpoint inhibitors have had promising results in patients with advanced hepatocellular carcinoma due to the contribution of inflammation and suppression of immune microenvironments to HCC pathogenesis, becoming essential in HCC management [7, 8].

In this chapter, we will review the major immunotherapy trials in patients with advanced HCC in both the firstline and subsequent line setting as well as discuss the mechanism of immune mediated side effects in these patients. We will also discuss the emerging role of immunotherapy in transplant patients.

## 2. Treatment of hepatocellular carcinoma with immunotherapy

### 2.1 Firstline treatment

#### *2.1.1 Bevacizumab with atezolizumab*

Immunotherapy agents alone or in combination with tyrosine kinase inhibitors (TKI's) or anti-vascular endothelial growth factor receptor (anti-VEGF) therapies have become the cornerstone of treatment for advanced HCC. **Table 1** shows a summary of the main clinical trials involving immune checkpoint inhibitors as both monotherapies and in combination with other systemic therapies used to treat HCC. The combination the PD-L1 monoclonal antibody atezolizumab and anti-VEGF antibody bevacizumab was initially studied in the phase 1b GO30140, which was a multicenter, multi-arm phase 1b study that enrolled patients for first line treatment in nonresectable HCC [9]. The combination of atezolizumab and bevacizumab was compared to atezolizumab alone. In the arm with no randomization (everyone received both atezolizumab and bevacizumab), the objective response rate (ORR) was 36% (95% confidence interval [CI] 26–46) at a median follow-up of 12.4 months with the median duration of response not reached (95% CI 11·8–not estimable), with responses of 6 months or longer observed in 23% of patients. In the comparison arm (atezolizumab and bevacizumab vs. atezolizumab alone), with a median follow-up of 6.6 months for the combination atezolizumab and bevacizumab group and 6.7 months for the atezolizumab alone group, median progression-free survival (PFS) was 5.6 vs. 3.4 months (hazard ratio [HR] 0.55; 80% CI 0.40–0.74; $p = 0.011$). The most common grade 3–4 treatment-related adverse events (TRAEs) were hypertension (5% in combination group, none in monotherapy group) and proteinuria (3% in combination group, none in monotherapy group) [9]. The combination of atezolizumab and bevacizumab in unresectable hepatocellular carcinoma was further studied in ImBrave 150, a phase III clinical trial [10]. In this study, patients with unresectable HCC who had not previously received systemic therapy were randomly assigned to receive either atezolizumab plus bevacizumab or sorafenib until unacceptable toxicity or disease progression. HR for death with atezolizumab and bevacizumab as compared to sorafenib was 0.58 (95% CI, 0.42–0.79; $p < 0.001$) with overall survival (OS) at 12 months 67.2% (95% CI, 61.3–73.1) with atezolizumab and bevacizumab and 54.6% (95% CI, 45.2–64.0) with sorafenib. Median PFS was 6.8 months (95% CI, 5.7–8.3) and 4.3 months (95% CI, 4.0–5.6) in the respective groups (HR for disease progression or death, 0.59; 95% CI, 0.47–0.76; $P < 0.001$). Grade 3 or 4 TRAEs occurred in 56.5% of 329 patients who received atezolizumab-bevacizumab and in 55.1% of 156 patients who received sorafenib. Grade 3 or 4 hypertension occurred

| Trial | Comparison and stage targeted | Outcomes | Adverse events |
|---|---|---|---|
| Monotherapy | | | |
| CheckMate 040 (Phase I/II) [13] | Nivolumab for advanced HCC, previously treated with or naïve/intolerant to sorafenib | Cohort 1 (dose escalation) = ORR 15%, median OS 15 months Cohort 2 (dose expansion) = ORR 20% | Cohort 1 (dose escalation) – grade 3/4 TRAE rate 25% Cohort 2 (dose expansion) – grade 3/4 TRAE rate 19% |
| CheckMate 459 (Phase III) [12] | Nivolumab vs. Sorafenib for advanced HCC, sorafenib naïve | ORR 15%, median OS 16.4 months (HR 0.85, p = 0.0752), median PFS 3.7 months | Grade 3/4 TRAE rate: nivolumab 34% vs. sorafenib 49% |
| KEYNOTE-224 (Phase II) [23] | Pembrolizumab for advanced HCC, previous sorafenib failure/intolerance | ORR 17%, median OS 12.9 months, median PFS 4.9 months | Grade 3/4 rate 26% |
| KEYNOTE-240 (Phase III) [24] | Pembrolizumab vs. placebo for advanced HCC, previous sorafenib failure/intolerance | ORR 18.3%, median OS 13.9 months, median PFS 3 months | Grade 3/4 TRAE rate pembrolizumab 18.6% vs. placebo 7.5% |
| KEYNOTE-394 (Phase III) [25] | Pembrolizumab vs. placebo for advanced HCC, previous sorafenib failure/intolerance | ORR 12.7%, median OS 14.6 months, median PFS 2.6 months | Grade 3/4 TRAE rate 14.4% vs. 5.9% |
| NCT02989922 (Phase II) [26] | Camrelizumab for advanced HCC, previous systemic therapy failure/intolerance | ORR 14.7%, median OS 13.8 months, median PFS 2.1 months | Grade 3/4 TRAE rate 22% |
| Combination therapy | | | |
| IMbrave150 (Phase III) [10] | Atezolizumab + Bevacizumab vs. Sorafenib for advanced HCC, sorafenib naïve | ORR 27.3%, median OS 19.2 months, median PFS 6.8 months | Grade 3/4 TRAE rate Atezolizumab + Bevacizumab 56.5% vs. Sorafenib 55.1% |
| CheckMate 040 (Phase I/II) [13] | Nivolumab + Ipilimumab (3 dosing arms) for advanced HCC, previous sorafenib failure/intolerance | Arm 1 = ORR 32%, median OS 22.8 months; Arm 2 = ORR 27%, median OS 12.5 months; Arm 3 = ORR 29%, median OS 12.7 months | Grade 3/4 TRAE rate arm 1 53%, arm 2 29%, arm 3 31% |
| HIMALAYA (Phase III) [14] | Durvalumab + Tremelimumab (D + T) vs. Durvalumab (D) vs. Sorafenib for unresectable HCC | Median OS 16.4 months D + T, 13.8 months in Sorafenib group, 16.6 months D | Grade 3/4 TRAEs in 25.8% (D + T), 12.9% (D), 36.8% Sorafenib |
| COSMIC-312 (Phase III) [15] | Cabozantinib + Atezolizumab vs. Sorafenib for advanced HCC, no prior therapy | Median PFS 6.8 months in Cabozantinib and Atezolizumab, 4.2 months in Sorafenib group, No statistically significant benefit for Cabozantinib and Atezolizumab vs. Sorafenib (HR 0.90, 96% CI 0.69–1.18, P = 0.438) | Grade 3 or 4 TRAEs 54% Cabozantinib and Atezolizumab, 32% Sorafenib |

| Trial | Comparison and stage targeted | Outcomes | Adverse events |
|---|---|---|---|
| NCT03006926 (Phase Ib) [18] | Pembrolizumab + Lenvatinib for unresectable HCC | Median OS 22 months, median PFS 8.6 months | Grade 3 or 4 TRAEs 67% |
| ORIENT-32 (Phase II/III) [21] | Sintilimab + IBI305 vs. Sorafenib for advanced HCC, no prior therapy | Median OS not reached vs. 10.4 months, median PFS 4.6 months vs. 2.8 months | TRAEs hypertension (14% combination, 6% Sorafenib), Palmar-plantar erythrodysaesthesia (none vs. 12%) |
| CheckMate 040 (Phase I/II) [27] | Cabozantinib + Nivolumab (arm 1) vs. Cabozantinib + Ipilimumab + Nivolumab (arm 2) for advanced HCC, no prior therapy | ORR 17% arm 1, 26% arm 2; median PFS 5.5 months arm 1, 6.8 months arm 2 | Grade 3/4 TRAEs 42% arm 1, 71% arm 2 |

*HCC, hepatocellular carcinoma; ORR, overall response rate; OS, overall survival; PFS, progression free survival; HR, hazard ratio; TRAE, treatment-related adverse event.*

**Table 1.**
*Immune checkpoint Inhibitor Clinical Trials in HCC.*

in 15.2% of patients in the atezolizumab-bevacizumab group vs. 12.2% in sorafenib group, grade 3 or 4 aspartate aminotransferase (AST) increase occurred in 7.0% of patients in the atezolizumab-bevacizumab group vs. 5.1% of patients in the sorafenib group; however, other high-grade toxic effects were infrequent [10]. Cheng et al. published updated efficacy and safety data from the IMbrave 150 trial. After a median follow-up of 15.6 months, the median OS was 19.2 months (95% CI 17.0–23.7) with atezolizumab and bevacizumab and 13.4 months (95% CI 11.4–16.9) with sorafenib (HR 0.66; 95% 0.52–0.85; descriptive $p < 0.001$). The median PFS was 6.9 (95% CI 5.7–8.6) and 4.3 (95% CI 4.0–5.6) months in the respective treatment groups (HR 0.65; 95% CI 0.53–0.81; descriptive $p < 0.001$). Grade 3/4 TRAEs occurred in 43% in the atezolizumab and bevacizumab group and 46% in the sorafenib group [11].

### 2.1.2 Nivolumab

The PD-1 inhibitor nivolumab as monotherapy was compared to sorafenib in the first line setting in the multicenter, phase 3 CheckMate 459 trial in patients with advanced HCC [12]. This was based on the results of CheckMate 040, which was a phase 1/2 non-comparative, dose escalation, and expansion trial with multiple arms for patients with advanced HCC [13]. There was an initial dose-escalation phase followed by dose-expansion for patients who had progressed on prior lines of therapy. During dose-escalation, nivolumab had a manageable safety profile—25% of patients had grade 3/4 TRAEs, 6% had treatment-related serious adverse events (pemphigoid, adrenal insufficiency, liver disorder). Nivolumab 3 mg/kg was chosen for dose-expansion. The ORR was 20% (95% CI 6–28) in the dose-expansion phase and 15% (95% CI 6–28) in the dose-escalation phase. Based on the results of CheckMate 040, CheckMate 459 sought to compare nivolumab monotherapy with sorafenib monotherapy in the first line setting. At a median follow-up for OS of 15.2 months in the nivolumab group and 13.4 months in the sorafenib group, median OS was

16.4 months (95% CI 13.9–18.4) with nivolumab and 14.7 months (95% CI 11.9–17.2) with sorafenib (HR 0.85, 95% CI 0.72–1.02, p = 0.075). ORR was 15% (95% CI 12–19) in nivolumab arm, 7% (95% CI 5–10) in sorafenib arm. The protocol defined significance level was not reached. The most common grade 3 or 4 TRAEs were palmar-plantar-erythrodysaesthesia (<1% in nivolumab group vs. 14% in sorafenib group), AST elevation (6% vs. 4%), and hypertension (0% vs. 7%) [12]. Although first line nivolumab monotherapy did not significantly improve overall survival compared with sorafenib, there was clinical benefit with a favorable safety profile that makes nivolumab monotherapy an option, especially for patients in whom tyrosine kinase inhibitors and antiangiogenic drugs are contraindicated or may have substantial risks.

#### *2.1.3 Other combination therapies*

The combination of durvalumab (anti-PD-L1) and tremelilumab (anti-CTLA-4) was compared to sorafenib for first line therapy in the HIMALAYA phase 3 clinical trial [14]. Patients with unresectable HCC were randomized to a single priming dose of tremelilumab with durvalumab (STRIDE), durvalumab monotherapy, sorafenib monotherapy, or tremelilumab and durvalumab. Recruitment to the arm with combination of tremelilumab and durvalumab ceased after a planned analysis showed that this did not differ from durvalumab. Thus, the primary objective was OS for the STRIDE regimen vs. sorafenib and secondary objective was OS noninferiority of durvalumab to sorafenib. Median OS was 16.4 months (95% CI 14.2–19.6) in the STRIDE group vs. 13.8 months in the sorafenib group (HR 0.78; 96% CI 0.65–0.92, p = 0.0035), meeting the primary endpoint. Durvalumab met the objective of OS noninferiority to sorafenib with median OS of 16.6 months (95% CI 14.1–19.1) in the durvalumab group vs. 13.8 months (95% CI 12.3–16.1) in the sorafenib group (HR 0.86; 96% CI 0.73–1.03). Grade 3 or 4 TRAEs occurred in 25.8% (STRIDE), 12.9% (durvalumab), and 36.8% (sorafenib) of patients [14]. This study showed that the STRIDE regimen with a priming dose of tremelilumab and durvalumab had improvements in outcomes with improved tolerability.

Immunotherapy agents have also been studied in combination with TKIs. In the phase III COSMIC-312 study, cabozantinib (multikinase TKI that inhibits MET, VEGFR, RET, etc) and atezolizumab (PD-L1 antagonist) was compared to sorafenib monotherapy and to cabozantinib monotherapy in the first line setting for patients with advanced HCC [15]. The study met the primary endpoint with improvement in PFS: 6.8 months in the cabozantinib and atezolizumab group vs. 4.2 months in the sorafenib group (HR 0.63, 99% CI 0.44–0.91; P = 0.0012. Interim analysis of OS did not show a statistically significant benefit for cabozantinib and atezolizumab vs. sorafenib (HR 0.90, 96% CI 0.69–1.18, P = 0.438). Grade 3 or 4 TRAEs occurred for 54% of patients who received cabozantinib and atezolizumab vs. 32% in patients who received sorafenib. The most common events were palmar-plantar-erythrodysaesthesia (7.9% in patients who received cabozantinib and atezolizumab vs. 8.2% in patients who received sorafenib), hypertension (7.0% vs. 6.3%), AST elevation (6.5% vs. 2.4%), and alanine transaminase increase (ALT) (6.3% vs. 1.9%) [15].

The multikinase inhibitor lenvatinib (inhibitor of VEGF receptors 1–3, FGF receptors 1–4, PDGF receptor alpha, RET, and KIT) is thought to have an immunomodulatory effect on tumor microenvironments and thought to contribute to antitumor activity when combined with immunotherapy. Lenvatinib can inhibit proneoangiogenic and immunosuppressive effects of tumor microenvironments, which would improve the benefit of immunotherapy agents [16, 17]. Finn et al. conducted a phase

1b trial with a combination of pembrolizumab and lenvatinib [18]. 100 out of 104 patients had no prior systemic treatment. At a median duration of follow-up of 10.6 months (95% CI, 9.2–11.5 months), median PFS was 8.6 months and median OS was 22 months. Grade 3 or higher TRAEs occurred in 67% of patients [18]. LEAP-002 is an ongoing clinical trial that is comparing the combination of Lenvatinib and pembrolizumab (PD-1 inhibitor) to lenvatinib plus placebo in the first line setting for advanced HCC [19]. This combination was well-tolerated with promising antitumor activity in patients with advanced HCC in the phase 1b KEYNOTE-524 trial [20].

ORIENT-32 study was a phase 2–3 randomized clinical trial in China that assessed the combination of sintilimab (a PD-1 inhibitor) and a IBI305 a bevacizumab biosimilar versus sorafenib as first-line treatment in advanced HCC [21]. At a median follow-up of 10.0 months, the combination group had a median PFS of 4.6 months (95% CI, 4.1–5.7) versus 2.8 months (95% CI, 2.7–3.2) in the sorafenib arm, HR 0.56, 95% CI 0.46–0.70, $p < 0.0001$. Median OS was not reached for the combination group versus 10.4 months (95% CI 8.5–not reached), HR 0.57, 95% CI, 0.43–0.75, $p < 0.0001$. The most common TRAEs were hypertension (14% of patients in combination group vs. 6% in sorafenib group and palmar-plantar erythrodysaesthesia (none vs. 12%). TRAEs leading to death occurred in 2% of patients in the combination group and 1% of patients receiving sorafenib [21].

## 2.2 Subsequent treatment

### *2.2.1 Nivolumab*

Immunotherapy agents have also been studied significantly in subsequent lines of therapy. As mentioned previously, CheckMate 040 was a phase 1/2 non-comparative, dose escalation, and expansion trial with multiple arms for patients with advanced HCC [13]. There was an initial dose-escalation phase followed by dose-expansion for patients who had progressed on prior lines of therapy. During dose-escalation, nivolumab had a manageable safety profile—25% of patients had grade 3/4 TRAEs, 6% had treatment-related serious adverse events (pemphigoid, adrenal insufficiency, liver disorder). Nivolumab 3 mg/kg was chosen for dose-expansion. The ORR was 20% (95% CI 6–28) in the dose-expansion phase and 15% (95% CI 6–28) in the dose-escalation phase [13].

Nivolumab (PD-1 inhibitor) monotherapy demonstrated manageable safety, ORR of 14%, duration of response of at least 12 months in 59% of patients, and promising long-term median OS of 15.1 months in patients with advanced HCC treated with sorafenib [13]. The Food and Drug Administration (FDA) granted accelerated approval to nivolumab in HCC based on this study. Further arms of CheckMate 040 then sought to assess the impact of the addition of CTLA-4 immune checkpoint inhibitor ipilimumab to nivolumab in patients with advanced HCC who were previously treated with sorafenib. Patients were randomized 1:1:1 to either nivolumab 1 mg/kg plus ipilimumab 3 mg/kg every 3 weeks for 4 doses followed by nivolumab 240 mg every 2 weeks (arm A); nivolumab 3 mg/kg plus ipilimumab 1 mg/kg followed by nivolumab 240 mg every 2 weeks (arm B); or nivolumab 3 mg/kg every 2 weeks plus ipilimumab 1 mg/kg every 6 weeks (arm C). Median follow-up was 30.7 months. Investigator-assessed ORR was 32% (95% CI, 20–47%) in arm A, 27% (95% CI 15–41%) in arm B, and 29% (95% CI 17–43%) in arm C. Median duration of response was not reached (8.3–33.7+) in arm A and was 15.2 months (4.2–29.9+) in arm B, and 21.7 months (2.8–32.7+) in arm C. Median OS was 22.8 months (95% CI,

9.4–not reached) in arm A, 12.5 months (95% CI, 7.6–16.4) in arm B, and 12.7 months (95% CI, 7.4–33.0) in arm C. Any-grade TRAEs were reported in 94% of patients in arm A, 71% in arm B, 79% in arm C, with similar types of events across arms. The FDA granted accelerated approval for this regimen based on this study [22].

#### *2.2.2 Pembrolizumab*

KEYNOTE-224, KEYNOTE 240, and KEYNOTE-394 evaluated pembrolizumab in the subsequent line setting in patients with advanced HCC. KEYNOTE-224 was a non-randomized phase 2 trial for patients with advanced HCC who had either progressed or were intolerant of sorafenib. Findings included an ORR of 17% (95% CI 11–26) in patients receiving pembrolizumab. TRAE's occurred in 73% of patients, with grade 3 in 24% and grade 4 in 1% of patients [23]. Based on this study, pembrolizumab was further studied in phase III trials.

KEYNOTE-240 was a randomized, phase III trial in multiple countries that enrolled patients with advanced HCC who had progressed on prior sorafenib to receive pembrolizumab vs. placebo [24]. Results were significant for median OS of 13.9 months (95% CI, 11.6–16.0 months) for pembrolizumab vs. 10.6 months (95% CI, 8.3–13.5) for placebo (HR 0.781; 95% CI 0.611–0.998, $p = 0.0238$). Median PFS for pembrolizumab was 3.0 months (95% CI, 2.8–4.1 months) vs. 2.8 months (95% CI, 1.6–3.0 months) with HR 0.718 (95% CI 0.570–0.904, $p = 0.0022$). Grade 3 or higher adverse events occurred in 52.7% vs. 46.3% for pembrolizumab vs. placebo, respectively. Primary end points in this study were OS and PFS, one-sided significance threshold, $P = 0.0174$ (final analysis) and $P = 0.002$ (first interim analysis). OS and PFS did not reach statistical significance per specified criteria, but the study showed a favorable risk benefit ratio for pembrolizumab in this population [24]. KEYNOTE-394 was a randomized, phase 3 study conducted in Asia that evaluated efficacy and safety of pembrolizumab vs. placebo as second-line therapy for previously treated advanced HCC [25]. At a median follow-up of 33.8 months (18.7–49.0), pembrolizumab significantly improved OS vs. placebo at 14.6 months for pembrolizumab (95% CI 12.6–18.0) vs. 13.0 (95% CI 10.5–15.1) for placebo (HR 0.79, 95% CI 0.63–0.99, $p = 0.0180$. Pembrolizumab significantly improved PFS, with median PFS 2.6 months (95% CI 1.5–2.8) for pembrolizumab vs. 2.3 months (95% 1.4–2.8) for placebo (HR 0.74, 95% CI 0.60–0.92, $P = 0.0032$). ORR was 12.7% vs. 1.3% (estimated difference 11.4%, 95% CI 6.7–16.0, $p = 0.00004$). TRAEs occurred in 66.9% of patients in the pembrolizumab arm and 49.7% in the placebo arm, including 14.4% vs. 5.9% with grade 3–5 events. This study supported pembrolizumab as a second line option in this patient population [25].

#### *2.2.3 Camrelizumab*

Camrelizumab is a PD-1 inhibitor that was investigated in a phase 2 trial in China in pretreated patients with advanced HCC. Patients were randomly assigned to receive camrelizumab every 2 or 3 weeks. With a median follow-up of 12.5 months, ORR was reported in 14.7% (95% CI 10.3–20.2) patients with overall survival probability at 6 months of 74.4% (95% CI 68.0–79.7%). Grade 3 or 4 treatment-related adverse events occurred in 22% of patients; with the most common increased AST (5%), decreased neutrophil count (3%) [26].

The combination of dual immune checkpoint inhibitors tremelimumab (anti-CTLA-4) and durvalumab (anti-PD-L1) was studied in the immunotherapy-naïve population who had progressed on, were intolerant to, or refused sorafenib [28].

Patients were randomized to one of two combinations (tremelimumab 300 mg + durvalumab 1500 mg 1 dose followed by durvalumab every 4 weeks or tremelimumab [arm 1] vs. durvalumab every 4 weeks for 4 doses followed by durvalumab every 4 weeks [arm 2]). These comparative arms were compared to durvalumab monotherapy [arm 3] or tremelimumab monotherapy [arm 4]. Median OS was 18.7 months (95% CI 10.8–NR) in arm 1, 11.3 months (95% CI 8.4–14.6) in arm 2, 11.7 months (95% CI 8.5–16.9) in arm 3, and 17.1 months (95% CI 10.9–NR) in arm 4. ORR was 22.7% (95% CI 13.8–33.8%) in arm 1, 9.5% (95% CI 4.2–17.9%) in arm 2, 9.6% (95% CI 4.7–17.0%) in arm 3, and 7.2% (95% CI 2.4–16.1%) in arm 4. Grade 3/4 treatment related adverse events occurred in 35.1% of patients in arm 1, 24.4% in arm 2, 17.8% in arm 3, and 42.0% in arm 4. This study showed encouraging clinical activity and tolerable safety profile especially with the arm 1 regimen [28].

Combination immunotherapy with TKI or anti-VEGF monoclonal antibody combinations have also been studied in the subsequent line setting in advanced HCC. One of the arms of CheckMate 040 compared the combination of cabozantinib (tyrosine kinase inhibitor that works on VEGF receptor as well as additional targets including c-MET and AXL) and nivolumab (arm 1) to nivolumab, ipilimumab, and cabozantinib (arm 2) [27]. ORR was 17% in arm 1 and 26% in arm 2, median PFS was 5.5 months in arm 1 and 6.8 months in arm 2. Grade 3–4 TRAEs were reported in 42% of patients in arm 1 and 71% of patients in arm 2 leading to treatment discontinuation in 3% of patients in arm 1 and 20% of patients in arm 2. Although the triplet regimen had a higher rate of TRAEs observed, the majority were manageable and reversible with this combination offering another treatment option for patients [27]. Immune checkpoint inhibitors have revolutionized the treatment of many solid tumors, including advanced HCC.

## 3. Immunotherapy and liver transplant

HCC is unique among solid organ malignancies in part due to the role of transplant in its management. For the select group of patients with unresectable HCC who are found to be appropriate candidates, liver transplant remains the only potentially curative treatment option. In all solid organ transplant patients, modulation of the immune system is necessary post-transplant to prevent graft rejection. Closely titrated and monitored immunosuppressant regimens are used to minimize the risks of both graft rejection and opportunistic infections. The use of both liver transplant and immunotherapy as treatment modalities for HCC gives rise to the question of whether these therapies could interact in a way that increases the risk of graft rejection, blunts the therapeutic effects of immunotherapy, or both. Although research into this field has only recently begun, some trends have begun to arise which may help elucidate the nature of these interactions and help guide future clinicians.

### 3.1 Treatment of HCC with liver transplant

Patients with locally advanced HCC can be potentially cured by liver transplant. In these cases, total liver resection with replacement of a functional liver acts to eradicate tumor that would otherwise have been unresectable. In order to ensure total removal with transplant is feasible, patients must fit a strict set of criteria to be considered. These criteria, as outlined by Mazzaferro et al. [29] and now known as the Milan criteria, define a subset of patients with more localized disease. According to the Milan criteria, patients must either one tumor less than or equal to 5.0 cm or up to three tumors none of which exceed 3.0 cm. Additionally, there must be no evidence of vascular invasion or extrahepatic disease. In the original study by Mazzaferro et al., the outcomes of 48 patients whose HCC adhered to these criteria were evaluated. 4-year overall survival following transplant was found to be 75% compared to historic 5-year overall survival rates of 30–40% [29]. 8% of the patients in this series developed recurrent HCC after transplant.

Another, more liberal, set of criteria known as the University of California, San Francisco (UCSF) criteria have been developed which consider patients eligible for orthotopic liver transplant if they had one tumor up to 6.5 cm or no more than three tumors, each 4.5 cm or smaller, with cumulative tumor 8 cm or less. The researchers who developed these criteria, Yao et al., found that patients who were transplanted under this framework had similar survival outcomes to those evaluated using the Milan criteria [30].

Since the development of more stringent criteria, liver transplant has become a mainstay of HCC treatment. Of the roughly 8000 liver transplants performed yearly, about 15–50% are performed on patients with HCC [31, 32]. Yoo et al. evaluated the outcomes of patients who had undergone liver transplant for HCC vs. other indications between 1988 and 2001 [33]. They found a 42.3% 5-year survival rate in patients transplanted for HCC compared to 71.7% in those transplanted for other reasons. However, over time the post-transplant 5-year survival rate in HCC patients had markedly improved from 25.3% between 1987 and 1991 to 46.6% between 1992 and 1996 and 61.1% between 1997 and 2001. A concurrent increase in survival was not demonstrated in patients transplanted for other reasons, supporting the hypothesis that this improvement in outcomes was driven by more stringent selection of patients for transplant rather than improvements in surgical techniques or postoperative management. Other studies have showed 5-year survival rates of roughly 60–80% in patients with HCC who underwent liver transplant, with similar rates seen in transplant patients without HCC [34–36].

### 3.2 Immunology of liver transplant rejection

Acute transplant rejection can be divided into T-cell mediated rejection (TCMR) and antibody-mediated rejection (AMR) [37]. Of these, TCMR is most common following liver transplant, occurring in 15–25% of patients even with proper use of immunosuppressive therapy [38]. TCMR is characterized by inflammatory infiltration of the portal tracts and perivenular areas with some extension into periportal areas in extreme cases [37]. The predominant cells found in these infiltrates are CD4+ and CD8+ T cells as well as macrophages [39]. In TCMR, alloantigen presentation and T-cell co-stimulation bring about T-cell activation. Activated T cells, mediated by the phosphatase calcineurin, upregulate expression of IL-2 which leads to T-cell proliferation and downstream inflammatory processes [40]. During periods of liver inflammation, MHC class II expression increases in liver endothelial cells, biliary epithelium, and hepatocytes, increasing antigen presentation and T-cell mediated damage at these sites [40]. Of note, there are several additional sources of antigen presenting cells specific to the liver. Liver sinusoidal endothelial cells appear to be capable of antigen presentation to CD4+ and CD8+ T cells. Additionally, the majority of the body's macrophages are present in the liver as Kupffer cells, which are also capable of antigen presentation [39].

Of note, there is some evidence to support the role of the PD-1/PD-L1 axis in preventing TCMR. In mouse models, PD-L1 expression on hepatic dendritic cells was shown to be necessary to prevent graft failure following liver transplant [41]. Shi et al. demonstrated that T cells which had previously infiltrated an allograft had increased rates of proliferation in response to PD-1/PD-L1 blockade [42]. Bone marrow stromal cells have been investigated as a potential therapy to prevent rejection following solid organ transplantation, owing in part to their expression of PD-L1 [43].

AMR following liver transplant is relatively rare compared to TCMR and is also less common than in other solid organ transplants [44]. AMR is primarily mediated by donor-specific antibodies against non-self class I and II MHC molecules on the surface of the transplanted liver's endothelial cells [40]. AMR is complement-mediated, and is graded by extent of C4d deposition in the portal microvascular endothelia [37].

The mainstay of immunosuppressive therapy for prevention of TCMR is treatment with a calcineurin inhibitor (CNI) [45]. The most commonly-used CNIs are tacrolimus and cyclosporine [46]. By inhibiting calcineurin, they prevent upregulation of IL-2 and therefore T-cell proliferation. In patients for whom CNI monotherapy is insufficient, it is recommended that patients additionally be started on antiproliferative therapy such as mycophenolate mofetil or mammalian target of rapamycin (mTOR) inhibitors such as everolimus [45]. Acute rejection is treated by either temporarily increasing the dose of the CNI in mild cases or with corticosteroids; in severe cases steroid-refractory rejection may be treated with anti-thymocyte globulin [45]. Acute rejection generally resolves with treatment without significant residual graft dysfunction [39].

### 3.3 Safety and efficacy of immunotherapy in liver transplant patients

Because liver transplant is reserved for patients with localized HCC, and because recurrence is uncommon post-transplant, the overlap of HCC patients who have received checkpoint inhibitor therapy and those who have undergone liver transplant is relatively small. However, for patients who do require both therapies, the simultaneous presence of allogeneic liver graft, chronic immunosuppressive therapy, and increased T-cell immune surveillance by checkpoint inhibitor therapy creates the potential for myriad clinical complications. The foremost concerns in this subpopulation of HCC patients are the prospect of increased risk of TCMR and decreased efficacy of immunotherapy.

#### *3.3.1 Post-transplant treatment with immunotherapy*

To date, the combination of immunotherapy and liver transplant is most likely to occur in post-transplant HCC patients who develop recurrence of HCC. While the rate of HCC recurrence post-transplant is low, it is nonzero; recent studies have found that recurrence occurs in about 15–20% of all patients who undergo transplant [47]. The risk of recurrence is elevated with increased immunosuppression with CNIs or corticosteroids, suggesting an effect of standard-of-care immunosuppression and decreased tumor surveillance following liver transplant [45, 48, 49]. Of note, mTOR inhibitors do not appear to confer the same risk [45].

Clinicians have generally been reticent to give immunotherapy in patients with recurrent HCC post-transplant out of concern for instigating TCMR. As such, descriptions of its use in this setting has largely been limited to case reports. In a recent comprehensive literature review, Yin et al. identified 28 patients who received checkpoint inhibitor therapy following liver transplant, 18 of whom were being treated for recurrent HCC [50] (see **Table 2**). Of these 18 patients, 6 (33%)

DOI: http://dx.doi.org/10.5772/intechopen.107097

| Author | Age (years) | Indication for LT | Indication for ICI post-LT | Time from LT to ICI (years) | ICI therapy used | Immune suppression at time of ICI | Best response to ICI | Liver toxicity | Time to develop toxicity | Treatment of toxicity | Response to treatment of toxicity |
|---|---|---|---|---|---|---|---|---|---|---|---|
| Kumar et al., 2019 [51] | 64 | HCC | HCC | 2 | Nivolumab | NA | NA | TCMR | 1 week | High dose steroids, ATG, PLEX | Improvement of rejection |
| Gomez et al., 2018 [52] | 61 | HCC | HCC | 2 | Nivolumab | NA | NA | TCMR | 1 month | Prednisone | Improvement of rejection |
| Anugwom et al., 2020 [53] | 62 | HCC | HCC | 5 | Nivolumab | Tacrolimus | POD | Immune hepatitis | 2 months | Steroids | Worsening of hepatitis |
| Varkaris et al., 2017 [54] | 70 | HCC | HCC | 8 | Pembrolizumab | Tacrolimus | POD | No | — | — | — |
| Friend et al., 2017 [55] | 20 | HCC | HCC | 3 | Nivolumab | Sirolimus | NA | TCMR + AMR | <1 month | Pulse high dose steroids, IVIG | No response, death |
| Friend et al., 2017 [55] | 14 | HCC | HCC | 2 | Nivolumab | Tacrolimus | NA | TCMR + AMR | <1 month | High dose steroids | No response, death |
| Rammohan et al., 2018 [56] | 57 | HCC | HCC | 4 | Pembrolizumab + sorafenib | mTor inhibitor, tacrolimus | CR | No | — | — | — |
| Amjad et al., 2020 [57] | 62 | HCC | HCC | 1.3 | Nivolumab | Tacrolimus | CR | No | — | — | — |
| DeLeon et al., 2018 [58] | 56 | HCC | HCC | 2.7 | Nivolumab | Tacrolimus | POD | No | — | — | — |
| DeLeon et al., 2018 [58] | 55 | HCC | HCC | 7.8 | Nivolumab | MMF, sirolimus | POD | No | — | — | — |
| DeLeon et al., 2018 [58] | 34 | HCC | HCC | 3.7 | Nivolumab | Tacrolimus | POD | No | — | — | — |

| Author | Age (years) | Indication for LT | Indication for ICI post-LT | Time from LT to ICI (years) | ICI therapy used | Immune suppression at time of ICI | Best response to ICI | Liver toxicity | Time to develop toxicity | Treatment of toxicity | Response to treatment of toxicity |
|---|---|---|---|---|---|---|---|---|---|---|---|
| DeLeon et al., 2018 [58] | 63 | HCC | HCC | 1.2 | Nivolumab | Tacrolimus | NA | No | — | — | — |
| DeLeon et al., 2018 [58] | 68 | HCC | HCC | 1.1 | Nivolumab | Sirolimus | POD | TCMR | <1 month | NA | NA (died due to POD) |
| Gassmann et al., 2018 [59] | 53 | HCC | HCC | 3 | Nivolumab | Everolimus | POD | TCMR | 2 weeks | Steroids, tacrolimus | No response, death |
| De Toni et al., 2017 [60] | 41 | HCC | HCC | 1 | Nivolumab | Tacrolimus | POD | No | — | — | — |
| Al Jarroudi et al., 2020 [61] | 70 | HCC | HCC | 3 | Nivolumab | Tacrolimus | NA | Autoimmune hepatitis vs. graft rejection | 2 months | High dose steroids | NA |
| Al Jarroudi et al., 2020 [61] | 62 | HCC | HCC | 2 | Nivolumab | Tacrolimus | POD | No | — | — | — |
| Al Jarroudi et al., 2020 [61] | 66 | HCC | HCC | 5 | Nivolumab | Tacrolimus | POD | No | — | — | — |
| Kuo et al., 2018 [62] | 62 | HCC | Melanoma | 4.5 | Ipilimumab then pembrolizumab | Sirolimus | PR | No | — | — | — |
| Schvartsman et al., 2017 [63] | 35 | Biliary atresia | Melanoma | 20 | Pembrolizumab | Steroids, MMF | CR | Immune hepatitis | 1 month | Steroids, MMF | Improvement of hepatitis |

| Author | Age (years) | Indication for LT | Indication for ICI post-LT | Time from LT to ICI (years) | ICI therapy used | Immune suppression at time of ICI | Best response to ICI | Liver toxicity | Time to develop toxicity | Treatment of toxicity | Response to treatment of toxicity |
|---|---|---|---|---|---|---|---|---|---|---|---|
| Ranganath et al., 2015 [64] | 59 | Cirrhosis | Melanoma | 8 | Ipilimumab | Tacrolimus | POD | No | — | — | — |
| Dueland et al., 2017 [65] | 67 | Melanoma | Melanoma | 1.5 | Ipilimumab | Prednisone | POD | TCMR | <1 month | High dose steroids, MMF, sirolimus | Improvement of rejection |
| DeLeon et al., 2018 [58] | 63 | Cholangiocarcinoma | Melanoma | 3.1 | Pembrolizumab | MMF, prednisone | NA | TCMR | <1 month | ATG, MMF, tacrolimus, prednisone | Improvement of rejection |
| Morales et al., 2015 [66] | 67 | HCC | Melanoma | 8 | Ipilimumab | Rapamycin | PR | Immune hepatitis | 2 months | None | Improvement of hepatitis |
| DeLeon et al., 2018 [58] | 54 | HCC | Melanoma | 5.5 | Pembrolizumab | Everolimus, MMF | CR | No | — | — | — |
| Chen et al., 2019 [67] | 61 | Cirrhosis | CRC | 2.5 | Pembrolizumab | Prednisone (1 mg/kg), tacrolimus | PR | No | — | — | — |
| Biondani et al., 2018 [68] | 54 | Cirrhosis | Metastatic squamous NSCLC | 13 | Nivolumab | Prednisone, tacrolimus, everolimus | POD | No | — | — | — |
| Lee et al., 2019 [69] | 73 | HCC | Cutaneous SCC | 12 | Nivolumab | Everolimus | NA | TCMR + AMR | 1 month | High dose steroids, everolimus, MMF | Improvement in TCMR but persistent AMR |

*Adapted with permission from Yin et al. [48]. HCC, hepatocellular carcinoma; CRC, colorectal carcinoma; NSCLC, non-small cell lung cancer; SCC, squamous cell carcinoma; LT, liver transplant; ICI, immune checkpoint inhibitor; NA, not available; MMF, mycophenolate mofetil; POD, progression of disease; CR, complete response; PR, partial response; TCMR, T-cell mediated rejection; AMR, antibody-mediated rejection; ATG, anti-thymocyte globulin; PLEX, plasma exchange; IVIG, intravenous immunoglobulin.*

**Table 2.**
*Characteristics of case reports of patients who received checkpoint inhibitor therapy post-transplant.*

experienced TCMR with an additional patient experiencing either acute graft rejection or immunotherapy-related hepatitis. All cases of TCMR occurred within 2 months of starting checkpoint inhibitor therapy. 2 of the 6 patients with proven TCMR also experienced AMR. 3 of 6 of the patients with TCMR died despite treatment with immunosuppressive regimens, including both patients with TCMR and AMR. All of the patients in the series with known PD-L1 positive tumors (4/28, 14%) developed TCMR, reinforcing the potential importance of the PD-1/PD-L1 axis in preventing rejection in liver transplant patients. In terms of mitigating factors, it was noted that the majority of patients who experienced graft rejection were 3 years or less post-transplant and that rejection was rare in late post-transplant patients. Additionally, graft rejection was not observed in any of the 3 patients treated with anti-CTLA-4 therapy alone. This finding is consistent with disruption of the PD-1/PD-L1 axis may be uniquely provocative of TCMR, but as the authors noted the sample size of was very small.

In the same series, of the 11 HCC patients with data regarding response, 2 of 11 (18%) had a complete response while the remaining 9 had progression of disease [50]. It is worth noting that all of these patients had previously received treatment with sorafenib and many had received other lines of therapy as well. The initiation of checkpoint inhibitor therapy after failure of other lines of treatment was likely due to concerns about causing graft rejection and may connote that the sample of patients presented here had more aggressive disease. It is therefore difficult to make definitive conclusions about the efficacy of checkpoint inhibitor therapy in this setting.

### *3.3.2 Treatment with immunotherapy as a bridge to transplant*

Another potential setting for treatment with both liver-transplant and checkpoint inhibitor therapy is in patients who receive immunotherapy as a bridge to transplant. It is not uncommon a patient with borderline tumor characteristics to undergo treatment with locoregional therapy such as trans-arterial chemoembolization or radiofrequency ablation in an attempt to shrink the tumor and qualify them for liver transplant [70]. The effects of these treatments go beyond their impact on tumor size. Extent of tumor necrosis post-therapy is associated with improved relapse-free and overall survival [71–73]. Systemic treatment modalities such as sorafenib have been tried as well. Recently, interest has been raised in the possibility of using immunotherapy to achieve more favorable tumor characteristics and increased tumor necrosis prior to transplant. However, checkpoint inhibitor therapy is characterized by its long duration of response and potential for enhancing immune surveillance long after treatment has been discontinued. Therefore, concerns persist that immunotherapy could cause TCMR post-transplant despite cessation prior to surgery.

In the aforementioned review, Yin et al. identified two cases of patients with HCC who had received immunotherapy as a bridge to transplant [50]. In one case, a patient failed sorafenib and received nivolumab for 2 years before being treated with TACE, at which time his tumor qualified him for transplant using the Milan criteria. He underwent transplant 8 days after his last dose of nivolumab and post-transplant rapidly developed graft rejection that progressed despite high-dose methylprednisolone and rabbit anti-thymocyte globulin before dying on postoperative day 10 [74]. In another case, a patient received 14 months of nivolumab following progression after 1 year of sorafenib at which time he was downstaged and met Milan criteria. He was transplanted 15 weeks after his last dose of nivolumab and at the time of the report, 1 year post-transplant, was doing well with no complications or evidence of recurrence [75].

A single-institution series of 9 cases was reported in which patients with HCC were treated with nivolumab prior to liver transplant [76]. Patients received between 2 and 32 cycles (median 9) of nivolumab with a range of 1–253 days (median 18) between last dose of nivolumab and transplant. Remarkably, only one patient experienced rejection, which was mild in nature and occurred in the setting of subtherapeutic tacrolimus level, and no patients had recurrence of their HCC. In one third of patients, explant showed >90% tumor necrosis. At the time of reporting, all patients were alive with a median of 16 months of follow-up (range 8–23 months) post-transplant [76]. These findings, while still stemming from a small treatment cohort, suggest potential promise in the use of immunotherapy as a bridge to transplant.

These data illustrate a wide spectrum of potential outcomes in patients who receive checkpoint inhibitor therapy either pre- or post-transplant for HCC. Further research is required to identify the subset of patients least likely to experience graft rejection, as well as those most likely to benefit from checkpoint inhibitor therapy despite being on immunosuppression.

## 4. Immune checkpoint inhibitor toxicity in HCC patients

Checkpoint inhibitors, while generally better-tolerated than conventional chemotherapy, can nonetheless have myriad complications due to autoimmune-mediated damage at various locations in the body. The characteristics of this toxicity profile and its management specific to HCC patients will be reviewed here, as will the clinical implications of checkpoint inhibitor toxicity in this population.

### 4.1 Challenges specific to HCC patients

Checkpoint inhibitor therapy can cause a number of different organ toxicities, including dermatologic complications, colitis, endocrine dysfunction, and hepatitis, among others. Some cancer types have higher associations with certain immune-related adverse events (irAEs). For instance, melanoma treatment with checkpoint inhibitor therapy is associated with a higher rate of dermatologic toxicities such as vitiligo, while renal cell carcinoma is associated with gastrointestinal toxicities following checkpoint inhibitor therapy [77]. Similarly, treatment of HCC with checkpoint inhibitors appears to be associated with increased rates of hepatitis compared with other cancer types [78]. A major contributing factor to this association is the high rates of underlying liver disease in patients with HCC. Concomitant liver disease such as HBV, HCV, and non-alcoholic steatohepatitis can provide an alternative cause of rising AST and ALT, increase the vulnerability of the liver to further damage, increasing the impact of irAE-related hepatitis when it does develop.

Chronic hepatitis B virus (HBV) and hepatitis C virus (HCV) infection are common contributors to the development of HCC, and concerns have been raised regarding the potential for both checkpoint inhibitor therapy and treatment of irAEs to cause viral reactivation. In a large recent cohort study, Yoo et al. evaluated rates of HBV reactivation 3465 patients who had received immunotherapy as part of cancer treatment [79]. Among patients positive for hepatitis B surface antigen (HBsAg), HBV reactivation was rarely seen in those with HCC, occurring in only 0.5% of cases. However, in all patients with positive HBsAg rate of HBV reactivation was higher in patients not taking antiviral prophylaxis (6.4%) compared to those who were (0.4%), emphasizing the importance of appropriate antiviral prophylaxis in this group regardless of HCC status. A literature review by Pu et al. of patients with HBV and/or HCV treated with checkpoint inhibitors identified 89 patients with HBV, 2 of whom (2.2%) experienced reactivation as well as 98 patients with HCV, 1 of whom (1.0%) had an increase in viral load following treatment [80].

While the risk of HBV and HCV reactivation appears to be low in patients treated with checkpoint inhibitor therapy, some of the immunosuppressive medications used to treat irAEs carry increased risk of viral reactivation. In the American Society for Clinical Oncology (ASCO) guidelines for management of irAEs, the use of TNF-alpha inhibitors such as infliximab is recommended for a number of grade III and/or IV toxicities such as colitis, pneumonitis, and inflammatory arthritis that are resistant to steroids [81]. TNF-alpha inhibitors are known to cause HBV reactivation but appear to be generally safe to use in patients with HCV [82, 83]. Mycophenolate has not been associated with HBV reactivation, and could be considered in many cases of patients with chronic HBV experiencing severe irAEs despite corticosteroid therapy [84].

### 4.2 Immunotherapy toxicity and outcomes in HCC patients

The development of irAEs with checkpoint inhibitor therapy is known to be associated with improved progression-free and overall survival across multiple cancer types [85]. Multiple studies have shown that this trend extends to patients with HCC [86–88]. The relationship between irAE development and prognosis extends to HCC patients who develop high-grade irAEs, and in some studies higher grade irAEs were an even greater predictor of overall survival [87]. Although patients with HCC may be at risk for increased morbidity from irAEs due to underlying liver disease, practitioners should generally attempt to continue treatment whenever feasible, in accordance with the established ASCO guidelines.

## 5. Conclusion

The landscape of treatment for HCC has been fundamentally changed with the advent of immunotherapy. Despite this shift, patients with HCC often have a unique set of circumstances which predisposes them to toxicities related to these drugs. Additionally, the dual roles for immunotherapy and liver transplant in this population can cause complex interactions and potentially devastating complications. Further research to identify other immunotherapeutic treatment modalities is underway. Additionally, more research will be required to better characterize the treatment toxicities and risks associated with transplant.

## Conflict of interest

The authors declare no conflict of interest.

## Author details

Jacob Zaemes[1*], Muneeb Rehman[1], Coleman Smith[2] and Ruth He[1]

1 Department of Hematology and Oncology, MedStar Georgetown University Hospital, Washington, DC, United States of America

2 Department of Transplant Hepatology, MedStar Georgetown University Hospital, Washington, DC, United States of America

*Address all correspondence to: jacob.p.zaemes@medstar.net

## References


[1] Bray F, Ferlay J, Soerjomataram I, Siegel RL, Torre LA, Jemal A. Global cancer statistics 2018: GLOBOCAN estimates of incidence and mortality worldwide for 36 cancers in 185 countries. CA: A Cancer Journal for Clinicians. 2018;**68**(6):394-424

[2] Llovet J, Zucman-Rossi J, Pikarsky E, Sangro B, Schwartz M, Sherman M, et al. Hepatocellular carcinoma. Nature Reviews. Disease Primers. 2016;**2**:16018

[3] Rabinovich GA, Gabrilovich D, Sotomayor EM. Immunosuppressive strategies that are mediated by tumor cells. Annual Review of Immunology. 2007;**25**:267

[4] Chen L, Flies DB. Molecular mechanisms of T cell co-stimulation and co-inhibition. Nature Reviews Immunology. 2013;**13**(4):227-242

[5] Ribas A, Wolchok JD. Cancer immunotherapy using checkpoint blockade. Science. 2018;**359**(6382):1350-1355

[6] He X, Xu C. Immune checkpoint signaling and cancer immunotherapy. Cell Research. 2020;**30**(8):660-669

[7] Prieto J, Melero I, Sangro B. Immunological landscape and immunotherapy of hepatocellular carcinoma. Nature Reviews Gastroenterology & Hepatology. 2015;**12**(12):681-700

[8] Ringelhan M, Pfister D, O'Connor T, Pikarsky E, Heikenwalder M. The immunology of hepatocellular carcinoma. Nature Immunology. 2018;**19**(3):222-232

[9] Lee MS, Ryoo B-Y, Hsu C-H, Numata K, Stein S, Verret W, et al. Atezolizumab with or without bevacizumab in unresectable hepatocellular carcinoma (GO30140): An open-label, multicentre, phase 1b study. The Lancet Oncology. 2020;**21**(6):808-820

[10] Finn RS, Qin S, Ikeda M, Galle PR, Ducreux M, Kim T-Y, et al. Atezolizumab plus bevacizumab in unresectable hepatocellular carcinoma. New England Journal of Medicine. 2020;**382**(20):1894-1905

[11] Cheng A-L, Qin S, Ikeda M, Galle PR, Ducreux M, Kim T-Y, et al. Updated efficacy and safety data from IMbrave150: Atezolizumab plus bevacizumab vs. sorafenib for unresectable hepatocellular carcinoma. Journal of Hepatology. 2022;**76**(4):862-873

[12] Yau T, Park J-W, Finn RS, Cheng A-L, Mathurin P, Edeline J, et al. Nivolumab versus sorafenib in advanced hepatocellular carcinoma (CheckMate 459): A randomised, multicentre, open-label, phase 3 trial. The Lancet Oncology. 2022;**23**(1):77-90

[13] El-Khoueiry AB, Sangro B, Yau T, Crocenzi TS, Kudo M, Hsu C, et al. Nivolumab in patients with advanced hepatocellular carcinoma (CheckMate 040): An open-label, non-comparative, phase 1/2 dose escalation and expansion trial. The Lancet. 2017;**389**(10088):2492-2502

[14] Abou-Alfa GK, Chan SL, Kudo M, Lau G, Kelley RK, Furuse J, et al. Phase 3 randomized, open-label, multicenter study of tremelimumab (T) and durvalumab (D) as first-line therapy in patients (pts) with unresectable hepatocellular carcinoma (uHCC):

HIMALAYA. American Society of Clinical Oncology. 2022

[15] Kelley R, Yau T, Cheng A-L, Kaseb A, Qin S, Zhu A, et al. VP10-2021: Cabozantinib (C) plus atezolizumab (A) versus sorafenib (S) as first-line systemic treatment for advanced hepatocellular carcinoma (aHCC): Results from the randomized phase III COSMIC-312 trial. Annals of Oncology. 2022;**33**(1):114-116

[16] Fukumura D, Kloepper J, Amoozgar Z, Duda DG, Jain RK. Enhancing cancer immunotherapy using antiangiogenics: Opportunities and challenges. Nature Reviews Clinical Oncology. 2018;**15**(5):325-340

[17] Kato Y, Tabata K, Kimura T, Yachie-Kinoshita A, Ozawa Y, Yamada K, et al. Lenvatinib plus anti-PD-1 antibody combination treatment activates CD8+ T cells through reduction of tumor-associated macrophage and activation of the interferon pathway. PLoS One. 2019;**14**(2):e0212513

[18] Finn RS, Ikeda M, Zhu AX, Sung MW, Baron AD, Kudo M, et al. Phase Ib study of lenvatinib plus pembrolizumab in patients with unresectable hepatocellular carcinoma. Journal of Clinical Oncology. 2020;**38**(26):2960

[19] Llovet JM, Kudo M, Cheng A-L, Finn RS, Galle PR, Kaneko S, et al. Lenvatinib (len) plus pembrolizumab (pembro) for the first-line treatment of patients (pts) with advanced hepatocellular carcinoma (HCC): Phase 3 LEAP-002 study. American Society of Clinical Oncology. 2019

[20] Zhu AX, Finn RS, Ikeda M, Sung MW, Baron AD, Kudo M, et al. A phase Ib study of lenvatinib (LEN) plus pembrolizumab (PEMBRO) in unresectable hepatocellular carcinoma (uHCC). American Society of Clinical Oncology. 2020

[21] Ren Z, Xu J, Bai Y, Xu A, Cang S, Du C, et al. Sintilimab plus a bevacizumab biosimilar (IBI305) versus sorafenib in unresectable hepatocellular carcinoma (ORIENT-32): A randomised, open-label, phase 2-3 study. The Lancet Oncology. 2021;**22**(7):977-990

[22] Yau T, Kang Y-K, Kim T-Y, El-Khoueiry AB, Santoro A, Sangro B, et al. Efficacy and safety of nivolumab plus ipilimumab in patients with advanced hepatocellular carcinoma previously treated with sorafenib: The CheckMate 040 randomized clinical trial. JAMA Oncology. 2020;**6**(11):e204564-e

[23] Zhu AX, Finn RS, Edeline J, Cattan S, Ogasawara S, Palmer D, et al. Pembrolizumab in patients with advanced hepatocellular carcinoma previously treated with sorafenib (KEYNOTE-224): A non-randomised, open-label phase 2 trial. The Lancet Oncology. 2018;**19**(7):940-952

[24] Finn RS, Ryoo B-Y, Merle P, Bouattour M, Lim H, Breder V, et al. Pembrolizumab as second-line therapy in patients with advanced hepatocellular carcinoma in KEYNOTE-240: A randomized, double-blind, phase III trial. 2020;**38**(3):193-202

[25] Qin S, Chen Z, Fang W, Ren Z, Xu R, Ryoo B-Y, et al. Pembrolizumab plus best supportive care versus placebo plus best supportive care as second-line therapy in patients in Asia with advanced hepatocellular carcinoma (HCC): Phase 3 KEYNOTE-394 study. American Society of Clinical Oncology. 2022

[26] Qin S, Ren Z, Meng Z, Chen Z, Chai X, Xiong J, et al. Camrelizumab in patients with previously treated

advanced hepatocellular carcinoma: A multicentre, open-label, parallel-group, randomised, phase 2 trial. The Lancet Oncology. 2020;**21**(4):571-580

[27] Yau T, Zagonel V, Santoro A, Acosta-Rivera M, Choo SP, Matilla A, et al. Nivolumab (NIVO) + ipilimumab (IPI) + cabozantinib (CABO) combination therapy in patients (pts) with advanced hepatocellular carcinoma (aHCC): Results from CheckMate 040. American Society of Clinical Oncology. 2020

[28] Kelley RK, Sangro B, Harris WP, Ikeda M, Okusaka T, Kang Y-K, et al. Efficacy, tolerability, and biologic activity of a novel regimen of tremelimumab (T) in combination with durvalumab (D) for patients (pts) with advanced hepatocellular carcinoma (aHCC). American Society of Clinical Oncology. 2020

[29] Mazzaferro V, Regalia E, Doci R, Andreola S, Pulvirenti A, Bozzetti F, et al. Liver transplantation for the treatment of small hepatocellular carcinomas in patients with cirrhosis. New England Journal of Medicine. 1996;**334**(11):693-700

[30] Yao FY, Ferrell L, Bass NM, Watson JJ, Bacchetti P, Venook A, et al. Liver transplantation for hepatocellular carcinoma: Expansion of the tumor size limits does not adversely impact survival. Hepatology. 2001;**33**(6):1394-1403

[31] Maynard E. Liver transplantation: Patient selection, perioperative surgical issues, and expected outcomes. Surgical Clinics. 2019;**99**(1):65-72

[32] Santopaolo F, Lenci I, Milana M, Manzia TM, Baiocchi L. Liver transplantation for hepatocellular carcinoma: Where do we stand? World journal of gastroenterology. 2019;**25**(21):2591

[33] Yoo HY, Patt CH, Geschwind J-F, Thuluvath PJ. The outcome of liver transplantation in patients with hepatocellular carcinoma in the United States between 1988 and 2001: 5-year survival has improved significantly with time. Journal of Clinical Oncology. 2003;**21**(23):4329-4335

[34] Figueras J, Jaurrieta E, Valls C, Benasco C, Rafecas A, Xiol X, et al. Survival after liver transplantation in cirrhotic patients with and without hepatocellular carcinoma: A comparative study. Hepatology. 1997;**25**(6):1485-1489

[35] Doyle MM, Vachharajani N, Maynard E, Shenoy S, Anderson C, Wellen JR, et al. Liver transplantation for hepatocellular carcinoma: Long-term results suggest excellent outcomes. Journal of the American College of Surgeons. 2012;**215**(1):19-28

[36] Wong SN, Reddy KR, Keeffe EB, Han SH, Gaglio PJ, Perrillo RP, et al. Comparison of clinical outcomes in chronic hepatitis B liver transplant candidates with and without hepatocellular carcinoma. Liver Transplantation. 2007;**13**(3):334-342

[37] Demetris AJ, Bellamy C, Hübscher S, O'leary J, Randhawa PS, Feng S, et al. 2016 comprehensive update of the Banff working group on liver allograft pathology: Introduction of antibody-mediated rejection. Wiley Online Library. 2016;**16**(10):2816-2835

[38] Choudhary NS, Saigal S, Bansal RK, Saraf N, Gautam D, Soin AS. Acute and chronic rejection after liver transplantation: What a clinician needs to know. Journal of Clinical and Experimental Hepatology. 2017;**7**(4):358-366

[39] Knechtle SJ, Kwun J, editors. Unique Aspects of Rejection and Tolerance in

Liver Transplantation. Seminars in Liver Disease. 2009;**29**(1):91-101

[40] Ronca V, Wootton G, Milani C, Cain O. The immunological basis of liver allograft rejection. Frontiers in Immunology. 2020;**11**(2155):1-17

[41] Liu H, Bakthavatsalam R, Meng Z, Li Z, Li W, Perkins J, et al., editors. PD-L1 signal on liver dendritic cells is critical for Foxp3+ CD4+ CD25+ Treg and liver tolerance induction in mice. Transplantation Proceedings. 2013;**45**(5):1853-1855

[42] Shi X-L, Mancham S, Hansen BE, de Knegt RJ, de Jonge J, van der Laan LJ, et al. Counter-regulation of rejection activity against human liver grafts by donor PD-L1 and recipient PD-1 interaction. Journal of Hepatology. 2016;**64**(6):1274-1282

[43] Chen Q, Zhou R, Zhang Y, Zhu S, Xiao C, Gong J, et al. Bone marrow mesenchymal stromal cells attenuate liver allograft rejection may via upregulation PD-L1 expression through downregulation of miR-17-5p. Transplant Immunology. 2018;**51**:21-29

[44] Abrol N, Jadlowiec CC, Taner T. Revisiting the liver's role in transplant alloimmunity. World Journal of Gastroenterology. 2019;**25**(25):3123

[45] Charlton M, Levitsky J, Aqel B, O'Grady J, Hemibach J, Rinella M, et al. International liver transplantation society consensus statement on immunosuppression in liver transplant recipients. Transplantation. 2018;**102**(5):727-743

[46] Haddad E, McAlister V, Renouf E, Malthaner R, Kjaer MS, Gluud LL. Cyclosporin versus tacrolimus for liver transplanted patients. Cochrane Database of Systematic Reviews. 2006;**4**:1-71

[47] Filgueira NA. Hepatocellular carcinoma recurrence after liver transplantation: Risk factors, screening and clinical presentation. World Journal of Hepatology. 2019;**11**(3):261

[48] Chen Z-S, He F, Zeng F-J, Jiang J-P, Du D-F, Liu B. Early steroid withdrawal after liver transplantation for hepatocellular carcinoma. World Journal of Gastroenterology: WJG. 2007;**13**(39):5273

[49] Rodríguez-Perálvarez M, Tsochatzis E, Naveas MC, Pieri G, García-Caparrós C, O'Beirne J, et al. Reduced exposure to calcineurin inhibitors early after liver transplantation prevents recurrence of hepatocellular carcinoma. Journal of Hepatology. 2013;**59**(6):1193-1199

[50] Yin C, Baba T, He AR, Smith C. Immune checkpoint inhibitors in liver transplant recipients-a review of current literature. Hepatoma Research. 2021;**7**:52

[51] Kumar S. 2235 nivolumab-induced severe allograft rejection in recurrent post-transplant hepatocellular carcinoma. Official Journal of the American College of Gastroenterology| ACG. 2019;**114**:S1251

[52] Gomez P, Naim A, Zucker K, Wong M. A case of hepatocellular carcinoma (HCC) immunotherapy inducing liver transplant rejection: 2416. Official Journal of the American College of Gastroenterology | ACG. 2018;**113**:S1347

[53] Anugwom C, Leventhal T. Nivolumab-induced autoimmune-like cholestatic hepatitis in a liver transplant recipient. ACG Case Reports Journal. 2020;**7**(7):1-4

[54] Varkaris A, Lewis DW, Nugent FW. Preserved liver transplant after PD-1

pathway inhibitor for hepatocellular carcinoma. Official Journal of the American College of Gastroenterology| ACG. 2017;**112**(12):1895-1896

[55] Friend BD, Venick RS, McDiarmid SV, Zhou X, Naini B, Wang H, et al. Fatal orthotopic liver transplant organ rejection induced by a checkpoint inhibitor in two patients with refractory, metastatic hepatocellular carcinoma. Pediatric Blood & Cancer. 2017;**64**(12):e26682

[56] Rammohan A, Reddy MS, Farouk M, Vargese J, Rela M. Pembrolizumab for metastatic hepatocellular carcinoma following live donor liver transplantation: The silver bullet? Hepatology. 2018;**67**(3):1166-1168

[57] Amjad W, Kotiah S, Gupta A, Morris M, Liu L, Thuluvath PJ. Successful treatment of disseminated hepatocellular carcinoma after liver transplantation with nivolumab. Journal of Clinical and Experimental Hepatology. 2020;**10**(2):185-187

[58] DeLeon TT, Salomao MA, Aqel BA, Sonbol MB, Yokoda RT, Ali AH, et al. Pilot evaluation of PD-1 inhibition in metastatic cancer patients with a history of liver transplantation: The Mayo Clinic experience. Journal of Gastrointestinal Oncology. 2018;**9**(6):1054

[59] Gassmann D, Weiler S, Mertens JC, Reiner CS, Vrugt B, Nägeli M, et al. Liver allograft failure after nivolumab treatment—A case report with systematic literature research. Transplantation Direct. 2018;**4**(8):1-7

[60] De Toni EN, Gerbes AL. Tapering of immunosuppression and sustained treatment with nivolumab in a liver transplant recipient. Gastroenterology. 2017;**152**(6):1631-1633

[61] Al Jarroudi O, Ulusakarya A, Almohamad W, Afqir S, Morere J-F. Anti-programmed cell death protein 1 (PD-1) immunotherapy for metastatic hepatocellular carcinoma after liver transplantation: A report of three cases. Cureus. 2020;**12**(10)

[62] Kuo JC, Lilly LB, Hogg D. Immune checkpoint inhibitor therapy in a liver transplant recipient with a rare subtype of melanoma: A case report and literature review. Melanoma Research. 2018;**28**(1):61-64

[63] Schvartsman G, Perez K, Sood G, Katkhuda R, Tawbi H. Immune checkpoint inhibitor therapy in a liver transplant recipient with melanoma. Annals of Internal Medicine. 2017;**167**(5):361-362

[64] Ranganath HA, Panella TJ. Administration of ipilimumab to a liver transplant recipient with unresectable metastatic melanoma. Journal of Immunotherapy. 2015;**38**(5):211

[65] Dueland S, Guren T, Boberg K, Reims H, Grzyb K, Aamdal S, et al. Acute liver graft rejection after ipilimumab therapy. Annals of Oncology. 2017;**28**(10):2619-2620

[66] Morales RE, Shoushtari AN, Walsh MM, Grewal P, Lipson EJ, Carvajal RD. Safety and efficacy of ipilimumab to treat advanced melanoma in the setting of liver transplantation. Journal for Immunotherapy of Cancer. 2015;**3**(1):1-4

[67] Chen JA, Esteghamat N, Kim EJ, Garcia G, Gong J, Fakih MG, et al. PD-1 blockade in a liver transplant recipient with microsatellite unstable metastatic colorectal cancer and hepatic impairment. Journal of the National Comprehensive Cancer Network. 2019;**17**(9):1026-1030

[68] Biondani P, De Martin E, Samuel D. Safety of an anti-PD-1 immune checkpoint inhibitor in a liver transplant recipient. Annals of Oncology. 2018;**29**(1):286-287

[69] Lee BT, Horwich BH, Chopra S, Ahearn A, Han HH. Checkpoint inhibitor–induced rejection of a liver allograft: A combination of acute T cell–mediated and antibody-mediated rejection. Liver Transplantation. 2019;**25**(12):1845-1848

[70] Coletta M, Nicolini D, Cacciaguerra AB, Mazzocato S, Rossi R, Vivarelli M. Bridging patients with hepatocellular cancer waiting for liver transplant: All the patients are the same? Translational Gastroenterology and Hepatology. 2017;**2**(9):1-7

[71] Chan K-M, Yu M-C, Chou H-S, Wu T-J, Lee C-F, Lee W-C. Significance of tumor necrosis for outcome of patients with hepatocellular carcinoma receiving locoregional therapy prior to liver transplantation. Annals of Surgical Oncology. 2011;**18**(9):2638-2646

[72] Haywood N, Gennaro K, Obert J, Sauer PF, Redden DT, Zarzour J, et al. Does the degree of hepatocellular carcinoma tumor necrosis following transarterial chemoembolization impact patient survival? Journal of Oncology. 2016;**2016**:1-8

[73] Kornberg A, Witt U, Küpper B, Wildgruber M, Friess H, editors. Postinterventional tumor necrosis predicts recurrence-free long-term survival in liver transplant patients with advanced hepatocellular carcinoma. Transplantation Proceedings. 2013;**45**(5):1913-1915

[74] Nordness MF, Hamel S, Godfrey CM, Shi C, Johnson DB, Goff LW, et al. Fatal hepatic necrosis after nivolumab as a bridge to liver transplant for HCC: Are checkpoint inhibitors safe for the pretransplant patient? American Journal of Transplantation. 2020;**20**(3):879-883

[75] Schwacha-Eipper B, Minciuna I, Banz V, Dufour JF. Immunotherapy as a downstaging therapy for liver transplantation. Hepatology. 2020;**72**(4):1488-1490

[76] Tabrizian P, Florman SS, Schwartz ME. PD-1 inhibitor as bridge therapy to liver transplantation? American Journal of Transplantation: Official Journal of the American Society of Transplantation and the American Society of Transplant Surgeons. 2021;**21**(5):1979-1980

[77] Rose LM, DeBerg HA, Vishnu P, Frankel JK, Manjunath AB, Flores JPE, et al. Incidence of skin and respiratory immune-related adverse events correlates with specific tumor types in patients treated with checkpoint inhibitors. Frontiers in Oncology. 2021;**10**:1-9

[78] Sangro B, Chan SL, Meyer T, Reig M, El-Khoueiry A, Galle PR. Diagnosis and management of toxicities of immune checkpoint inhibitors in hepatocellular carcinoma. Journal of Hepatology. 2020;**72**(2):320-341

[79] Yoo S, Lee D, Shim JH, Kim KM, Lim Y-S, Lee HC, et al. Risk of hepatitis B virus reactivation in patients treated with immunotherapy for anti-cancer treatment. Clinical Gastroenterology and Hepatology. 2022;**20**(4):898-907

[80] Pu D, Yin L, Zhou Y, Li W, Huang L, Cai L, et al. Safety and efficacy of immune checkpoint inhibitors in patients with HBV/HCV infection and advanced-stage cancer: A systematic review. Medicine. 2020;**99**(5):1-6

[81] Brahmer JR, Lacchetti C, Schneider BJ, Atkins MB, Brassil KJ, Caterino JM, et al. Management of immune-related adverse events in patients treated with immune checkpoint inhibitor therapy: American Society of Clinical Oncology Clinical Practice Guideline. Journal of Clinical Oncology: Official Journal of the American Society of Clinical Oncology. 2018;**36**(17):1714

[82] Sayar S, Kürbüz K, Kahraman R, Öztürk O, Çalışkan Z, Doğanay HL, et al. Risk of hepatitis B reactivation during anti-TNF therapy; evaluation of patients with past hepatitis B infection. The Turkish Journal of Gastroenterology. 2020;**31**(7):522

[83] Pompili M, Biolato M, Miele L, Grieco A. Tumor necrosis factor-α inhibitors and chronic hepatitis C: A comprehensive literature review. World Journal of Gastroenterology: WJG. 2013;**19**(44):7867

[84] Koutsianas C, Thomas K, Vassilopoulos D. Reactivation of hepatitis B virus infection in rheumatic diseases: Risk and management considerations. Therapeutic Advances in Musculoskeletal Disease. 2020;**12**:1759720X20912646

[85] Matsuoka H, Hayashi T, Takigami K, Imaizumi K, Shiroki R, Ohmiya N, et al. Correlation between immune-related adverse events and prognosis in patients with various cancers treated with anti PD-1 antibody. BMC Cancer. 2020;**20**(1):1-8

[86] Xu S, Lai R, Zhao Q, Zhao P, Zhao R, Guo Z. Correlation between immune-related adverse events and prognosis in hepatocellular carcinoma patients treated with immune checkpoint inhibitors. Frontiers in Immunology. 2021;**12**:794099

[87] Ng KYY, Tan SH, Tan JJE, Tay DSH, Lee AWX, Ang AJS, et al. Impact of immune-related adverse events on efficacy of immune checkpoint inhibitors in patients with advanced hepatocellular carcinoma. Liver Cancer. 2021;**10**(6):1-13

[88] Lu L, Xing K, Wei W, Ling Y, Li P, Li S, et al. Immune-related adverse events predict responses to PD-1 blockade immunotherapy in hepatocellular carcinoma. International Journal of Cancer. 2021;**149**(4):959-966

Section 3

# Current Advances and Techniques

Chapter 7

# Current Advances in Immune Checkpoint Therapy

*Bonnie L. Russell, Sibusiso T. Malindisa, Selisha A. Sooklal and Monde Ntwasa*

## Abstract

Although immune checkpoint inhibitors (ICIs) have shown survival benefits for patients with metastatic cancers, some challenges have been under intense study in recent years. The most critical challenges include the side effects and the emergence of resistance. Potential opportunities exist to develop personalized immune checkpoint inhibitor therapy based on biomarker discovery. Combinational therapy involving immune checkpoint inhibitors and other forms of anticancer therapies has varied success. This chapter reviews drugs currently undergoing Phase III clinical trials and others that are FDA-approved. We take a critical look at the combinational strategies and address the ever-present challenge of resistance. Moreover, we review and evaluate the discovery of biomarkers and assess prospects for personalized immune checkpoint therapy.

**Keywords:** immune checkpoint inhibitors, PD-1, PD-L1, CTLA-4, FDA-approved, ICI resistance, combinational therapy, biomarkers

## 1. Introduction

Immunotherapy including the use of immune checkpoint inhibitors (ICIs) exploits the immune system's components to fight cancer progression. The use of immunotherapy on its own or in combination with conventional cancer treatments such as chemotherapy or radiation has been relatively successful in many cancers [1]. Immune checkpoint proteins are co-inhibitory receptors that are responsible for keeping the immune system in check. Cancer cells exploit these receptor proteins in order to induce tumor tolerance and T cell exhaustion [1, 2]. The FDA has approved treatments for several cancers with immune checkpoint inhibitors that target cytotoxic T lymphocyte antigen 4 (CTLA-4), programmed cell death 1 (PD-1), programmed cell death ligand 1 (PD-L1), and most recently, lymphocyte activation gene-3 (LAG-3). However, there are several additional molecules in clinical trials (Phases I, II, and III) that target immune checkpoint proteins as monotherapy or in combination with other ICIs or different kinds of therapy such as small molecule drugs, chemotherapy, or radiotherapy. Although some adverse reactions occur after treatment with immune checkpoint inhibitors, the main issue encountered is resistance [3]. The most promising strategy to overcome resistance is the use of combination therapies. However, the identification of reliable biomarkers that can predict resistance and response to ICIs may assist in guiding patient selection and identifying those that will indeed benefit from treatment. Numerous biomarkers have been developed in this regard; however, current biomarkers are challenged with technical limitations. In this review, we present FDA-approved ICIs and novel ICIs in clinical trials. In addition, we address ICI resistance and the use of combinational therapy strategies to overcome it, as well as discuss some of the most extensively studied biomarkers and the limitations associated with each.

## 2. Approved immune checkpoint inhibitors

T cell activation is critical for normal physiology to suppress carcinogenesis. During carcinogenesis, tumor cells present neoantigens which, in complex with the major histocompatibility complex (MHC), and together with various costimulatory signals, activate naïve T cells through intracellular signals. This process is balanced by signaling through inhibitory molecules called checkpoint inhibitors on the tumor and T cells [4]. However, cancer cells have developed mechanisms to antagonize T cell activation, thereby promoting carcinogenesis. Strategies have been developed to exploit events at the checkpoint synapse to design anticancer therapeutic drugs. In **Figure 1**, the schematic diagram shows the points at which various immunotherapeutic drugs intervene in cancer progression. Currently, approved immune checkpoint drugs target CTLA-4, PD-1, PD-L1, and LAG-3 (**Table 1**). Significantly, all the approved ICIs are indicated for solid tumors, but few are effective against hematological cancers. We discuss their success and current limitations. We consider success to be associated with the overall response rate (ORR), which is generally defined as the proportion of patients who achieve a complete or partial response per RECIST (Response Evaluation Criteria in Solid Tumors) or WHO (World Health Organization) criteria.

### 2.1 CTLA4 inhibitors

Cytotoxic T-lymphocyte-associated protein 4 (CTLA-4 or CD152) is a membrane glycoprotein expressed exclusively on the surface of effector T cells. Despite sharing only 30% sequence similarity with the T cell surface receptor CD28, CTLA-4 has similar structural and functional properties [57]. CTLA-4 and CD28 regulate T cell responses, with CD28 having a stimulatory effect and CTLA-4 having an inhibitory effect. Both receptors bind to B7 ligands (CD80 and CD86) found on antigen-presenting cells (APCs). However, CTLA-4 has been shown to have a higher affinity for these molecules and competes for binding to common ligands [58]. CTLA-4 usually aids in maintaining self-antigen immunity by preventing T cell activation (**Figure 1A**). However, when CTLA-4 binds to B7 ligands present on cancer cells, it exerts an antagonistic effect on T cell activation and results in the evasion of immune responses. Blockade of the CTLA-4/B7 axis invigorates T cell activation and proliferation and therefore presented a unique therapeutic opportunity for cancer patients [59].

Ipilimumab (Yervoy®) is the first immune checkpoint inhibitor that the FDA approved for the treatment of human cancers. Ipilimumab is a humanized IgG1 antibody developed by Bristol-Myers Squibb, and targets CTLA-4, thereby preventing its interaction with B7 ligands (**Figure 1B**). Ipilimumab was initially approved by the FDA for the treatment of late-stage unresectable melanomas in 2011 (**Table 1**). In 2015, it was further approved for cutaneous melanomas [5, 60]. In melanomas,

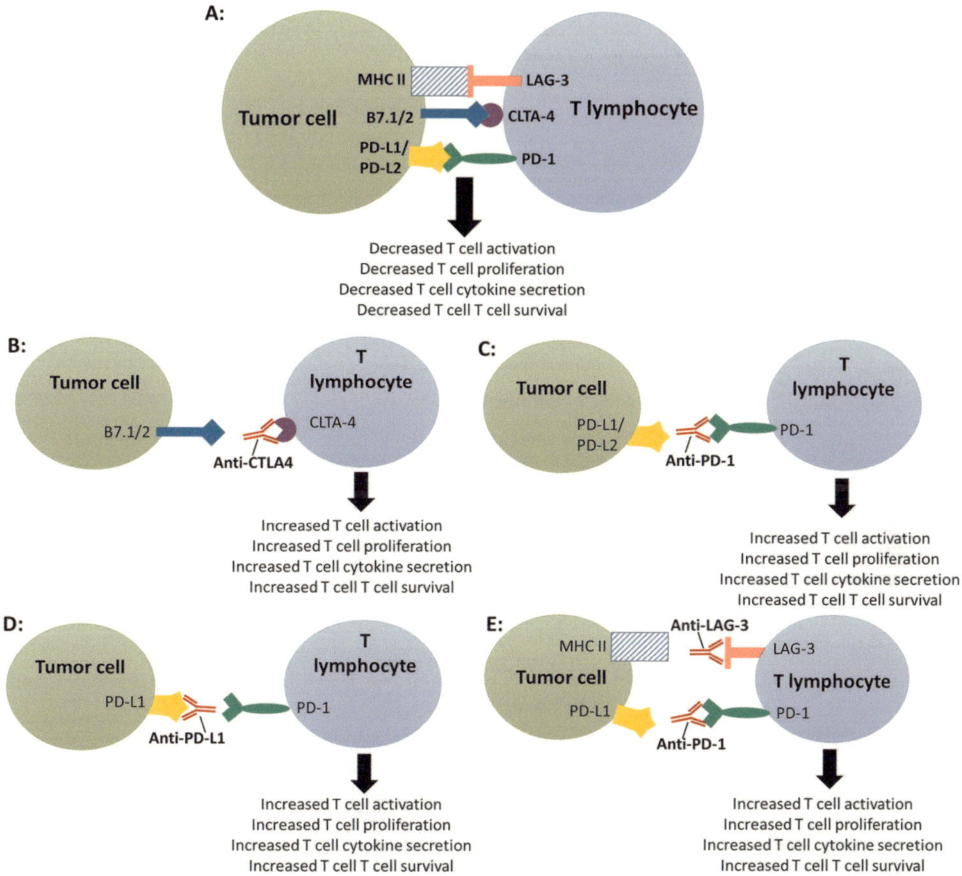


**Figure 1.**
*Mechanism of immune checkpoint inhibitors. (A) Immune checkpoint proteins present on T lymphocytes interact with corresponding ligands on tumor cells, which leads to an alteration in normal T cell phenotypes. The main outcome is the suppression of T cell activation and the resultant decrease in the immune response. (B) Immunotherapy targeting CTLA-4 that disrupts the binding of the B7 family and subsequent signaling. (C) Anti-PD-1 immunotherapy disrupting the interaction with PD-L1/2. (D) The PD-1 and PD-L1 pathway being inhibited by an antibody against PD-L1. (E) The dual blocking of the LAG-3/MHC II pathway and PD-1/PD-L1 pathway, using antibodies that target LAG-3 and PD-1 simultaneously. Blocking these interactions between immune checkpoint proteins and their ligands, using the targeted antibodies, results in a reversal of T cell inhibition.*

Ipilimumab exhibited an ORR of 10.9%. In 2018, Ipilimumab received approval for the treatment of renal cell carcinoma (RCC) (ORR 40.4%) and metastatic colorectal cancer (ORR 49%) in conjunction with Nivolumab [7, 61]. More recently, Ipilimumab was approved in conjunction with Nivolumab for non-small cell lung cancer (ORR 36%), malignant pleural mesothelioma (ORR 40%), and hepatocellular carcinoma (ORR 32%) in 2020 (**Table 1**) [40, 62, 63].

Although not yet approved, Tremelimumab is in the final stages of approval. Tremelimumab is a human IgG2 monoclonal antibody that also targets the CTLA-4 receptor. Following the promising results obtained from the HIMALAYA Phase III trial [64] Tremelimumab in combination with Durvalumab (STRIDE (Single T Regular Interval D) regimen) was accepted under Priority Review by the FDA for patients with unresectable hepatocellular carcinoma. The clinical trial demonstrated that patients experienced an improved median overall survival (OS) (16.4 months) and

| Drug | Combination | Cancer and reference | Approval year | ORR (95% CI) |
|---|---|---|---|---|
| **CTLA-4 inhibitors** | | | | |
| Ipilimumab | NA | Melanoma [5] | 2011 | 10.9% (6.3–17.4) |
| | NA | Colorectal cancer [6] | 2018 | 49% (39–58) |
| | Nivolumab | Renal cell carcinoma [7] | 2018 | 40.4% (26.4–55.7) |
| | Nivolumab | Hepatocellular carcinoma (HCC) [8] | 2020 | 32%; (9–38) |
| | Nivolumab | Non-small cell lung cancer [39] | 2020 | 36% (31–41) |
| | Nivolumab | Pleural mesothelioma [40] | 2020 | 40% (34.1–45.4) |
| **PD-1 inhibitors** | | | | |
| Pembrolizumab | NA | Melanoma [41, 42] | 2014 | 24% (15–34) |
| | NA | Metastatic non-small [43] cell lung cancer | 2015 | 44.8% (36.8–53.0) |
| | NA | Head and neck squamous cell carcinoma [44] | 2016 | 16% (11–22) |
| | NA | Hodgkin's lymphoma [45] | 2017 | 69% (62–75) |
| | NA | Urothelial carcinoma [46] | 2017 | 24% (20–29) |
| | Pemetrexed-platinum | Non-squamous NSCLC [47] | 2017 | 47.6% (39.2–56.0) |
| | NA | Solid tumor with MSI-H or dMMR [9] | 2017 | 39.6% (31.7–47.9) |
| | NA | Gastric cancer [10] | 2017 | 11.6% (8.0–16.1) |
| | NA | Cervical cancer [11] | 2018 | 12.2% (6.5–20.4) |
| | NA | Primary mediastinal large B-cell lymphoma (PMBCL) [12] | 2018 | 45% (32–60) |
| | Platinum-based chemotherapy | Squamous NSCLC [13] | 2018 | 57.9% (51.9–63.8) |
| | NA | Hepatocellular carcinoma (HCC) [14] | 2018 | 17% (11–26) |
| | NA | Merkel cell carcinoma (MCC) [15] | 2018 | 56% (41–70) |
| | Axitinib | Renal cell carcinoma (RCC) [16] | 2019 | 59% (54–64) |
| | NA | Esophageal squamous cell cancer [17] | 2019 | 22% (14–33) |
| | Lenvatinib | Endometrial carcinoma [18] | 2019 | 38.0% (28.8–47.8) |
| | NA | Non-muscle-invasive bladder cancer (NMIBC) [19] | 2020 | 41% (31–51) |
| | NA | MSI-R or dMMR colorectal cancer [20] | 2020 | 43.8% (35.8–52.0) |
| | NA | Cutaneous squamous cell carcinoma (cSCC) [21] | 2021 | 50.0% (36.1–63.9) (localized) 35.2% (26.2–45.2) (metastatic) |

| Drug | Combination | Cancer and reference | Approval year | ORR (95% CI) |
|---|---|---|---|---|
| Nivolumab | NA | Melanoma [22] | 2014 | 31·7% (23.5–40.8) |
| | NA | Squamous NSCLC [23] | 2015 | 20% (14–28) |
| | NA | Renal cell carcinoma [24] | 2015 | 25% (3.68–9.72) |
| | NA | Hodgkin's lymphoma [25] | 2016 | 65% (55–75) |
| | NA | Head and neck squamous cell carcinoma [26] | 2016 | 13.3% (9.3–18.3) |
| | NA | Urothelial carcinoma [27] | 2017 | 19.6% (15.1–24.9) |
| | NA | Colorectal cancer (MSI-H) [6] | 2017 | 31·1% (20.8–42.9) |
| | NA | Hepatocellular carcinoma [28] | 2017 | 20% (15–26) |
| | NA | Small cell lung cancer [29] | 2017 | 12% (5–23) |
| | Ipilimumab | Malignant pleural mesothelioma [30, 40] | 2020 | 40% (34.1–45.4) |
| | Platinum–based chemotherapy or Ipilimumab | Esophageal squamous cell carcinoma [31] | 2022 | 47% (42–53)<br>28% (23–33) |
| Cemiplimab | NA | Cutaneous squamous cell carcinoma [32] | 2018 | 49% (31–67) (localized)<br>47% (35–59) (metastatic) |
| | NA | Advanced basal cell carcinoma [33] | 2021 | 31% (21–42) |
| | NA | Non-small cell lung cancer [34] | 2021 | 39% (34–45) |
| Dostarlimab | NA | Mismatch repair deficient (dMMR) recurrent or advanced solid tumors [35] | 2021 | 41.6% (34.9–48.6), |
| **PD-L1 inhibitors** | | | | |
| Atezolizumab | NA | Urothelial carcinoma [36] | 2016 | 14.8% (11.1–19.3) |
| | NA | Non-small cell lung cancer [37] | 2016 | 17% (11.0–23.8) |
| | Nab-paclitaxel | Triple negative breast cancer | 2019 | 56% (51.3–60.6) |
| | Carboplatin and etoposide | Extensive-stage small cell lung cancer ES-SCLC [38] | 2019 | 60.2% (53.1–67.0) |
| | Bevacizumab | Hepatocellular carcinoma [20] | 2020 | 33.3% (28.3–38.7) |
| | Vemurafenib and cobimetinib | Melanoma [48] | 2020 | 66.·3% (60.1–72.1) |
| Avelumab | NA | Merkel cell carcinoma [49] | 2017 | 31·8% (21.9–43.1) |
| | NA | Urothelial cancer [50] | 2017 | 18.2% (8.2–32.7) |
| | Axitinib | Renal cell carcinoma [51] | 2019 | 55.2% (49.0–61.2) |
| Durvalumab | NA | Urothelial carcinoma [52] | 2017 | 17.0% (11.9–23.3) |
| | NA | Non-small cell lung cancer [53] | 2018 | 28.4% (24.3–32.9) |

| Drug | Combination | Cancer and reference | Approval year | ORR (95% CI) |
|---|---|---|---|---|
| | Platinum-etoposide chemotherapy | Extensive-stage small cell lung cancer [54, 55] | 2020 | 68% (62–73) |
| **LAG-3 inhibitor** | | | | |
| Relatlimab | Nivolumab | Melanoma [56] | 2022 | 43.1% (37.9–48.4) |

**Table 1.**
*FDA-approved immune checkpoint inhibitors.*

overall response rate (20.1%) when compared to Sorafenib treatment (13.8 months and 5.1%, respectively). An approval decision in the fourth quarter of 2022 is expected. These data suggest that a combination of an ant-CTLA-4 and an anti-PD-L1 as a strategy may be a feasible approach.

## 2.2 PD-1 inhibitors

Programmed cell Death 1 (PD-1) (also known as CD279) is a co-inhibitory trans-membrane protein that is expressed on antigen-stimulated T and B lymphocytes, natural killer (NK) cells, and myeloid suppressor dendritic cells (MDSCs). PD-1 is activated via antigen recognition or cytokine stimulation and results in the modulation of immune response intensity [65]. PD-1 ligands, namely, programmed death ligands 1 and 2 (PD-L1 (B7-H1) and PD-L2 (B7-DC)), are widely expressed on antigen-presenting cells. The interaction between PD-1 and its ligands results in the inhibition of lymphocyte proliferation or activation, culminating in T cell exhaustion (**Figure 1A**) [65–68]. To date, the FDA approved four PD-1 immune checkpoint inhibitors for the treatment of human cancers, namely Pembrolizumab (Keytruda®), Nivolumab (Opdivo®), Cemiplimab (Libtayo®), and Dostarlimab-gxly.

Pembrolizumab (MK-3475 or Lambrolizumab, Keytruda) is a humanized IgG4 antibody against PD-1, developed by Merck. The FDA initially approved it for the treatment of patients with unresectable or metastatic melanoma in September 2014 after the KEYNOTE-001 clinical trial (NCT01295827) [69]. These patients had to have had prior unsuccessful treatment with Ipilimumab. Pembrolizumab binds to the PD-1 receptor, thereby disrupting the PD-1 pathway and resulting in the restoration of the antitumor immune response of T lymphocyte cells (**Figure 1C**) [70–72]. Pembrolizumab has subsequently been approved for treatment predominantly as monotherapy and occasionally as part of a combinational therapy for an additional 16 cancer types (**Table 1**). The overall/objective response rates to Pembrolizumab ranges from 12 to 69% in these various cancers. The adverse reactions to Pembrolizumab include both immune-related adverse effects (irAEs) and infusion-related reactions. irAEs include encephalopathy, pneumonia, nephritis, hepatitis, myocarditis, and colitis. However, the most common adverse effects (reported in ≥20% of patients) are fatigue, musculoskeletal pain, decreased appetite, pruritus, diarrhea, nausea, rash, pyrexia, cough, dyspnea, constipation, pain, and abdominal pain [65, 69].

Nivolumab (Opdivo, ONO4538, MDX-1106, or BMS-936,558) is a genetically engineered, fully humanized IgG4 mAb against PD-1 developed by Bristol-Myers Squibb. Like Pembrolizumab, the FDA-approved Nivolumab for the treatment of unresectable or metastatic melanoma, which had progressed after prior treatment with

Ipilimumab. Nivolumab was approved in December 2014 after the CheckMate-037 trial, which tested its efficacy when combined with chemotherapy. Nivolumab selectively inhibits the interaction between the PD-1 and its ligands, PD-L1, and PD-L2. It achieves this by binding to the PD-1 receptor and interfering with the negative regulation of T lymphocyte activation and proliferation caused by the PD-1 pathway, including the antitumor immune response [73, 74]. Since Nivolumab was first approved for the treatment of melanoma in 2014 [22], it has subsequently been approved by the FDA for the treatment of an additional seven cancer types, either in monotherapy or as part of combination therapy (**Table 1**). The overall/objective response rates to Nivolumab ranges from 12 to 65% in the various cancers. Nivolumab is also the most used ICI for combination with CTLA-4 inhibitors and most recently a LAG-3 inhibitor. Serious adverse effects to Nivolumab include increased risk of severe immune-mediated inflammation in the lungs, the colon, the liver, and the kidneys, immune-mediated hypothyroidism and hyperthyroidism and autoimmune diabetes [75–77].

Cemiplimab (REGN2810, SAR439684, Libtayo) is a human IgG4 anti-PD-1 mAb developed by Sanofi/Regeneron. It was approved in September 2018 for the treatment of metastatic cutaneous squamous cell carcinoma (cSCC) or locally advanced cSCC in patients who did not qualify for surgery or radiation [32, 78]. cSCC has a high mutational burden and is therefore hard to treat. Cemiplimab binds to the PD-1 receptor and blocks its interaction with PD-L1, resulting in the upregulation of cytotoxic T cells and an increase in the antitumor activity of the immune system (**Figure 1C**) [78–80]. After its first approval in 2018, it was further approved by the FDA in 2021 for the treatment of two additional cancers, namely basal cell carcinoma and non-small cell lung cancer (**Table 1**). The overall/objective response rate to Cemiplimab ranges from 31 to 49% in the three cancer types. Reported adverse effects of Cemiplimab include severe and fatal immune-mediated adverse reactions in any organ, system, or tissue, including pneumonia, colitis, hepatitis, endocrine disorders, adverse skin reactions, nephritis, and renal dysfunction. In addition, severe infusion-related reactions (Grade 3) can also occur. However, the most common adverse reactions are fatigue, rash, and diarrhea [65, 78, 79].

Recently, in August 2021, the FDA accelerated the approval of the novel PD-1-humanized IgG4 monoclonal antibody known as Dostarlimab-gxly (Jemperli, GlaxoSmithKline LLC) for patients with mismatch repair deficient (dMMR) recurrent or advanced solid tumors after clinical trial NCT02715284 [81]. The overall response rate was 41.6% (95% CI: 34.9, 48.6), with a 9.1% complete response rate and a 32.5% partial response rate. The most reported adverse reactions in patients with dMMR solid tumors were fatigue, anemia, diarrhea, and nausea. Most common Grade 3 or 4 adverse reactions included anemia, fatigue, increased transaminases, sepsis, and acute kidney injury. In a few patients, immune-mediated adverse reactions are associated with Dostarlimab. These include pneumonitis, colitis, hepatitis, endocrinopathies, nephritis, and dermatologic toxicity. In 2022, Dostarlimab was preferred for treating colon cancer, as a small group of 12 patients in clinical Phase II responded positively to the drug, with a 100% complete response rate. This is a rare phenomenon in clinical trials (NCT04165772) [82]. In addition, no adverse events of Grade 3 or higher or relapse were reported. However, the FDA has not yet approved Dostarlimab for the treatment of colon cancer.

### 2.3 PD-L1 inhibitors

The Programmed Death receptor Ligand 1 (PD-L1) plays a vital role in the downregulation of T cell activation in the tumor microenvironment (TME). PD-L1

(B7-H1) and PD-L2 (B7-DC) are the two ligands known to bind to the PD-1 receptor described earlier [66, 83, 84]. Under normal physiological conditions, the PD-1/PD-L1 interaction moderates excessive immune cell activity, thereby preventing the development of autoimmunity and tissue destruction due to hyperactivation of the immune system. Cancer cells in the TME exploit this regulatory mechanism by overexpressing PD-L1 on their surface. The interaction between PD-L1 on tumor cells and PD-1 on cells (T cells) negatively regulates T-cell-mediated immune responses in the TME, resulting in T cell exhaustion and limitation of effector T cell responses [66, 84, 85]. Consequently, cancer development and progression are enhanced by maintaining tumor cell proliferation and survival. Therefore, the PD-L1 signaling represents an attractive target for novel anticancer therapy.

The development and clinical application of immune checkpoint inhibitors targeting the PD-1/PD-L1 axis have significantly enhanced antitumor immunity, produced durable responses, and prolonged survival in cancer patients. Currently, there are three FDA-approved PD-L1 inhibitors, namely, Atezolizumab, Durvalumab, and Avelumab, for treating several solid cancers such as non-small cell lung cancer and metastatic melanoma [85] (**Table 1**). Atezolizumab was the first PD-L1 immune checkpoint inhibitor to be approved by the FDA in 2016 for the treatment of advanced or metastatic urothelial carcinoma (UC) [46]. Studies from clinical trial results revealed that treatment with Atezolizumab increased the ORR and was linked to the PD-L1 status of patients. Patients with less than 5% PD-L1 expression detected saw 9.5% ORR compared to 26% in patients with PD-L1 expression greater than 5% after the 14.4 month follow-up.

Atezolizumab (MPDL3280 or Tecentriq®, Genentech) is a fully humanized IgG1 monoclonal antibody. Its mechanism of action involves binding to PD-L1, thereby blocking PD-L1 interaction with the PD-1 receptor. The disruption of this interaction between immune (PD-1) and PD-L1-expressing tumor cells in the TME results in the reactivation of T-cell-mediated antitumor cytotoxicity. Clinical data have demonstrated that Atezolizumab is safe and efficacious in a wide range of solid tumors and hematologic malignancies [20, 46, 86]. Following its approval for the treatment of UC, the drug has been further approved for the treatment of non-small-cell and extensive stage lung cancer [87, 88]. The treatment of NSCLC and ES-SCLC with Atezolizumab improved the ORR by 17% compared to conventional chemotherapy.

Durvalumab (MEDI4736 or ImfinziTM, AstraZeneca) is another fully humanized IgG1 monoclonal antibody like Atezolizumab that binds with high affinity and specificity to PD-L1, blocking the interaction with PD-1. The US FDA first approved the immune checkpoint inhibitor in 2017 to treat locally advanced or metastatic urothelial carcinoma (UC) [89]. Following its approval, Durvalumab received further accelerated approval for treating unresectable stage III NSCLC following platinum-based chemotherapy and radiotherapy [90]. The introduction of Durvalumab in the treatment of UC and NSCLC improved the ORRs by 17% and 28.4%, respectively. In 2020, the drug was approved to treat extensive stage small cell lung cancer [54]. Currently, Durvalumab is being tested in combination with targeted therapies, chemotherapy, and immunotherapy to maximize its activity and improve patient survival rates.

Avelumab (MSB0010718C or Banvecio®, Merck and Pfizer) is another fully humanized IgG1 monoclonal antibody that binds to PD-L1. Banvecio® binds and blocks PD-L1 expressed in tumor cells resulting in T-cell-mediated antitumor immune response, particularly T cell reactivation and cytokine production [91]. The FDA accelerated the approval of Avelumab for treating 12-year-old and older patients with metastatic Merkel cell carcinoma (MCC) in March 2017 [49]. The approval was based on the observed improved ORRs by 31.8% compared to chemotherapy. Avelumab was further approved in May 2017 for the treatment of locally advanced or metastatic UC with disease progression during or following platinum-based chemotherapy [50]. The treatment improved ORR by 18.2%. Avelumab's most recent approval is for the treatment of renal cell carcinoma [51]. Avelumab is currently being tested in combination with traditional cancer therapies in emerging new small molecules (that have synergistic or complementary functions) in clinical trials. Several other PD-L1 immune checkpoint inhibitors are currently in preclinical and early-phase clinical trials [83].

### 2.4 LAG-3 inhibitors

The lymphocyte activation gene-3 (LAG-3) (CD223) is a membrane receptor protein that is predominately expressed by activated CD4+ and CD8+ T cells, regulatory T cells (Tregs), and natural killer (NK) cells. LAG-3 can also be expressed to a lower extent by B cells and plasmacytoid dendritic cells (DCs) [92]. It interacts with its primary ligand, the major histocompatibility complex class II (MHC-II) (**Figure 1A**), as well as other ligands, including galectin-3, liver sinusoidal endothelial cell lectin (LSECtin), α-synuclein, and fibrinogen-like protein 1 (FGL1). These interactions result in immune cell exhaustion and decreased cytokine secretion [92–95]. Blocking LAG-3 alone cannot reverse T cell exhaustion; however, combining it with a PD-1 inhibitor has been shown to decrease tumor size [96]. Therefore, in March 2022, the combination of Relatlimab (anti-LAG-3) and Nivolumab (anti-PD-1) was approved by the FDA for the treatment of advanced or metastatic melanoma (**Figure 1E**) [56]. The most common adverse reactions (≥20%) were musculoskeletal pain, fatigue, rash, pruritus, and diarrhea. The most common laboratory abnormalities (≥20%) were decreased hemoglobin, decreased lymphocytes, increased aspartate aminotransferase (AST), increased alanine aminotransferase (ALT), and decreased sodium. Currently, there are 17 small molecule drugs targeting LAG-3 in clinical trials comprising of mono and combination treatments (**Table 2**). Furthermore, Tebotelimab (MGD013) is a bispecific DART molecule designed to independently or coordinately block PD-1 and LAG-3 and is being investigated in patients with HER2-positive gastric cancer or gastroesophageal junction cancer (GEJ) (NCT04082364).

## 3. Immune checkpoint inhibitors in phase III clinical trials

Clinical trials are underway on novel immune checkpoint inhibitors and new combinations of already FDA-approved ICIs. Novel emerging immune checkpoint inhibitors include drugs that target lymphocyte activation gene-3 (LAG-3), T cell immunoglobulin and ITIM domain (TIGIT), T cell immunoglobulin and mucin domain containing-3 (TIM-3), V-domain immunoglobulin suppressor of T cell activation (VISTA), B7 homolog 3 protein (B7-H3), inducible T cell costimulatory (ICOS), and B and T lymphocyte attenuator (BTLA). Currently, at least nine novel ICIs have reached Phase III clinical trials (**Table 2**). We note that in addition to the drugs listed in **Table 2**, there are more than 50 other agents (antibodies and small molecules) targeting immune checkpoint proteins that are in Phase I and II [106].

| Target | Drug, clinical trial number, and year | Cancer | Protocol |
|---|---|---|---|
| CTLA-4 [97] | Tremelimumab NCT03298451 2017 | Advanced hepatocellular carcinoma (HCC) | Durvalumab + Tremelimumab vs. Durvalumab monotherapy vs. Sorafenib |
| LAG-3 [98] | Relatlimab NCT03470922 2018 | Advanced melanoma | Relatlimab + Nivolumab vs. Nivolumab monotherapy |
| LAG-3 [99] | MGD013 NCT04082364 2019 | Gastric cancer (GC) or gastroesophageal junction cancer (GEJ) | Margetuximab, Retifanlimab, Tebotelimab, and Chemotherapy |
| TIGHT [100] | Tiragolumab NCT04294810 2020 | Non-small cell lung cancer (NSCLC) | Tiragolumab + Atezolizumab Versus Placebo + Atezolizumab |
| TIGHT [101] | Tiragolumab NCT04256421 2020 | Extensive-stage small cell lung cancer (ES-SCLC) | Atezolizumab + Carboplatin and Etoposide (with or without Tiragolumab) |
| TIM-3 [102] | Sabatolimab NCT04266301 2020 | Myelodysplastic syndrome (MDS) or chronic myelomonocytic leukemia-2 (CMML-2) | MBG453+ Azacitidine |
| B7-H3 [103] | Enoblituzumab NCT04129320 2019 | Head and neck squamous cell carcinoma (HNSCC) | Enoblituzumab + MGA012 or MGD013 |
| B7-H3 [104] | 131I-Omburtamab NCT03275402 2017 | Neuroblastoma, central nervous system, or leptomeningeal metastases | 131I-omburtamab + Radioimmunotherapy |
| ICOS [105] | GSK3359609 NCT04128696 2019 | Head and neck squamous cell carcinoma (HNSCC) | GSK3359609 + Pembrolizumab |

**Table 2.**
*Immune checkpoint inhibitors in phase III clinical trials.*

## 4. Resistance to immune checkpoint inhibitors

One of the most significant challenges in immune checkpoint therapy is the development of resistance, whether it is primary (the patient never responds to treatment) or acquired (the patient initially responds to treatment but stops responding after the commencement of therapy). Resistance can also be intrinsic or extrinsic to tumor cells [107]. Intrinsic resistance occurs when cancer cells alter processes related to immune recognition, cell signaling, gene expression, and DNA damage response. Resistance to immune checkpoint inhibitors is associated with loss of immunogenic neoantigens, an increase of immunosuppressive cells, and the upregulation of alternate immune checkpoint receptors [27, 108]. Response to ICIs can also vary by tumor type, with the highest response rates found in tumors with a high mutational burden, such as melanoma, lung, and bladder cancers.

In contrast, tumors with lower tumor mutational burden (TMB), such as prostate and pancreas, show a lower response [109]. However, ICI response can vary among tumors with a similar TMB, thus suggesting that response to ICI is influenced by several other factors [110]. These factors may include PD-L1 expression or induction, deficiencies in DNA mismatch repair (MMR), levels of tissue-specific neoantigens and tumor-infiltrating lymphocytes (TILs), endogenous retroviruses (RVs) epigenetic alterations, and oncogenic alterations [27, 108, 111, 112]. Extrinsic resistance occurs external to tumor cells throughout the T cell activation process. Tumors can have different immunophenotypes, such as variation in type, density, and location of immune infiltrates, and these differences can affect the response to ICI therapy. In general, inflamed tumors generally respond better to ICI therapy [113, 114]. In addition, the tumor microenvironment (TME) also plays a big role in treatment response, contributing to both primary and acquired resistance. The TME is complex and comprises various immune and stromal cells, the extracellular matrix, surrounding vasculature, and cytokines [114, 115]. This scenario further complicates the development of drug resistance.

Resistance can also be attributed to contextual factors, which include the gut microbiome, expression of human endogenous retroviruses, and gender. The response to ICI therapy influenced by gut microbiomes is thought to involve the activation of dendritic cells, upregulation of MHC-II, and the increased levels of effector T cells [107, 116–118]. High expression of human endogenous retroviruses (RVs) in tumors resulted in a phenotype consistent with immune checkpoint activation in various cancer types. Furthermore, the abnormal expression of ERVs appears to activate epigenetic changes such as histone methylation [111, 119]. Overall, the abnormal expression of ERVs indicates a positive response to ICI treatment.

With overall response rates for most cancers to FDA-approved drugs generally being between 10 and 50%, this indicates that in at least 50% of patients, either primary or acquired resistance is occurring. Two of the most promising strategies by which we can overcome resistance are combinational therapy and identifying predictive biomarkers of ICI therapy.

## 5. Combinational therapy as a strategy to overcome resistance

In the past decades, patients diagnosed with various cancers that did not respond well to traditional methods such as chemotherapy and radiotherapy received very poor prognoses. Moreover, these conventional cancer therapy methods are also known to cause damage to healthy normal cells. Since then, various cancer therapies targeting disordered proteins, immune cells, and components of the tumor microenvironment (TME) have been developed to improve prognosis. Small molecules and immunotherapy have drastically improved the prognosis for some patients. Despite that, a limited number of patients obtain benefits from the treatment. This is attributed mainly to low response and acquired resistance during the treatment, and severe side effects also lead to unfavorable outcomes. To overcome this, researchers are investigating the potential of combining ICIs with various other treatments, including chemo/radiotherapy and targeted therapies. Immunotherapy based on single targets often results in serious side effects, unresponsiveness, or overreaction. In contrast, combinational immunotherapies show synergistic outcomes with higher efficacy and safety. Strategies combining immunotherapy and conventional therapies like radiotherapy and/or chemotherapy have demonstrated promising clinical and basic research results. However, the underlying mechanisms are still unclear.

### 5.1 Combination of two or more immune checkpoint inhibitors

Checkpoint inhibitors that target CTLA-4 and the PD-1/PD-L1 axis are promising candidates for combination immunotherapy. The rationale behind the dual checkpoint inhibitor treatment is the synergy of inhibiting both CTLA-4 and PD-1 with Nivolumab plus Ipilimumab which was the first combination immunotherapy to be licensed in the US and Europe and has been used in the treatment of melanoma for several years [120]. Clinical studies have shown that the combination of Ipilimumab with Nivolumab significantly improved overall survival rates to 57% compared to Nivolumab (43%) and Ipilimumab (25%) alone in melanoma patients after a 6.5-year follow-up to assess efficacy and safety [120]. Following its first approval for the treatment of advanced melanoma in 2017, the combination is now used for the treatment of advanced RCC, HCC microsatellite instability-high (MSI-H), or mismatch repair deficient (dMMR) metastatic colorectal carcinoma (CRC), NSCLC, and malignant pleural mesothelioma (MPM) as shown in **Table 1** [61, 63, 121, 122]. Combination therapy has significantly improved the clinical outcomes for most patients. Long-term follow-up (42 months) in RCC patients revealed an improved overall response rate of 42% (Nivolumab + Ipilimumab) versus 26% in patients treated with Sunitinib, a small molecule monotherapy [123]. Furthermore, durable long-term efficacy was observed, especially among patients with more than 1% PD-L1 expression [62].

More recently, the combination of Relatlimab and Nivolumab, known as Opdualag, was approved by the FDA for treating advanced or metastatic melanoma in patients aged 12 years and older. The approval was based on results from the RELATIVITY-047 clinical trials [98]. The combination treatment with Relatlimab +Nivolumab was at 47.7% compared to 36% in the Nivolumab monotherapy group after 12 months of follow-up. As described in the introduction, Relatlimab inhibits LAG-3 while Nivolumab inhibits PD-1, which are both often expressed by immune cells in the TME (**Figure 1E**). The expression of PD-1 and LAG-3 negatively regulates T cell tumor infiltration and proliferation, respectively. Combination immunotherapy has become an attractive avenue for the treatment of resistant cancers following the Ipilimumab + Nivolumab treatment of various cancers. Currently, several Phase III/IV clinical trials are ongoing to test the safety and efficacy of dual checkpoint inhibitor therapy combining two or more ICIs as listed in **Table 3**.

### 5.2 Combination of immune checkpoint inhibitors with conventional therapies (chemotherapy/radiotherapy and small molecules)

In some instances, chemotherapeutic agents have appeared to impact the immune system positively. The positive effects of standard chemotherapy on tumor immunity are mainly reflected in inducing immunogenic cell death and disrupting tumor escape strategies. Experimental data have shown that some anticancer chemotherapeutic agents can stimulate naïve immune cells to induce immunogenic cancer cell death [133]. For this reason, chemotherapy in combination with immune checkpoint inhibitors is an attractive strategy for synergistic combination treatment in cancer. Several studies using murine models have shown that chemotherapeutic agents such as cyclophosphamide, fluorouracil (5-FU), and Gemcitabine can reduce Tregs, improve circulating NK cells, and augment tumor-infiltrating T cells, respectively [134, 135]. Indeed, a combination of PD-L1 inhibitor (Nivolumab) plus Gemcitabine and Cisplatin significantly improved the ORR over monotherapy in a Japanese Phase I clinical trial [136]. Since then, several ICI and chemotherapy combination treatments have been investigated to improve patient response rate and survival.

To date, there are several ICI and chemotherapy/radiation combination therapies that have been approved by the FDA. Others are currently in Phase III/IV clinical trials as listed in **Table 3**. Pembrolizumab combined with standard chemotherapy has

| Protocol | Disease (refs) | ORR (95% CI) |
|---|---|---|
| Ipilimumab + Nivolumab | Unresectable stage III or IV melanoma [124] | No data available |
| | EDSCLC + after completion of platinum-based chemotherapy (CheckMate 451) [125, 126] | 9.1% (5.9–13.2) |
| | NSCLC combined with two cycles of chemotherapy [62] | 45.4% (38.4–52.4) |
| | Esophageal squamous cell carcinoma [31] | 42% (34–50) |
| Pembrolizumab + Ipilimumab | Metastatic NSCLC [127] | 45.4% (39.5–51.4) |
| Chemoradiotherapy + Temozolomide (chemo) + Nivolumab | Glioblastoma [128] | ORR not measured |
| Ipilimumab + Paclitaxel and Carboplatin | Squamous NSLC [129] | 44% (39–49) |
| Nivolumab + chemotherapy (capecitabine and oxaliplatin every 3 weeks or leucovorin, fluorouracil, and oxaliplatin every 2 weeks) | Advanced gastric, gastroesophageal junction, and esophageal adenocarcinoma [130] | 57.1% (34.0–78.2) |
| Ipilimumab + Etoposide and Platinum chemotherapy | Extensive-stage small cell lung cancer [131] | 62% (58–67) |
| Spartalizumab + Dabrafenib and Trametinib | BRAF V600-mutant unresectable or metastatic melanoma [132] | 69% (62.6–74.1) |

**Table 3.**
*Current combination therapies.*

become the first such combination therapy to be licensed for first-line use in patients with metastatic non-squamous NSCLC in the US and Europe after a trial showed that the combination enhanced overall survival at 12 months by 69.2% compared to 49.4% in the monotherapy group [137]. Since then, Pembrolizumab in combination with Axitinib, a vascular endothelial growth factor (VEGF) inhibitor has been further approved for the treatment of RCC. The ORR favored the Pembrolizumab/Axitinib group (59.3%) over the sunitinib group (35.7%). Atezolizumab and Durvalumab, both targeting the PD-L1, have been FDA-approved in combination with chemotherapy as a first-line treatment for advanced SCLC [138]. The approval was based on the IMpower133 and CASPIAN clinical trials which both evaluated Atezolizumab and Durvalumab, respectively, in combination with etoposide and carboplatin-based chemotherapy. Both studies revealed improved overall survival (OS) by Atezolizumab + chemotherapy (12.3 months); Durvalumab + chemotherapy (13 months) compared to chemotherapy alone (10 months) [54, 139].

## 6. Predictive biomarkers of therapy dynamics

### 6.1 Genomic biomarkers

#### *6.1.1 Tumor mutational burden*

Tumor mutational burden (TMB) refers to the frequency of non-synonymous mutations and is directly related to the neoantigen load. A high frequency of mutations generally results in a high rate of neoantigen production, thereby increasing the probability of an immune response [140]. Therefore, TMB has been investigated and validated as a predictive biomarker for ICI response by numerous studies.

The association between TMB and a response to ICI has been extensively studied in NSCLC patients, however, with variable outcomes. After whole-exome sequencing (WES), a high mutational burden (>178 mutations per sample) observed in NSCLC patients treated with Pembrolizumab correlated to better ORR (68%) compared to patients with a low mutational burden (0%). Therefore, low TMB was correlated with poor efficacy in patients and is considered a marker of primary resistance to ICI treatment [140]. Similarly, a study with 4064 NSCLC patients showed that a high TMB had a significantly higher OS compared to a low TMB [141]. Numerous other studies have also shown a similar association between TMB and ICI response [142–144]. In contrast to these observations, a study whereby NSCLC patients were treated with Pembrolizumab and chemotherapy showed that TMB with >175 mutations per exome was not able to predict a response [145]. It is important to note that some tumors with a low TMB are still capable of responding to ICI. This highlights that, although TMB is a good indicator of ICI response, it is not the only determinant factor. On a broader scale, the correlation between TMB and response to ICI has been demonstrated across 27 tumor types [146]. The KEYNOTE-158 study with 750 participants showed that TMB-high tumors were associated with better overall response rates (28%) and progression-free survival (24%) compared to TMB-low tumors (7% and 14%, respectively). Interestingly, 12.5% of the TMB-high cohort were also mismatch repair deficient and were even more likely to respond to ICIs [147]. These studies provided compelling evidence for the use of TMB as a biomarker to determine benefit from ICIs.

Despite the association between TMB and ICI response, there are challenges that complicate the use of TMB as a biomarker in the clinic. TMB is typically measured using whole-genome sequencing (WGS), whole-exome sequencing (WES), or targeted next-generation sequencing (NGS). WES has been the standard method of choice but is resource-intensive and time-consuming and is most often used in a research setting. Therefore, in a drive for a more feasible detection method, multiple NGS panel assays were developed which targets specific sites of the genome [148]. The current challenge is the standardization of the method in terms of the regions that are targeted and sequencing depth [149]. The definition of TMB and sampling methods also limit its use. Variations in cancer types means there is no standard cut point in the definition for a high TMB or low TMB, and each tumor type may have its own optimal threshold to predict a response [150]. In addition, the sampling methods are invasive, and single biopsies can often lead to misclassification of the TMB due to tumor and intratumor heterogeneity. A study showed that 20% of NSCLC and 52% of urothelial cancers were misrepresented as a high TMB. Further multi-sample analysis revealed a low TMB [151]. Lastly, it would be useful to test the effect of TMB on a protein level for neoantigens, since only a subset of mutated genes result in potent neoantigens that are able to elicit an immune response [152]. Although numerous studies have provided supportive evidence for TMB as a predictive biomarker for ICI response, assessment of combination or multiple biomarkers in conjunction with TMB may have a stronger predictive value.

#### *6.1.2 Mismatch repair deficiency and microsatellite instability*

Mismatch repair genes such MLH-1, MSH-2, MSH-6, and PMS-2 are responsible for DNA repair. Loss of function in these genes is referred to as mismatch repair deficiency (MMR-D). It leads to the accumulation of mutations during replication at a significantly higher rate than normal as well as the development of microsatellite instability (MSI) [153]. MMR-D/MSI is especially common in pancreatic, endometrial, cervical, prostate, and gastrointestinal cancers, including colorectal, gastric, and small intestinal cancer [154]. These tumors are particularly rich in frameshift mutations resulting in a high neoantigen load. Additionally, these tumors have also been found to contain a high level of infiltrating immune cells. These factors frequently enhance the immune response. Therefore, MMR-D can be used as a predictive biomarker for determining ICI response.

Clinical trials have shown that Pembrolizumab has durable outcomes in patients with MMR-D/MSI tumors. A study evaluating the efficacy of Pembrolizumab in colorectal cancer patients with and without MMR-D as well as MMR-D non-colorectal cancer patients showed promising results. For colorectal cancer with MMR-D, an overall response rate of 40% was observed whereas, for non-colorectal cancers with MMR-D, an overall response rate of 71% was observed. In contrast, patients without MMR-D exhibited an ORR of 0%. These results demonstrated that MMR-D patients produce a more favorable response to ICI treatment and are ideal candidates. This study led to the recommendation for MMR-D testing in metastatic colorectal cancer. In 2017, the FDA approved Pembrolizumab for patients with solid MMR-D/MSI tumors. This represents the first FDA approval for cancer treatment based on a genetic biomarker alone [155].

### *6.1.3 IFN pathway profiles*

Activated CD8+ T cells secrete IFN-γ following binding to the MHC–peptide complex. IFN-γ is a cytokine that activates immune cells and stimulates an immune response. In the tumor cell, JAK/STAT signaling is activated by IFN-γ which results in the release of chemokines to promote an anticancer response. Moreover, IFN-γ triggers the upregulation of MHC-1 and PD-L1 expression promoting antigen presentation in APCs. IFN-γ expression was found to predict a positive response to PD-1 immune checkpoint inhibitors in melanomas and NSCLC. Conversely, mutations in IFN pathway genes such as IFNGR1/IFNGR2, JAK1/JAK2, STAT, and IRF1 have been associated with poor outcomes and resistance in patients receiving ICI therapy [156, 157]. In melanomas and MMR-D colorectal cancers, the loss of function in JAK1 and JAK2 have also been identified as mechanisms of both primary and secondary resistance to ICIs [158, 159].

A study including NSCLC and melanoma patients treated with Nivolumab and Pembrolizumab, respectively, indicated that increased expression of IFN-γ correlated with improved OS and PFS [160]. Similarly, another study investigating a four-gene IFN-γ signature (IFN-γ, CD274, LAG3, and CXCL9) in NSCLC patients treated with Durvalumab revealed that a positive signature for the gene set was associated with higher ORRs, PFS, and OS in comparison with signature-low patients [161]. It has also become increasingly common to assess IFN-γ in combination with other biomarkers such as TMB. A study in melanoma patients assessed both inflammatory gene profiles and the TMB. Patients treated with Pembrolizumab exhibiting high levels of both biomarkers had an ORR of 54% compared to an ORR of 14% in patients with low expression levels [162]. Furthermore, in melanoma patients treated with neoadjuvant Ipilimumab and Nivolumab, tumors with high IFN gene signatures and TMB displayed a 100% response rate, while tumors with low expression profiles of both had a 37% response rate [163, 164]. Similar results have been observed for NSCLC and renal cell carcinoma [165]. These studies demonstrate the emerging role of inflammatory gene expression profiles as a predictive biomarker for ICI response. Challenges associated with the use of such gene panels arise from the replication of results due to intratumor heterogeneity and sampling methods, once again highlighting the limitations of single region sampling.

## 6.2 Tumor-immune microenvironment biomarkers

### *6.2.1 PD-L1*

ICIs that target PD-1 or PD-L1 aim to disrupt the PD-1/PD-L1 axis, allowing cells to mount an antitumor response by preventing T cell downregulation [166]. Consequently, PD-L1 expression is one of the most extensively studied predictive biomarkers for response to ICI therapy. In the KEYNOTE-001 study, patients with PD-L1 expression of more than 50% had an ORR of 45% and improved PFS and OS. In comparison, patients who displayed 1–49% PD-L1 expression had an ORR of only 17% [167]. This study ultimately led to the approval of Pembrolizumab in NSCLC patients who display more than 50% PD-L1 and established the expression of PD-L1 as a companion predictive biomarker for patient selection. Positive correlations have also been seen for gastric cancer, colorectal cancer, and hepatocellular carcinoma [17, 168, 169]. Subsequent trials for PD-L1 as a predictive biomarker led to approvals by the FDA for urothelial, triple-negative breast cancer (TNBC), head and neck, gastric, esophageal cancers, and cervical cancer at various cut points.

PD-L1 expression has significant spatial and temporal heterogeneity. Expression varies between sites of the same tumor and between metastatic sites. Given this, the use of PD-L1 as a predictive biomarker has limitations. Detection is usually carried out using immunohistochemistry, but it is not adequately standardized. Even in the same cancer type, there are variations in thresholds. There are five main PD-L1 diagnostic antibodies that are available for detection. These antibodies have only been validated in the context of its companion drug trial: Pembrolizumab (Dako 22c3), Nivolumab (Dako 28–8), Durvalumab (Ventana SP263), Avelumab (Dako 73–10), and Atezolizumab (Ventana SP142). Variations in detection between assays have been noted. Dako 73–10 scores more cells as positive and Ventana SP142 scores more as negative leading to misinterpretations [170]. Detection of PD-L1 is frequently observed in patients who respond to anti-PD-1/ PD-L1 immunotherapies. However, [43] reported that even when NSCLC tumors displayed more than 50% PD-L1 staining, approximately half of the subset of patients still had primary resistance to Pembrolizumab. This study suggested that PD-L1 expression alone may be insufficient at predicting resistance. As with TMB, it is critical to note that PD-L1 does not preclude response to treatment. In the study mentioned earlier, although PD-L1-positive patients had a higher response rate, 15% of PD-L1-negative patients still responded [171].

### *6.2.2 Tumor infiltrating lymphocytes*

Tumor-infiltrating lymphocytes (TILs) encompass lymphatic cell populations that invade the tumor tissue. TILs may promote an antitumor response (CD4+), exert cytotoxic antitumor activity (CD8+), or even limit a response (FOXP3+ Treg). These cells have therefore been associated with prognosis and response to ICI in many cancer types, including NSCLC, TNBC, colorectal cancer, and melanoma. The density, location as well as phenotype of TILs give an indication of the response. In melanoma patients treated with Pembrolizumab, the spatiotemporal dynamics of TILs showed that the presence of CD4+ and CD8+ T cells at the infiltrative margin of the tumor was associated with patients who respond to treatment. The high density of cells allowed for increased infiltration into the tumor parenchyma of responders [172]. Another study revealed that responders had high levels of stromal TILs (50%) in comparison with non-responders (15%) for TNBC patients treated with Pembrolizumab [173]. An investigation into the temporal dynamics of TILs showed that an increase in TILs at 3 weeks, compared to the baseline reading, was correlated with response in melanoma patients treated with Ipilimumab [174]. Furthermore, the phenotype of TILs may also be used as a prognostic biomarker. A study showed that CD69+ CD103+ tumor resident CD8+ T cells were associated with improved survival in melanoma [175]. In contrast, FOXP3 tregs have been associated with poor survival in numerous cancer types [176]. The prognostic value of TILs has also been demonstrated by combining detection with PD-L1 expression to allow for better accuracy in determining response. Patients who exhibited high CD8+ TILs and low PD-L1 had an OS of approximately 93% in comparison with patients with low CD8+ TILs and high PD-L1 (61%). The authors suggested that CD8+ TIL combined with PD-L1 expression was better at predicting response than each biomarker alone [177].

### 6.3 Blood-based biomarkers

#### *6.3.1 Circulating tumor DNA and tumor cells*

The noninvasive nature of blood biopsies reduces patient suffering and provides certain advantages such as overcoming the heterogeneity issues of single sample tissue biopsies. It also allows multiple sampling throughout the disease progression and acquisition of real-time data. Therefore, there it is imperative to develop reliable blood-based biomarkers [178]. Emerging studies have linked circulating DNA (ctDNA) and circulating tumor cells (CTCs) found in the peripheral blood with response to ICI. In a study with melanoma patients, detectable baseline ctDNA that persist during treatment correlated with a poor response of only 6%. However, when ctDNA was initially detectable and became undetectable at 12 weeks, the response rate was 77% and when ctDNA was undetectable at both the baseline and 12 weeks, the response rate was 72% [179]. Thus, ctDNA may serve as a biomarker of response. Studies went further to assess TMB from the ctDNA. In NSCLC, it was shown that blood TMB correlated with tissue TMB and was associated with ICI response [180]. CTCs have also been suggested as prognostic biomarkers. In NSCLC patients, blood sampled before and after treatment with Nivolumab showed that high levels of CTCs before treatment was associated with an increased risk of disease progression and death [181].

#### *6.3.2 Soluble biomarkers*

Some indicators such as neutrophil-to-lymphocyte ratio (NLR), lactate dehydrogenase (LDH), and various cytokines (IL-6 and IL-8) have been studied as biomarkers of response to ICI in a variety of tumors [182]. Neutrophils that express PD-L1 attenuate the antitumor response by binding to PD-1 T cells. Therefore, NLR has been suggested to have a predictive role for response to ICIs in melanoma and NSCLC. A study of melanoma patients treated with Ipilimumab demonstrated that patients with an NLR > 3 had a poor OS and PFS [183]. Similar results were shown in another study where an NLR >5 was also associated with a lower OS and PFS [184]. In advanced solid tumors, the OS of high NLR patients was 8.5 months, while the OS of patients with a low NLR was 19.4 months [185]. Changes in LDH during ICI treatment correlates with patient response. A study showed that patients who displayed an elevated baseline serum LDH value had a shorter OS at 12 months (44%) compared to patients with normal LDH values (71%). Moreover, a 10% increase from the baseline level during ICI treatment also indicated poor ICI efficacy [186]. Lower levels of the cytokine IL-6 at the baseline and on treatment have been correlated with improved response, while higher levels of IL-6 correlate with a shorter OS [187]. Additionally, in NSCLC and melanoma, it was reported that lower levels of IL-8 were associated with improved treatment responses, while higher baseline IL-8 levels were associated with poorer OS [188].

### 6.4 Biomarkers associated with the gut

Studies have suggested the association of the bacterial species in the gut with ICI responses. Bacterial species such as *Akkermansia muciniphila* have been observed and correlated with ICI response, whereas species such as *Ruminococcus obeum* have been correlated with resistance [189, 190]. The use of antibiotics prior to ICI treatment was also associated with a shorter overall survival and progression-free survival. As such, it has been suggested that careful consideration should be given when prescribing antibiotics in patients starting ICI treatment [190]. This is still an emerging field of study and further evidence is needed (**Table 4**).

| Biomarker (Ref) | Method of detection | Indication |
|---|---|---|
| **Biomarkers associated with the tumor genome** | | |
| TMB [146, 147] | WES and NGS gene panels on tissue and blood samples | High mutational burden correlates with high response rates and improved OS and PFS.<br>Low TMB associated with primary resistance. |
| MMR-D and MSI [155] | WES on tissue samples | Somatic MMR-D and MSI correlates with high response rates. FDA approved genetic biomarker for patient selection. |
| IFN pathway profiles [160, 161] | Gene panels and transcriptome on tumor sample | Increased expression of IFN-γ correlated with improved OS and PFS.<br>Mutations in the IFN pathway associated with poor outcomes and resistance. |
| **Biomarkers associated with the tumor immune microenvironment** | | |
| PD-L1 [167] | IHC staining of tumor cells and immune cells | High PD-L1 density (> 50% expression) predicts improved response rates, OS, and PFS. FDA approved biomarker for patient selection. |
| TILs [172] | Anti-CD4 and anti-CD8 IHC staining on tissue samples | High CD4 and CD8 density or increase in density correlates with higher response rates.<br>FOXP3 Tregs associated with poor survival. |

| Biomarker (Ref) | Method of detection | Indication |
|---|---|---|
| **Biomarkers associated with the peripheral blood** | | |
| ctDNA and CTCs [179, 181] | FACS on blood sample | Detectable and persistent ctDNA correlates with poor response.<br>High CTCs prior to treatment associated with disease progression and death. |
| Soluble biomarkers [183, 186] | IHC, FACS, and enzymatic assays | High NLR associated with poor response, OS, and PFS.<br>Increase in LDH correlates with poor response. |
| **Biomarkers associated with the gut** | | |
| Microbiota [189, 190] | Shotgun metagenomic analysis of feces | Distinct species profiles correlate with responses.<br>*Ruminococcus* correlated with resistance. |

**Table 4.**
*Biomarkers associated with the tumor genome, tumor-immune microenvironment, peripheral blood, and gut that predict response to ICI.*

## 7. Conclusions

The heterogeneity of tumors has introduced a profound complexity in our understanding of carcinogenesis and the numerous challenges in developing strategies for the treatment of cancer. The recent developments in immunotherapy enable us to devise interventions that promise to improve cancer therapy. Immune checkpoint inhibitors (ICIs) are recently developed drugs that promise to increase overall response. Our evaluation of ICIs shows that the PD-1-PD-L1/L2 pathway is the most targeted pathway. With PD-1 inhibitors in particular having been FDA-approved for the largest variety of cancers. PD-1 inhibitors have been found to have a good response in monotherapy but have recently been frequently tested as part of combinational therapy with other ICIs, such as CTLA-4 and LAG-3. This dual targeting of immune checkpoint proteins has resulted in some of the most promising outcomes. Despite these successes, there are challenges of serious adverse events and the development of resistance. The serious adverse events must be addressed because they are of Grade 3–4. Attempts to overcome them are in progress. Resistance occurs in a significant percentage of patients and therefore urgently needs to be addressed. The two main strategies targeting resistance are the use of combinational therapies and biomarker identification.

## Acknowledgements

BR is funded by Buboo (Pty) Ltd., The Innovation Hub, Hatfield, Gauteng, Pretoria, 0200, South Africa.

STM is funded by the National Research Foundation of South Africa (GUN 121878) and the University of South Africa.

## Conflict of interest

The authors declare no conflict of interest.

## Author details

Bonnie L. Russell[1,2†], Sibusiso T. Malindisa[1†], Selisha A. Sooklal[1†] and Monde Ntwasa[1*]

1 Department of Life and Consumer Sciences, University of South Africa, Johannesburg, South Africa

2 Buboo (Pty) Ltd., The Innovation Hub, Gauteng, Pretoria, South Africa

*Address all correspondence to: ntwasmm@unisa.ac.za

† These authors contributed equally.

## References

[1] Sadeghi Rad H, Monkman J, Warkiani ME, Ladwa R, O'Byrne K, Rezaei N, et al. Understanding the tumor microenvironment for effective immunotherapy. Medicinal Research Reviews. 2021;**41**(3):1474-1498

[2] Barbari C, Fontaine T, Parajuli P, Lamichhane N, Jakubski S, Lamichhane P, et al. Immunotherapies and combination strategies for Immuno-oncology. International Journal of Molecular Sciences. 2020;**21**(14):1-28

[3] Paucek RD, Baltimore D, Li G. The cellular immunotherapy revolution: Arming the immune system for precision therapy. Trends in Immunology. 2019; **40**(4):292-309

[4] Russell BL, Sooklal SA, Malindisa ST, Daka LJ, Ntwasa M. The tumor microenvironment factors that promote resistance to immune checkpoint blockade therapy. Frontiers in Oncology. 2021;**11**:641428

[5] Hodi FS, O'Day SJ, McDermott DF, Weber RW, Sosman JA, Haanen JB, et al. Improved survival with ipilimumab in patients with metastatic melanoma. The New England Journal of Medicine. 2010; **363**(8):711-723

[6] Overman MJ, McDermott R, Leach JL, Lonardi S, Lenz HJ, Morse MA, et al. Nivolumab in patients with metastatic DNA mismatch repair-deficient or microsatellite instability-high colorectal cancer (CheckMate 142): An open-label, multicentre, phase 2 study. The Lancet Oncology. 2017;**18**(9): 1182-1191

[7] Hammers HJ, Plimack ER, Infante JR, Rini BI, McDermott DF, Lewis LD, et al. Safety and efficacy of nivolumab in combination with ipilimumab in metastatic renal cell carcinoma: The CheckMate 016 study. Journal of Clinical Oncology. 2017;**35**(34):3851-3858

[8] Saung MT, Pelosof L, Casak S, Donoghue M, Lemery S, Yuan M, et al. FDA approval summary: Nivolumab plus ipilimumab for the treatment of patients with hepatocellular carcinoma previously treated with sorafenib. The Oncologist. 2021;**26**(9):797-806

[9] Marcus L, Lemery SJ, Keegan P, Pazdur R. FDA approval summary: Pembrolizumab for the treatment of microsatellite instability-high solid tumors. Clinical Cancer Research. 2019; **25**(13):3753-3758

[10] Fuchs CS, Doi T, Jang RW, Muro K, Satoh T, Machado M, et al. Safety and efficacy of pembrolizumab monotherapy in patients with previously treated advanced gastric and gastroesophageal junction cancer: Phase 2 clinical KEYNOTE-059 trial. JAMA Oncology. 2018;**4**(5):e180013

[11] Chung HC, Ros W, Delord JP, Perets R, Italiano A, Shapira-Frommer R, et al. Efficacy and safety of pembrolizumab in previously treated advanced cervical cancer: Results from the phase II KEYNOTE-158 study. Journal of Clinical Oncology. 2019; **37**(17):1470-1478

[12] Armand P, Rodig S, Melnichenko V, Thieblemont C, Bouabdallah K, Tumyan G, et al. Pembrolizumab in relapsed or refractory primary mediastinal large B-cell lymphoma. Journal of Clinical Oncology. 2019; **37**(34):3291-3299

[13] Paz-Ares L, Luft A, Vicente D, Tafreshi A, Gümüş M, Mazières J, et al. Pembrolizumab plus chemotherapy for

squamous non-small-cell lung cancer. The New England Journal of Medicine. 2018;**379**(21):2040-2051

[14] Zhu AX, Finn RS, Edeline J, Cattan S, Ogasawara S, Palmer D, et al. Pembrolizumab in patients with advanced hepatocellular carcinoma previously treated with sorafenib (KEYNOTE-224): A non-randomised, open-label phase 2 trial. The Lancet Oncology. 2018;**19**(7):940-952

[15] Nghiem P, Bhatia S, Lipson EJ, Sharfman WH, Kudchadkar RR, Brohl AS, et al. Three-year survival, correlates and salvage therapies in patients receiving first-line pembrolizumab for advanced Merkel cell carcinoma. Journal for Immunotherapy of Cancer. 2021;**9**(4):e002478. Available from: https://jitc.bmj.com/content/jitc/9/4/e002478.full.pdf

[16] Rini BI, Plimack ER, Stus V, Gafanov R, Hawkins R, Nosov D, et al. Pembrolizumab plus Axitinib versus sunitinib for advanced renal-cell carcinoma. The New England Journal of Medicine. 2019;**380**(12):1116-1127

[17] Kojima T, Muro K, Francois E, Hsu CH, Moriwaki T, Kim SB, et al. Pembrolizumab versus chemotherapy as second-line therapy for advanced esophageal cancer: Phase III KEYNOTE-181 study. Journal of Clinical Oncology. 2019;**37**(4_suppl):2. Available from: h ttps://ascopubs.org/doi/abs/10.1200/JCO.2019.37.4_suppl.2

[18] Makker V, Taylor MH, Aghajanian C, Oaknin A, Mier J, Cohn AL, et al. Lenvatinib plus pembrolizumab in patients with advanced endometrial cancer. Journal of Clinical Oncology. 2020;**38**(26):2981-2992

[19] Balar AV, Kamat AM, Kulkarni GS, Uchio EM, Boormans JL, Roumiguié M, et al. Pembrolizumab monotherapy for the treatment of high-risk non-muscle-invasive bladder cancer unresponsive to BCG (KEYNOTE-057): An open-label, single-arm, multicentre, phase 2 study. The Lancet Oncology. 2021;**22**(7): 919-930

[20] Casak SJ, Marcus L, Fashoyin-Aje L, Mushti SL, Cheng J, Shen YL, et al. FDA approval summary: Pembrolizumab for the first-line treatment of patients with MSI-H/dMMR advanced unresectable or metastatic colorectal carcinoma. Clinical Cancer Research. 2021;**27**(17): 4680-4684

[21] Hughes BGM, Munoz-Couselo E, Mortier L, Bratland Å, Gutzmer R, Roshdy O, et al. Pembrolizumab for locally advanced and recurrent/metastatic cutaneous squamous cell carcinoma (KEYNOTE-629 study): An open-label, nonrandomized, multicenter, phase II trial. Annals of Oncology. 2021;**32**(10):1276-1285

[22] Weber JS, D'Angelo SP, Minor D, Hodi FS, Gutzmer R, Neyns B, et al. Nivolumab versus chemotherapy in patients with advanced melanoma who progressed after anti-CTLA-4 treatment (CheckMate 037): A randomised, controlled, open-label, phase 3 trial. The Lancet Oncology. 2015; **16**(4):375-384

[23] Brahmer J, Reckamp KL, Baas P, Crinò L, Eberhardt WE, Poddubskaya E, et al. Nivolumab versus docetaxel in advanced squamous-cell non-small-cell lung cancer. The New England Journal of Medicine. 2015;**373**(2):123-135

[24] Motzer RJ, Escudier B, McDermott DF, George S, Hammers HJ, Srinivas S, et al. Nivolumab versus Everolimus in advanced renal-cell carcinoma. The New England Journal of Medicine. 2015;**373**(19):1803-1813

[25] Kasamon YL, de Claro RA, Wang Y, Shen YL, Farrell AT, Pazdur R. FDA approval summary: Nivolumab for the treatment of relapsed or progressive classical Hodgkin lymphoma. The Oncologist. 2017;**22**(5):585-591

[26] Ferris RL, Blumenschein G Jr, Fayette J, Guigay J, Colevas AD, Licitra L, et al. Nivolumab for recurrent squamous-cell carcinoma of the head and neck. The New England Journal of Medicine. 2016;**375**(19):1856-1867

[27] Sharma P, Retz M, Siefker-Radtke A, Baron A, Necchi A, Bedke J, et al. Nivolumab in metastatic urothelial carcinoma after platinum therapy (CheckMate 275): A multicentre, single-arm, phase 2 trial. The Lancet Oncology. 2017;**18**(3):312-322

[28] El-Khoueiry AB, Sangro B, Yau T, Crocenzi TS, Kudo M, Hsu C, et al. Nivolumab in patients with advanced hepatocellular carcinoma (CheckMate 040): An open-label, non-comparative, phase 1/2 dose escalation and expansion trial. Lancet. 2017;**389**(10088):2492-2502

[29] Janjigian YY, Bendell J, Calvo E, Kim JW, Ascierto PA, Sharma P, et al. CheckMate-032 study: Efficacy and safety of nivolumab and nivolumab plus ipilimumab in patients with metastatic esophagogastric cancer. Journal of Clinical Oncology. 2018;**36**(28):2836-2844

[30] Nowak AK, Lesterhuis WJ, Kok PS, Brown C, Hughes BG, Karikios DJ, et al. Durvalumab with first-line chemotherapy in previously untreated malignant pleural mesothelioma (DREAM): A multicentre, single-arm, phase 2 trial with a safety run-in. The Lancet Oncology. 2020;**21**(9):1213-1223

[31] Doki Y, Ajani JA, Kato K, Xu J, Wyrwicz L, Motoyama S, et al. Nivolumab combination therapy in advanced esophageal squamous-cell carcinoma. The New England Journal of Medicine. 2022;**386**(5):449-462

[32] Migden MR, Rischin D, Schmults CD, Guminski A, Hauschild A, Lewis KD, et al. PD-1 blockade with Cemiplimab in advanced cutaneous squamous-cell carcinoma. The New England Journal of Medicine. 2018; **379**(4):341-351

[33] Stratigos AJ, Sekulic A, Peris K, Bechter O, Prey S, Kaatz M, et al. Cemiplimab in locally advanced basal cell carcinoma after hedgehog inhibitor therapy: An open-label, multi-centre, single-arm, phase 2 trial. The Lancet Oncology. 2021;**22**(6):848-857

[34] Sezer A, Kilickap S, Gümüş M, Bondarenko I, Özgüroğlu M, Gogishvili M, et al. Cemiplimab monotherapy for first-line treatment of advanced non-small-cell lung cancer with PD-L1 of at least 50%: A multicentre, open-label, global, phase 3, randomised, controlled trial. Lancet. 2021;**397**(10274):592-604

[35] Berton D, Banerjee SN, Curigliano G, Cresta S, Arkenau HT, Abdeddaim C, et al. Antitumor activity of dostarlimab in patients with mismatch repair-deficient/microsatellite instability–high tumors: A combined analysis of two cohorts in the GARNET study. Journal of Clinical Oncology. 2021;**39**(15_suppl):2564. Available from: https://ascopubs.org/doi/abs/10.1200/JCO.2021.39.15_suppl.2564

[36] Rosenberg JE, Hoffman-Censits J, Powles T, van der Heijden MS, Balar AV, Necchi A, et al. Atezolizumab in patients with locally advanced and metastatic urothelial carcinoma who have progressed following treatment with platinum-based chemotherapy: A single-arm, multicentre, phase 2 trial. Lancet. 2016;**387**(10031):1909-1920

[37] Fehrenbacher L, Spira A, Ballinger M, Kowanetz M, Vansteenkiste J, Mazieres J, et al. Atezolizumab versus docetaxel for patients with previously treated non-small-cell lung cancer (POPLAR): A multicentre, open-label, phase 2 randomised controlled trial. Lancet. 2016;**387**(10030):1837-1846

[38] Liu SV, Reck M, Mansfield AS, Mok T, Scherpereel A, Reinmuth N, et al. Updated overall survival and PD-L1 subgroup analysis of patients with extensive-stage small-cell lung cancer treated with atezolizumab, carboplatin, and etoposide (IMpower133). Journal of Clinical Oncology. 2021;**39**(6):619-630

[39] Hellmann MD, Paz-Ares L, Bernabe Caro R, Zurawski B, Kim SW, Carcereny Costa E, et al. Nivolumab plus ipilimumab in advanced non-small-cell lung Cancer. The New England Journal of Medicine. 2019;**381**(21):2020-2031

[40] Baas P, Scherpereel A, Nowak AK, Fujimoto N, Peters S, Tsao AS, et al. First-line nivolumab plus ipilimumab in unresectable malignant pleural mesothelioma (CheckMate 743): A multicentre, randomised, open-label, phase 3 trial. Lancet. 2021;**397**(10272): 375-386

[41] Robert C, Ribas A, Wolchok JD, Hodi FS, Hamid O, Kefford R, et al. Anti-programmed-death-receptor-1 treatment with pembrolizumab in ipilimumab-refractory advanced melanoma: A randomised dose-comparison cohort of a phase 1 trial. The Lancet. 2014;**384**(9948):1109-1117. DOI: 10.1016/S0140-6736(14)60958-2

[42] Chuk MK, Chang JT, Theoret MR, Sampene E, He K, Weis SL, et al. FDA approval summary: Accelerated approval of pembrolizumab for second-line treatment of metastatic melanoma. Clinical Cancer Research. 2017;**23**(19): 5666-5670. DOI: 10.1158/1078-0432. CCR-16-0663

[43] Reck M, Rodríguez-Abreu D, Robinson AG, Hui R, Csőszi T, Fülöp A, et al. Pembrolizumab versus chemotherapy for PD-L1-positive non-small-cell lung cancer. The New England Journal of Medicine. 2016;**375**(19):1823-1833

[44] Larkins E, Blumenthal GM, Yuan W, He K, Sridhara R, Subramaniam S, et al. FDA approval summary: Pembrolizumab for the treatment of recurrent or metastatic head and neck squamous cell carcinoma with disease progression on or after platinum-containing chemotherapy. The Oncologist. 2017;**22**(7):873-878

[45] Chen R, Zinzani PL, Fanale MA, Armand P, Johnson NA, Brice P, et al. Phase II study of the efficacy and safety of pembrolizumab for relapsed/refractory classic Hodgkin lymphoma. Journal of Clinical Oncology. 2017;**35**(19):2125-2132

[46] Balar AV, Castellano D, O'Donnell PH, Grivas P, Vuky J, Powles T, et al. First-line pembrolizumab in cisplatin-ineligible patients with locally advanced and unresectable or metastatic urothelial cancer (KEYNOTE-052): A multicentre, single-arm, phase 2 study. The Lancet Oncology. 2017;**18**(11):1483-1492

[47] Gadgeel S, Rodríguez-Abreu D, Speranza G, Esteban E, Felip E, Dómine M, et al. Updated analysis from KEYNOTE-189: Pembrolizumab or placebo plus pemetrexed and platinum for previously untreated metastatic nonsquamous non-small-cell lung cancer. Journal of Clinical Oncology. 2020;**38**(14):1505-1517

[48] Gutzmer R, Stroyakovskiy D, Gogas H, Robert C, Lewis K, Protsenko S, et al. Atezolizumab,

vemurafenib, and cobimetinib as first-line treatment for unresectable advanced BRAF(V600) mutation-positive melanoma (IMspire150): Primary analysis of the randomised, double-blind, placebo-controlled, phase 3 trial. Lancet. 2020;**395**(10240):1835-1844

[49] Kaufman HL, Russell J, Hamid O, Bhatia S, Terheyden P, D'Angelo SP, et al. Avelumab in patients with chemotherapy-refractory metastatic Merkel cell carcinoma: A multicentre, single-group, open-label, phase 2 trial. The Lancet Oncology. 2016;**17**(10):1374-1385

[50] Apolo AB, Infante JR, Balmanoukian A, Patel MR, Wang D, Kelly K, et al. Avelumab, an anti-programmed death-ligand 1 antibody, In patients with refractory metastatic urothelial carcinoma: Results from a multicenter, Phase Ib Study. Journal of Clinical Oncology. 2017;**35**(19):2117-2124

[51] Motzer RJ, Penkov K, Haanen J, Rini B, Albiges L, Campbell MT, et al. Avelumab plus Axitinib versus sunitinib for advanced renal-cell carcinoma. The New England Journal of Medicine. 2019; **380**(12):1103-1115

[52] Powles T, O'Donnell PH, Massard C, Arkenau HT, Friedlander TW, Hoimes CJ, et al. Efficacy and safety of durvalumab in locally advanced or metastatic urothelial carcinoma: Updated results from a phase 1/2 open-label study. JAMA Oncology. 2017;**3**(9):e172411

[53] Antonia SJ, Villegas A, Daniel D, Vicente D, Murakami S, Hui R, et al. Durvalumab after chemoradiotherapy in stage III non-small-cell lung cancer. The New England Journal of Medicine. 2017; **377**(20):1919-1929

[54] Paz-Ares L, Dvorkin M, Chen Y, Reinmuth N, Hotta K, Trukhin D, et al. Durvalumab plus platinum-etoposide versus platinum-etoposide in first-line treatment of extensive-stage small-cell lung cancer (CASPIAN): A randomised, controlled, open-label, phase 3 trial. Lancet. 2019;**394**(10212): 1929-1939

[55] Al-Salama ZT. Durvalumab: A review in extensive-stage SCLC. Targeted Oncology. 2021;**16**(6):857-864

[56] FDA approves anti-LAG3 checkpoint. Nature Biotechnology. 2022; **40**(5):625. DOI: 10.1038/s41587-022-01331-0

[57] Zhao Y, Yang W, Huang Y, Cui R, Li X, Li B. Evolving roles for targeting CTLA-4 in cancer immunotherapy. Cellular Physiology and Biochemistry. 2018;**47**(2):721-734

[58] Yokosuka T, Kobayashi W, Takamatsu M, Sakata-Sogawa K, Zeng H, Hashimoto-Tane A, et al. Spatiotemporal basis of CTLA-4 costimulatory molecule-mediated negative regulation of T cell activation. Immunity. 2010;**33**(3):326-339

[59] Ramagopal UA, Liu W, Garrett-Thomson SC, Bonanno JB, Yan Q, Srinivasan M, et al. Structural basis for cancer immunotherapy by the first-in-class checkpoint inhibitor ipilimumab. Proceedings of the National Academy of Sciences of the United States of America. 2017;**114**(21):E4223-e4232

[60] Zimmer L, Eigentler TK, Kiecker F, Simon J, Utikal J, Mohr P, et al. Open-label, multicenter, single-arm phase II DeCOG-study of ipilimumab in pretreated patients with different subtypes of metastatic melanoma. Journal of Translational Medicine. 2015; **13**:351

[61] Motzer RJ, Tannir NM, McDermott DF, Arén Frontera O,

Melichar B, Choueiri TK, et al. Nivolumab plus ipilimumab versus sunitinib in advanced renal-cell carcinoma. The New England Journal of Medicine. 2018;**378**(14):1277-1290

[62] Paz-Ares L, Ciuleanu TE, Cobo M, Schenker M, Zurawski B, Menezes J, et al. First-line nivolumab plus ipilimumab combined with two cycles of chemotherapy in patients with non-small-cell lung cancer (CheckMate 9LA): An international, randomised, open-label, phase 3 trial. The Lancet Oncology. 2021;**22**(2):198-211

[63] Yau T, Kang YK, Kim TY, El-Khoueiry AB, Santoro A, Sangro B, et al. Efficacy and safety of nivolumab plus ipilimumab in patients with advanced hepatocellular carcinoma previously treated with sorafenib: The CheckMate 040 randomized clinical trial. JAMA Oncology. 2020;**6**(11): e204564

[64] Abou-Alfa GK, Chan SL, Kudo M, Lau G, Kelley RK, Furuse J, et al. Phase 3 randomized, open-label, multicenter study of tremelimumab (T) and durvalumab (D) as first-line therapy in patients (pts) with unresectable hepatocellular carcinoma (uHCC): HIMALAYA. Journal of Clinical Oncology. 2022;**40**(4_suppl):379-379. DOI: 101200/JCO2022404_suppl379

[65] Sun C, Mezzadra R, Schumacher TN. Regulation and function of the PD-L1 checkpoint. Immunity. 2018;**48**(3): 434-452

[66] Freeman GJ, Long AJ, Iwai Y, Bourque K, Chernova T, Nishimura H, et al. Engagement of the PD-1 immunoinhibitory receptor by a novel B7 family member leads to negative regulation of lymphocyte activation. The Journal of Experimental Medicine. 2000; **192**(7):1027-1034

[67] Davis AA, Patel VG. The role of PD-L1 expression as a predictive biomarker: An analysis of all US Food and Drug Administration (FDA) approvals of immune checkpoint inhibitors. Journal for Immunotherapy of Cancer. 2019; **7**(1):278

[68] Amarnath S, Mangus CW, Wang JC, Wei F, He A, Kapoor V, et al. The PDL1-PD1 axis converts human TH1 cells into regulatory T cells. Science Translational Medicine. 2011;**3**(111):111ra120

[69] Kwok G, Yau TC, Chiu JW, Tse E, Kwong YL. Pembrolizumab (Keytruda). Human Vaccines & Immunotherapeutics. 2016;**12**(11): 2777-2789

[70] du Rusquec P, de Calbiac O, Robert M, Campone M, Frenel JS. Clinical utility of pembrolizumab in the management of advanced solid tumors: An evidence-based review on the emerging new data. Cancer Management and Research. 2019;**11**: 4297-4312

[71] Agata Y, Kawasaki A, Nishimura H, Ishida Y, Tsubata T, Yagita H, et al. Expression of the PD-1 antigen on the surface of stimulated mouse T and B lymphocytes. International Immunology. 1996;**8**(5):765-772

[72] Ni D, AlZahrani F, Smylie M. AIHA and pancytopenia as complications of pembrolizumab therapy for metastatic melanoma: A case report. Case Reports in Oncology. 2019;**12**(2):456-465

[73] Wang C, Thudium KB, Han M, Wang XT, Huang H, Feingersh D, et al. In vitro characterization of the anti-PD-1 antibody nivolumab, BMS-936558, and in vivo toxicology in non-human primates. Cancer Immunology Research. 2014;**2**(9):846-856

[74] Robert C, Long G, Brady B, Dutriaux C, Maio M, Mortier L, et al. Nivolumab in previously untreated melanoma without BRAF mutation. The New England Journal of Medicine. 2015; **372**(4):320-330

[75] Gettinger SN, Horn L, Gandhi L, Spigel DR, Antonia SJ, Rizvi NA, et al. Overall survival and Long-term safety of nivolumab (anti-programmed death 1 antibody, BMS-936558, ONO-4538) in patients with previously treated advanced non-small-cell lung cancer. Journal of Clinical Oncology. 2015;**33**(18):2004-2012

[76] Hellmann MD, Rizvi NA, Goldman JW, Gettinger SN, Borghaei H, Brahmer JR, et al. Nivolumab plus ipilimumab as first-line treatment for advanced non-small-cell lung cancer (CheckMate 012): Results of an open-label, phase 1, multicohort study. The Lancet Oncology. 2017;**18**(1):31-41

[77] Iwai Y, Hamanishi J, Chamoto K, Honjo T. Cancer immunotherapies targeting the PD-1 signaling pathway. Journal of Biomedical Science. 2017; **24**(1):26

[78] Markham A, Duggan S. Cemiplimab: First global approval. Drugs. 2018; **78**(17):1841-1846

[79] Ahmed SR, Petersen E, Patel R, Migden MR. Cemiplimab-rwlc as first and only treatment for advanced cutaneous squamous cell carcinoma. Expert Review of Clinical Pharmacology. 2019;**12**(10):947-951

[80] Kaplon H, Reichert JM. Antibodies to watch in 2018. MAbs. 2018;**10**(2): 183-203

[81] Patnaik A, Weiss GJ, Rasco DW, Blaydorn L, Mirabella A, Beeram M, et al. Safety, antitumor activity, and pharmacokinetics of dostarlimab, an anti-PD-1, in patients with advanced solid tumors: A dose-escalation phase 1 trial. Cancer Chemotherapy and Pharmacology. 2022;**89**(1):93-103

[82] Cercek A, Lumish M, Sinopoli J, Weiss J, Shia J, Lamendola-Essel M, et al. PD-1 blockade in mismatch repair-deficient, locally advanced rectal cancer. The New England Journal of Medicine. 2022;**386**(25):2363-2376

[83] Akinleye A, Rasool Z. Immune checkpoint inhibitors of PD-L1 as cancer therapeutics. Journal of Hematology & Oncology. 2019;**12**(1):92. DOI: 10.1186/s13045-019-0779-5

[84] Keir ME, Butte MJ, Freeman GJ, Sharpe AH. PD-1 and its ligands in tolerance and immunity. Annual Review of Immunology. 2008;**26**:677-704

[85] Vafaei S, Zekiy AO, Khanamir RA, Zaman BA, Ghayourvahdat A, Azimizonuzi H, et al. Combination therapy with immune checkpoint inhibitors (ICIs); a new frontier. Cancer Cell International. 2022;**22**(1):2

[86] Socinski MA, Jotte RM, Cappuzzo F, Orlandi F, Stroyakovskiy D, Nogami N, et al. Atezolizumab for first-line treatment of metastatic nonsquamous NSCLC. The New England Journal of Medicine. 2018;**378**(24):2288-2301

[87] Horn L, Mansfield AS, Szczęsna A, Havel L, Krzakowski M, Hochmair MJ, et al. First-line atezolizumab plus chemotherapy in extensive-stage small-cell lung cancer. The New England Journal of Medicine. 2018;**379**(23): 2220-2229

[88] Rittmeyer A, Barlesi F, Waterkamp D, Park K, Ciardiello F, von Pawel J, et al. Atezolizumab versus docetaxel in patients with previously treated non-small-cell lung cancer

(OAK): A phase 3, open-label, multicentre randomised controlled trial. Lancet. 2017;**389**(10066):255-265

[89] Syed YY. Durvalumab: First global approval. Drugs. 2017;**77**(12):1369-1376

[90] Antonia SJ, Villegas A, Daniel D, Vicente D, Murakami S, Hui R, et al. Overall survival with durvalumab after chemoradiotherapy in stage III NSCLC. The New England Journal of Medicine. 2018;**379**(24):2342-2350

[91] Butte MJ, Keir ME, Phamduy TB, Sharpe AH, Freeman GJ. Programmed death-1 ligand 1 interacts specifically with the B7-1 costimulatory molecule to inhibit T cell responses. Immunity. 2007; **27**(1):111-122

[92] Huard B, Tournier M, Hercend T, Triebel F, Faure F. Lymphocyte-activation gene 3/major histocompatibility complex class II interaction modulates the antigenic response of CD4+ T lymphocytes. European Journal of Immunology. 1994; **24**(12):3216-3221

[93] Baixeras E, Huard B, Miossec C, Jitsukawa S, Martin M, Hercend T, et al. Characterization of the lymphocyte activation gene 3-encoded protein. A new ligand for human leukocyte antigen class II antigens. The Journal of Experimental Medicine. 1992;**176**(2): 327-337

[94] Anderson AC, Joller N, Kuchroo VK. Lag-3, Tim-3, and TIGIT: Co-inhibitory receptors with specialized functions in immune regulation. Immunity. 2016; **44**(5):989-1004

[95] Wang J, Sanmamed MF, Datar I, Su TT, Ji L, Sun J, et al. Fibrinogen-like protein 1 is a major immune inhibitory ligand of LAG-3. Cell. 2019;**176**(1–2): 334-347.e12

[96] Woo SR, Turnis ME, Goldberg MV, Bankoti J, Selby M, Nirschl CJ, et al. Immune inhibitory molecules LAG-3 and PD-1 synergistically regulate T-cell function to promote tumoral immune escape. Cancer Research. 2012;**72**(4): 917-927

[97] Kelley R, Kudo M, Harris W, Ikeda M, Okusaka T, Kang Y, et al. O-6 the novel regimen of tremelimumab in combination with durvalumab provides a favorable safety profile and clinical activity for patients with advanced hepatocellular carcinoma. Annals of Oncology. 2020;**31**:233-234. DOI: 10.1016/j.annonc.2020.04.059

[98] Tawbi HA, Schadendorf D, Lipson EJ, Ascierto PA, Matamala L, Castillo Gutiérrez E, et al. Relatlimab and nivolumab versus nivolumab in untreated advanced melanoma. The New England Journal of Medicine. 2022; **386**(1):24-34

[99] Catenacci DV, Rosales M, Chung HC, Yoon HH, Shen L, Moehler M, et al. MAHOGANY: Margetuximab combination in HER2+ unresectable/metastatic gastric/ gastroesophageal junction adenocarcinoma. Future Oncology. 2021; **17**(10):1155-1164

[100] Cho BC, Abreu DR, Hussein M, Cobo M, Patel AJ, Secen N, et al. Tiragolumab plus atezolizumab versus placebo plus atezolizumab as a first-line treatment for PD-L1-selected non-small-cell lung cancer (CITYSCAPE): Primary and follow-up analyses of a randomised, double-blind, phase 2 study. The Lancet Oncology. 2022;**23**(6):781-792

[101] Rudin CM, Liu SV, Lu S, Soo RA, Hong MH, Lee JS, et al. SKYSCRAPER-02: Primary results of a phase III, randomized, double-blind, placebo-controlled study of atezolizumab (atezo)

+ carboplatin + etoposide (CE) with or without tiragolumab (tira) in patients (pts) with untreated extensive-stage small cell lung cancer (ES-SCLC). Journal of Clinical Oncology. 2022;**40** (17_suppl):LBA8507-LBA8507. Available from: https://ascopubs.org/doi/abs/10.1200/JCO.2022.40.17_suppl.LBA8507

[102] Zeidan AM, Esteve J, Giagounidis A, Kim HJ, Miyazaki Y, Platzbecker U, et al. The STIMULUS program: Clinical trials evaluating Sabatolimab (MBG453) combination therapy in patients (pts) with higher-risk myelodysplastic syndromes (HR-MDS) or acute myeloid Leukemia (AML). Blood. 2020;**136**(Supplement 1):45-46. DOI: 10.1182/blood-2020-134718

[103] Yuan X, Yi M, Zhang W, Xu L, Chu Q, Luo S, et al. The biology of combination immunotherapy in recurrent metastatic head and neck cancer. The International Journal of Biochemistry & Cell Biology. 2021;**136**: 106002

[104] Kramer K, Khan O, Haque S. Central nervous system neuroblastoma metastases pseudoprogression following intraventricular anti-B7-H3 radioimmunotherapy. Journal of Neuro-Oncology. 2019;**144**(1):227-229

[105] Hansen AR, Stanton TS, Hong MH, Cohen EEW, Mehanna HM, Chisamore MJ, et al. INDUCE-3: A randomized, double-blind study of GSK3359609 (GSK609), an inducible T-cell co-stimulatory (ICOS) agonist antibody, plus pembrolizumab (PE) versus placebo (PL) plus PE for first-line treatment of PD-L1-positive recurrent/metastatic head and neck squamous cell carcinoma (R/M HNSCC). Journal of Clinical Oncology. 2020;**38**(15_suppl): TPS6591-TPS6591. Available from: https://ascopubs.org/doi/abs/10.1200/JCO.2020.38.15_suppl.TPS6591

[106] Twomey JD, Zhang B. Cancer immunotherapy update: FDA-approved checkpoint inhibitors and companion diagnostics. The AAPS Journal. 2021; **23**(2):39

[107] Pitt JM, Vétizou M, Daillère R, Roberti MP, Yamazaki T, Routy B, et al. Resistance mechanisms to immune-checkpoint blockade in cancer: Tumor-intrinsic and -extrinsic factors. Immunity. 2016;**44**(6):1255-1269

[108] Fares CM, van Allen EM, Drake CG, Allison JP, Hu-Lieskovan S. Mechanisms of resistance to immune checkpoint blockade: Why does checkpoint inhibitor immunotherapy not work for all patients? American Society of Clinical Oncology Educational Book. 2019;**39**:147-164

[109] Maleki VS. High and low mutational burden tumors versus immunologically hot and cold tumors and response to immune checkpoint inhibitors. Journal for Immunotherapy of Cancer. 2018;**6**(1):157

[110] Hu-Lieskovan S, Malouf GG, Jacobs I, Chou J, Liu L, Johnson ML. Addressing resistance to immune checkpoint inhibitor therapy: An urgent unmet need. Future Oncology. 2021; **17**(11):1401-1439

[111] Smith CC, Beckermann KE, Bortone DS, de Cubas AA, Bixby LM, Lee SJ, et al. Endogenous retroviral signatures predict immunotherapy response in clear cell renal cell carcinoma. The Journal of Clinical Investigation. 2018;**128**(11):4804-4820

[112] Duruisseaux M, Martínez-Cardús A, Calleja-Cervantes ME, Moran S, Castro de Moura M, Davalos V, et al. Epigenetic prediction of response to anti-PD-1 treatment in non-small-cell lung cancer: A multicentre, retrospective

analysis. Lancet Respiratory Medicine. 2018;**6**(10):771-781

[113] Galon J, Bruni D. Approaches to treat immune hot, altered and cold tumours with combination immunotherapies. Nature Reviews. Drug Discovery. 2019;**18**(3): 197-218

[114] Liu D, Jenkins RW, Sullivan RJ. Mechanisms of resistance to immune checkpoint blockade. American Journal of Clinical Dermatology. 2019;**20**(1): 41-54

[115] Anderson NM, Simon MC. The tumor microenvironment. Current Biology. 2020;**30**(16):R921-r925

[116] Fessler J, Matson V, Gajewski TF. Exploring the emerging role of the microbiome in cancer immunotherapy. Journal for Immunotherapy of Cancer. 2019;**7**(1):108

[117] Gopalakrishnan V, Helmink BA, Spencer CN, Reuben A, Wargo JA. The influence of the gut microbiome on cancer, immunity, and cancer immunotherapy. Cancer Cell. 2018; **33**(4):570-580

[118] Frankel AE, Deshmukh S, Reddy A, Lightcap J, Hayes M, McClellan S, et al. Cancer immune checkpoint inhibitor therapy and the gut microbiota. Integrative Cancer Therapies. 2019;**18**: 1534735419846379

[119] Panda A, de Cubas AA, Stein M, Riedlinger G, Kra J, Mayer T, et al. Endogenous retrovirus expression is associated with response to immune checkpoint blockade in clear cell renal cell carcinoma. JCI Insight. 2018;**3**(16):1-12

[120] Wolchok JD, Chiarion-Sileni V, Gonzalez R, Rutkowski P, Grob JJ, Cowey CL, et al. Overall survival with combined nivolumab and ipilimumab in advanced melanoma. The New England Journal of Medicine. 2017;**377**(14): 1345-1356

[121] Overman MJ, Lonardi S, Wong KYM, Lenz HJ, Gelsomino F, Aglietta M, et al. Durable clinical benefit with nivolumab plus ipilimumab in DNA mismatch repair-deficient/microsatellite instability-high metastatic colorectal cancer. Journal of Clinical Oncology. 2018;**36**(8):773-779

[122] Scherpereel A, Mazieres J, Greillier L, Lantuejoul S, Dô P, Bylicki O, et al. Nivolumab or nivolumab plus ipilimumab in patients with relapsed malignant pleural mesothelioma (IFCT-1501 MAPS2): A multicentre, open-label, randomised, non-comparative, phase 2 trial. The Lancet Oncology. 2019;**20**(2): 239-253

[123] Sheng IY, Ornstein MC. Ipilimumab and nivolumab as first-line treatment of patients with renal cell carcinoma: The evidence to date. Cancer Management and Research. 2020;**12**:4871-4881

[124] Larkin J, Chiarion-Sileni V, Gonzalez R, Grob JJ, Cowey CL, Lao CD, et al. Combined nivolumab and ipilimumab or monotherapy in untreated melanoma. The New England Journal of Medicine. 2015;**373**(1):23-34

[125] Owonikoko TK, Kim HR, Govindan R, Ready NE, Reck M, Peters S, et al. Nivolumab (nivo) plus ipilimumab (ipi), nivo, or placebo (pbo) as maintenance therapy in patients (pts) with extensive disease small cell lung cancer (ED-SCLC) after first-line (1L) platinum-based chemotherapy (chemo): Results from the double-blind, randomized phase III CheckMate 451 study. Annals of Oncology. 2019;**30** (Suppl. 2):ii77

[126] Owonikoko TK, Park K, Govindan R, Ready N, Reck M, Peters S, et al. Nivolumab and ipilimumab as maintenance therapy in extensive-disease small-cell lung cancer: CheckMate 451. Journal of Clinical Oncology. 2021;**39**(12):1349-1359

[127] Boyer M, Şendur MAN, Rodríguez-Abreu D, Park K, Lee DH, Çiçin I, et al. Pembrolizumab plus ipilimumab or placebo for metastatic non-small-cell lung cancer with PD-L1 tumor proportion score ≥ 50%: Randomized, double-blind phase III KEYNOTE-598 study. Journal of Clinical Oncology. 2021;**39**(21):2327-2338

[128] Lim M, Weller M, Idbaih A, Steinbach J, Finocchiaro G, Raval RR, et al. Phase III trial of chemoradiotherapy with temozolomide plus nivolumab or placebo for newly diagnosed glioblastoma with methylated MGMT promoter. Neuro-Oncology. 2022:1-15. [Epub ahead of print]. Available from: https://academic.oup.com/neuro-oncology/advance-article/doi/10.1093/neuonc/noac116/6577049

[129] Govindan R, Szczesna A, Ahn MJ, Schneider CP, Gonzalez Mella PF, Barlesi F, et al. Phase III trial of ipilimumab combined with paclitaxel and carboplatin in advanced squamous non-small-cell lung cancer. Journal of Clinical Oncology. 2017;**35**(30):3449-3457

[130] Janjigian YY, Shitara K, Moehler M, Garrido M, Salman P, Shen L, et al. First-line nivolumab plus chemotherapy versus chemotherapy alone for advanced gastric, gastro-oesophageal junction, and oesophageal adenocarcinoma (CheckMate 649): A randomised, open-label, phase 3 trial. Lancet. 2021; **398**(10294):27-40

[131] Reck M, Luft A, Szczesna A, Havel L, Kim SW, Akerley W, et al. Phase III randomized trial of ipilimumab plus etoposide and platinum versus placebo plus etoposide and platinum in extensive-stage small-cell lung cancer. Journal of Clinical Oncology. 2016; **34**(31):3740-3748

[132] Dummer R, Long GV, Robert C, Tawbi HA, Flaherty KT, Ascierto PA, et al. Randomized phase III trial evaluating spartalizumab plus dabrafenib and trametinib for BRAF V600-mutant unresectable or metastatic melanoma. Journal of Clinical Oncology. 2022;**40**(13):1428-1438

[133] Zitvogel L, Apetoh L, Ghiringhelli F, Kroemer G. Immunological aspects of cancer chemotherapy. Nature Reviews. Immunology. 2008;**8**(1):59-73

[134] Orecchioni S, Talarico G, Labanca V, Calleri A, Mancuso P, Bertolini F. Vinorelbine, cyclophosphamide and 5-FU effects on the circulating and intratumoural landscape of immune cells improve anti-PD-L1 efficacy in preclinical models of breast cancer and lymphoma. British Journal of Cancer. 2018;**118**(10): 1329-1336

[135] Salewski I, Henne J, Engster L, Schneider B, Lemcke H, Skorska A, et al. Combined gemcitabine and immune-checkpoint inhibition conquers anti-PD-L1 resistance in low-immunogenic mismatch repair-deficient tumors. International Journal of Molecular Sciences. 2021;**22**(11):1-16

[136] Ueno M, Ikeda M, Morizane C, Kobayashi S, Ohno I, Kondo S, et al. Nivolumab alone or in combination with cisplatin plus gemcitabine in Japanese patients with unresectable or recurrent biliary tract cancer: A non-randomised, multicentre, open-label, phase 1 study. The Lancet Gastroenterology & Hepatology. 2019;**4**(8):611-621

[137] Gandhi L, Rodríguez-Abreu D, Gadgeel S, Esteban E, Felip E, de Angelis F, et al. Pembrolizumab plus chemotherapy in metastatic non-small-cell lung cancer. The New England Journal of Medicine. 2018;**378**(22): 2078-2092

[138] Mathieu L, Shah S, Pai-Scherf L, Larkins E, Vallejo J, Li X, et al. FDA approval summary: Atezolizumab and durvalumab in combination with platinum-based chemotherapy in extensive stage small cell lung cancer. The Oncologist. 2021;**26**(5):433-438

[139] Reck M, Liu SV, Mansfield AS, Mok TSK, Scherpereel A, Reinmuth N, et al. IMpower133: Updated overall survival (OS) analysis of first-line (1L) atezolizumab (atezo) + carboplatin + etoposide in extensive-stage SCLC (ES-SCLC). Annals of Oncology. 2019;**30**: v710-v711. DOI: 10.1093/annonc/mdz264

[140] Rizvi NA, Hellmann MD, Snyder A, Kvistborg P, Makarov V, Havel JJ, et al. Mutational landscape determines sensitivity to PD-1 blockade in non-small cell lung cancer. Science (1979). 2015; **348**(6230):124-128

[141] Singal G, Miller PG, Agarwala V, Li G, Kaushik G, Backenroth D, et al. Association of patient characteristics and tumor genomics with clinical outcomes among patients with non-small cell lung cancer using a clinicogenomic database. JAMA. 2019;**321**(14):1391-1399. Available from: https://pubmed.ncbi.nlm.nih.gov/30964529/

[142] Carbone DP, Reck M, Paz-Ares L, Creelan B, Horn L, Steins M, et al. First-line nivolumab in stage IV or recurrent non-small-cell lung cancer. The New England Journal of Medicine. 2017; **376**(25):2415. Available from: /pmc/articles/PMC6487310/

[143] Fang W, Ma Y, Yin JC, Hong S, Zhou H, Wang A, et al. Precision medicine and imaging comprehensive genomic profiling identifies novel genetic predictors of response to anti-PD-(L)1 therapies in non-small cell lung cancer. Clinical Cancer Research. 2019; **25**(16):5015-5026. Available from: http://clincancerres.aacrjournals.org/

[144] Hellmann MD, Callahan MK, Awad MM, Calvo E, Ascierto PA, Atmaca A, et al. Tumor mutational burden and efficacy of nivolumab monotherapy and in combination with ipilimumab in small-cell lung cancer. Cancer Cell. 2018;**33**(5):853-861.e4

[145] Paz-Ares L, Langer CJ, Novello S, Halmos B, Cheng Y, Gadgeel SM, et al. Pembrolizumab (pembro) plus platinum-based chemotherapy (chemo) for metastatic NSCLC: Tissue TMB (tTMB) and outcomes in KEYNOTE-021, 189, and 407. Annals of Oncology. 2019;**30**:v917-v918

[146] Yarchoan M, Hopkins A, Jaffee EM. Tumor mutational burden and response rate to PD-1 inhibition. New England Journal of Medicine. 2017;**377**(25): 2500-2501

[147] Marabelle A, Fakih M, Lopez J, Shah M, Shapira-Frommer R, Nakagawa K, et al. Association of tumour mutational burden with outcomes in patients with advanced solid tumours treated with pembrolizumab: Prospective biomarker analysis of the multicohort, open-label, phase 2 KEYNOTE-158 study. The Lancet Oncology. 2020;**21**(10):1353-1365. Available from: http://www.thelancet.com/article/S1470204520304459/fulltext

[148] Rizvi H, Sanchez-Vega F, La K, Chatila W, Jonsson P, Halpenny D, et al. Molecular determinants of response to anti-programmed cell death (PD)-1 and

anti-programmed death-ligand 1 (PD-L1) blockade in patients with non-small-cell lung cancer profiled with targeted next-generation sequencing. Journal of Clinical Oncology. 2018;**36**(7):633-641

[149] Fancello L, Gandini S, Pelicci PG, Mazzarella L. Tumor mutational burden quantification from targeted gene panels: Major advancements and challenges. Journal for Immunotherapy of Cancer. 2019;**7**(1):1-13. Available from: https://pubmed.ncbi.nlm.nih.gov/31307554/

[150] Addeo A, Friedlaender A, Banna GL, Weiss GJ. TMB or not TMB as a biomarker: That is the question. Critical Reviews in Oncology/Hematology. 2021;**163**:103374

[151] Litchfield K, Stanislaw S, Spain L, Gallegos LL, Rowan A, Schnidrig D, et al. Representative sequencing: Unbiased sampling of solid tumor tissue. Cell Reports. 2020;**31**(5):1-13. Available from: https://pubmed.ncbi.nlm.nih.gov/32375028/

[152] Topalian SL, Taube JM, Anders RA, Pardoll DM. Mechanism-driven biomarkers to guide immune checkpoint blockade in cancer therapy. Nature Reviews. Cancer. 2016;**16**(5):275. Available from: /pmc/articles/PMC5381938/

[153] Williams DS, Bird MJ, Jorissen RN, Yu YL, Walker F, Zhang HH, et al. Nonsense mediated decay resistant mutations are a source of expressed mutant proteins in colon cancer cell lines with microsatellite instability. PLoS One. 2010;**5**(12):1-16

[154] Salem ME, Puccini A, Grothey A, Raghavan D, Goldberg RM, Xiu J, et al. Landscape of tumor mutation load, mismatch repair deficiency, and PD-L1 expression in a large patient cohort of gastrointestinal cancers. Molecular Cancer Research. 2018;**16**(5):805. Available from: /pmc/articles/PMC6833953/

[155] Le DT, Uram JN, Wang H, Bartlett BR, Kemberling H, Eyring AD, et al. PD-1 blockade in tumors with mismatch-repair deficiency. The New England Journal of Medicine. 2015;**372**(26):2509. Available from: /pmc/articles/PMC4481136/

[156] Garcia-Diaz A, Shin DS, Moreno BH, Saco J, Escuin-Ordinas H, Rodriguez GA, et al. Interferon receptor signaling pathways regulating PD-L1 and PD-L2 expression. Cell Reports. 2017;**19**(6):1189. Available from: /pmc/articles/PMC6420824/

[157] Zaretsky JM, Garcia-Diaz A, Shin DS, Escuin-Ordinas H, Hugo W, Hu-Lieskovan S, et al. Mutations associated with acquired resistance to PD-1 blockade in melanoma. The New England Journal of Medicine 2016;**375**(9):819. Available from: /pmc/articles/PMC5007206/

[158] Shin DS, Zaretsky JM, Escuin-Ordinas H, Garcia-Diaz A, Hu-Lieskovan S, Kalbasi A, et al. Primary resistance to PD-1 blockade mediated by JAK1/2 mutations. Cancer Discovery. 2017;**7**(2):188. Available from: /pmc/articles/PMC5296316/

[159] Marabelle A, Aspeslagh S, Postel-Vinay S, Soria JC. JAK mutations as escape mechanisms to anti-PD-1 therapy. Cancer Discovery. 2017;**7**(2):128-130. Available from: https://pubmed.ncbi.nlm.nih.gov/28167612/

[160] Karachaliou N, Gonzalez-Cao M, Crespo G, Drozdowskyj A, Aldeguer E, Gimenez-Capitan A, et al. Interferon gamma, an important marker of response to immune checkpoint

blockade in non-small cell lung cancer and melanoma patients Therapeutic Advances in Medical Oncology. 2018;**10**: 1-23. Available from: /pmc/articles/ PMC5784541/

[161] Higgs BW, Morehouse CA, Streicher K, Brohawn PZ, Pilataxi F, Gupta A, et al. Interferon gamma messenger RNA signature in tumor biopsies predicts outcomes in patients with non–small cell lung carcinoma or urothelial cancer treated with durvalumab. Clinical Cancer Research. 2018;**24**(16): 3857-3866. Available from: https://aacrjournals.org/clincancerres/article/24/16/3857/277387/Interferon-Gamma-Messenger-RNA-Signature-in-Tumor

[162] Ribas A, Robert C, Schachter J, Long GV, Arance A, Carlino MS, et al. Abstract 4217: Tumor mutational burden (TMB), T cell-inflamed gene expression profile (GEP) and PD-L1 are independently associated with response to pembrolizumab (Pembro) in patients with advanced melanoma in the KEYNOTE (KN)-006 study. Cancer Research. 2019; **79**(13_Supplement):4217-4217. Available from: https://aacrjournals.org/cancerres/article/79/13_Supplement/4217/635974/Abstract-4217-Tumor-mutational-burden-TMB-T-cell

[163] Rozeman EA, Menzies AM, Krijgsman O, Hoefsmit EP, van de Wiel BA, Sikorska K, et al. 18-months relapse-free survival (RFS) and biomarker analyses of OpACIN-neo: A study to identify the optimal dosing schedule of neoadjuvant (neoadj) ipilimumab (IPI) + nivolumab (NIVO) in stage III melanoma. Annals of Oncology. 2019;**30**:v910

[164] Rozeman EA, Reijers ILM, Hoefsmit EP, Sikorska K, Krijgsman O, van de Wiel BA, et al. Twenty-four months RFS and updated toxicity data from OpACIN-neo: A study to identify the optimal dosing schedule of neoadjuvant ipilimumab (IPI) and nivolumab (NIVO) in stage III melanoma. Journal of Clinical Oncology. 2020;**38**(15_suppl):10015-10015. DOI: 101200/JCO20203815_suppl10015

[165] McDermott DF, Huseni MA, Atkins MB, Motzer RJ, Rini BI, Escudier B, et al. Clinical activity and molecular correlates of response to atezolizumab alone or in combination with bevacizumab versus sunitinib in renal cell carcinoma. Nature Medicine. 2018;**24**(6):749-757. Available from: https://mayoclinic.pure.elsevier.com/en/publications/clinical-activity-and-molecular-correlates-of-response-to-atezoli

[166] Doroshow DB, Bhalla S, Beasley MB, Sholl LM, Kerr KM, Gnjatic S, et al. PD-L1 as a biomarker of response to immune-checkpoint inhibitors. Nature Reviews Clinical Oncology. 2021;**18**(6):345-362. Available from: https://www.nature.com/articles/s41571-021-00473-5

[167] Garon EB, Rizvi NA, Hui R, Leighl N, Balmanoukian AS, Eder JP, et al. Pembrolizumab for the treatment of non-small-cell lung cancer. The New England Journal of Medicine. 2015; **372**(21):2018-2028

[168] Burtness B, Harrington KJ, Greil R, Soulières D, Tahara M, de Castro G, et al. Pembrolizumab alone or with chemotherapy versus cetuximab with chemotherapy for recurrent or metastatic squamous cell carcinoma of the head and neck (KEYNOTE-048): A randomised, open-label, phase 3 study. The Lancet. 2019;**394**(10212):1915-1928. Available from: http://www.thelancet.com/article/S0140673619325917/fulltext

[169] Schmid P, Adams S, Rugo HS, Schneeweiss A, Barrios CH, Iwata H,

et al. Atezolizumab and nab-paclitaxel in advanced triple-negative breast cancer. The New England Journal of Medicine. 2018;**379**(22):2108-2121

[170] O'Donnell PH, Balar AV, Vuky J, Castellano DE, Bellmunt J, Powles T, et al. KEYNOTE-052: Phase 2 study evaluating first-line pembrolizumab (pembro) in cisplatin-ineligible advanced urothelial cancer (UC)—Updated response and survival results. Journal of Clinical Oncology. 2019;**37** (15_suppl):4546-4546. DOI: 101200/JCO20193715_suppl4546

[171] Hirsch FR, McElhinny A, Stanforth D, Ranger-Moore J, Jansson M, Kulangara K, et al. PD-L1 immunohistochemistry assays for lung cancer: Results from phase 1 of the blueprint PD-L1 IHC assay comparison project. Journal of Thoracic Oncology. 2017;**12**(2):208-222. Available from: http://www.jto.org/article/S1556086416335365/fulltext

[172] Tumeh PC, Harview CL, Yearley JH, Shintaku IP, Taylor EJM, Robert L, et al. PD-1 blockade induces responses by inhibiting adaptive immune resistance. Nature. 2014; **515**(7528):568. Available from: /pmc/articles/PMC4246418/

[173] Loi S, Adams S, Schmid P, Cortés J, Cescon DW, Winer EP, et al. Relationship between tumor infiltrating lymphocyte (TIL) levels and response to pembrolizumab (pembro) in metastatic triple-negative breast cancer (mTNBC): Results from KEYNOTE-086. Annals of Oncology. 2017;**28**:v608. Available from: http://www.annalsofoncology.org/article/S0923753420391055/fulltext

[174] Hamid O, Schmidt H, Nissan A, Ridolfi L, Aamdal S, Hansson J, et al. A prospective phase II trial exploring the association between tumor microenvironment biomarkers and clinical activity of ipilimumab in advanced melanoma. Journal of Translational Medicine. 2011;**9**(1):204. Available from: /pmc/articles/PMC3239318/

[175] Savas P, Virassamy B, Ye C, Salim A, Mintoff CP, Caramia F, et al. Single-cell profiling of breast cancer T cells reveals a tissue-resident memory subset associated with improved prognosis. Nature Medicine. 2018;**24**(7):986-993. Available from: https://www.nature.com/articles/s41591-018-0078-7

[176] Shang B, Liu Y, Jiang SJ, Liu Y. Prognostic value of tumor-infiltrating FoxP3+ regulatory T cells in cancers: A systematic review and meta-analysis. Scientific Reports. 2015;**5**:1-9. Available from::/pmc/articles/PMC4604472/

[177] Xiao B, Peng J, Wang Y, Deng Y, Ou Q, Wu X, et al. Prognostic value of tumor infiltrating lymphocytes combined with PD-L1 expression for patients with solitary colorectal cancer liver metastasis. Annals of Translational Medicine. 2020; **8**(19):1221–1221. Available from: /pmc/articles/PMC7607072/

[178] Poulet G, Massias J, Taly V. Liquid biopsy: General concepts. Acta Cytologica. 2019;**63**(6):449-455. Available from: https://www.karger.com/Article/FullText/499337

[179] Lee JH, Long GV, Boyd S, Lo S, Menzies AM, Tembe V, et al. Circulating tumour DNA predicts response to anti-PD1 antibodies in metastatic melanoma. Annals of Oncology. 2017;**28**(5): 1130-1136. Available from: http://www.annalsofoncology.org/article/S0923753419320058/fulltext

[180] Wang Z, Duan J, Cai S, Han M, Dong H, Zhao J, et al. Assessment of blood tumor mutational burden as a potential biomarker for immunotherapy

in patients with non–small cell lung cancer with use of a next-generation sequencing cancer gene panel. JAMA Oncology 2019;5(5):696. Available from: /pmc/articles/PMC6512308/

[181] Guibert N, Delaunay M, Lusque A, Boubekeur N, Rouquette I, Clermont E, et al. PD-L1 expression in circulating tumor cells of advanced non-small cell lung cancer patients treated with nivolumab. Lung Cancer. 2018;**120**: 108-112. Available from: http://www.lungcancerjournal.info/article/S0169500218303179/fulltext

[182] Li L, Yu R, Cai T, Chen Z, Lan M, Zou T, et al. Effects of immune cells and cytokines on inflammation and immunosuppression in the tumor microenvironment. International Immunopharmacology. 2020;**88**:106939

[183] Ferrucci PF, Ascierto PA, Pigozzo J, del Vecchio M, Maio M, Antonini Cappellini GC, et al. Baseline neutrophils and derived neutrophil-to-lymphocyte ratio: Prognostic relevance in metastatic melanoma patients receiving ipilimumab. Annals of Oncology. 2016; **27**(4):732-738. Available from: http://www.annalsofoncology.org/article/S0923753419357655/fulltext

[184] Bagley SJ, Kothari S, Aggarwal C, Bauml JM, Alley EW, Evans TL, et al. Pretreatment neutrophil-to-lymphocyte ratio as a marker of outcomes in nivolumab-treated patients with advanced non-small-cell lung cancer. Lung Cancer. 2017;**106**:1-7. Available from: http://www.lungcancerjournal.info/article/S0169500217300247/fulltext

[185] Ameratunga M, Chénard-Poirier M, Moreno Candilejo I, Pedregal M, Lui A, Dolling D, et al. Neutrophil-lymphocyte ratio kinetics in patients with advanced solid tumours on phase I trials of PD-1/PD-L1 inhibitors. European Journal of Cancer. 2018;**89**:56-63. Available from: http://www.ejcancer.com/article/S0959804917314090/fulltext

[186] Diem S, Kasenda B, Spain L, Martin-Liberal J, Marconcini R, Gore M, et al. Serum lactate dehydrogenase as an early marker for outcome in patients treated with anti-PD-1 therapy in metastatic melanoma. British Journal of Cancer. 2016;**114**(3):256. Available from: /pmc/articles/PMC4742588/

[187] Weber JS, Tang H, Hippeli L, Qian M, Wind-Rotolo M, Larkin JMG, et al. Serum IL-6 and CRP as prognostic factors in melanoma patients receiving single agent and combination checkpoint inhibition. Journal of Clinical Oncology. 2019;**37**(15_suppl):100-100. DOI: 101200/JCO20193715_suppl100

[188] Sanmamed MF, Perez-Gracia JL, Schalper KA, Fusco JP, Gonzalez A, Rodriguez-Ruiz ME, et al. Changes in serum interleukin-8 (IL-8) levels reflect and predict response to anti-PD-1 treatment in melanoma and non-small-cell lung cancer patients. Annals of Oncology. 2017;**28**(8):1988-1995. Available from: http://www.annalsofoncology.org/article/S0923753419321386/fulltext

[189] Elkrief A, Derosa L, Zitvogel L, Kroemer G, Routy B. The intimate relationship between gut microbiota and cancer immunotherapy. Gut Microbes 2019;**10**(3):424. Available from: /pmc/articles/PMC6546322/

[190] Routy B, le Chatelier E, Derosa L, Duong CPM, Alou MT, Daillère R, et al. Gut microbiome influences efficacy of PD-1-based immunotherapy against epithelial tumors. Science (1979). 2018;**359**(6371): 91-97. Available from: https://www.science.org/doi/10.1126/science.aan3706

Chapter 8

# Recent Developments in Application of Multiparametric Flow Cytometry in CAR-T Immunotherapy

*Hui Wang and Man Chen*


## Abstract

In recent years, chimeric antigen receptor (CAR) modified T-cell (CAR-T) immunotherapy has achieved great success in cancer treatment, especially in some hematologic malignancies. Multiparametric flow cytometry (MFC) is a key immunologic tool and plays an important role in every step of CAR-T design, development, and clinical trials. This chapter discusses the application and new developments of MFC in CAR-T, including the selection of CAR-T targets, the enrollment of patients, the detection of minimal/measurable residual disease (MRD), the quality evaluation of CAR-T product, the detection of immune cell subsets and cytokines, and the study of immune checkpoint and immune suppressive microenvironment.


**Keywords:** chimeric antigen receptor, immunotherapy, multiparametric flow cytometry, hematological malignancies, immune

## 1. Introduction

Chimeric antigen receptor (CAR) modified T-cell (CAR-T) has been a remarkable achievement in the field of cancer therapy in recent years [1–7], especially for the treatment of refractory and relapsed B-cell acute lymphoblastic leukemia (ALL) [1–3]. CD19-CAR-T alone or bridging allogeneic hematopoietic stem cell transplantation (allo-HSCT) can greatly improve the complete remission (CR) rate and overall survival (OS) rate. CAR-T therapy for other malignancies is being explored as well [4–7]. However, the main problem with CAR-T therapy is its high relapse rate, which involves a variety of mechanisms. Current researches focus on improving CAR-T structure, selecting new targets, and eliminating the inhibitory immune microenvironment [8–14].

Multiparametric flow cytometry (MFC) is an immunological technique developed in the 1970s and has become an indispensable methodology for clinical diagnosis and basic research [15, 16]. CAR-T is one kind of immunotherapy, and MFC plays a pivotal role in the entire process of CAR-T [3, 17–29]. These applications involve multiple aspects of MFC, and basically can be divided into two categories, that is, protocols

 IntechOpen

| Phage | Aim | Specimen type | Tumor or target-related assays | Immune-related assays | Important parameters | Optional parameters |
|---|---|---|---|---|---|---|
| CAR-T design | Selection of target and prediction of side effects. | Patient specimens or cell lines. | Immunophenotype or MRD. | Lymphocyte activity and function, immune cell subsets, and cytokines | Coverage, expression intensity, and specificity of target antigen in certain diseases. Killing efficiency related to CAR-T design. | |
| Enrollment | The expression rate and intensity of target antigens on tumor cells. Function and activity of patient's lymphocytes. Enrollment possibility. The choice of raw material. | BM, PB, or other sites from patient. | Immunophenotype or MRD. | Above and optionally TME and immune checkpoint. | The proportion of tumor cells in nuclear cells, the immunophenotype of tumor cells, the expression rate, expression intensity, and specificity of potential targets in tumor cells. | The killing efficacy of CAR-T cells was evaluated by coculture with tumor cells, and the inhibitory signal in the immune microenvironment was evaluated. |
| CAR-T product | Quality control of CAR-T product. | CAR-T product | MRD | CAR positive cells, immune cell subsets, and cytokines. | Percentages and absolute counts of CAR-expressing cells, CAR-T cell components (lymphocyte and functional subsets), and residual tumor and other cells in the product were assessed. | Evaluation of inhibitory and activating signals, cytokine release ability. |

| Phage | Aim | Specimen type | Tumor or target-related assays | Immune-related assays | Important parameters | Optional parameters |
|---|---|---|---|---|---|---|
| After CAR-T infusion | Efficacy evaluation and kinetic detection of target recovery. | BM, PB, or other sites from patient. | MRD | Kinetics of target antigen recovery. | MRD was used to evaluate the efficacy and recovery of CAR-T target expression in normal cells. | Expression curves of CAR-T target antigens in normal and tumor cells at each time point before and after infusion. |
| | Immune cell subsets. | PB or CSF from patient. | | CAR T-cell detection, basic T-lymphocyte subsets, individualized immune cell subsets, and cytokine detection. | Proportion and absolute count of CAR-expressing cells, CAR-T cell component, relationship between CAR-T cell peak and clinical response, basic T-lymphocyte subsets. | Individualized immune cell subset, functional cytokines, immune activation or exhaustion, and aging marker expression. |
| | Study on relapse mechanism and re-selection of targets. | BM, PB, or other sites from patient. | Selection of target. | TME and immune checkpoint. | Target positive and negative relapse, and selection of new CAR-T targets after relapse. | Evaluation of TME and immune checkpoint. |

*Note. CAR: chimeric antigen receptor, CSF: cerebrospinal fluid, MRD: minimal residual/measurable diseases, and TME: tumor microenvironment.*

**Table 1.**
*Application of MFC in CAR-T development and study.*

to detect tumor cells and/or target antigen-positive cells and those to evaluate the immune system. The previous category includes tumor cell immunophenotyping to select promising targets [17, 18], minimal residual/measurable diseases (MRD) detection [3, 19, 20], and recovery kinetics of target antigen-positive cells [3, 21, 22]. The latter category includes lymphocyte activity and function evaluation, CAR-positive cell assay [21–25], immune cell subsets detection [21–31], lymphocyte killing function assay [27], cytokines detection [26–29], tumor microenvironment (TME) evaluation, and immunosuppressive signals detection [23, 26].

If according to time points, the application progress of MFC in CAR-T can be divided into four stages: CAR-T research and development, patient enrollment of clinical research, quality evaluation after product preparation, and posttreatment evaluation.

These tests involve almost all aspects of MFC, including routine clinical testing items and special research items, and are carried out repeatedly at different time points, even with some overlaps. See **Table 1**.

However, even in routine items, the special nature of CAR-T brings technical challenges. The analysis of the immunophenotype of tumor cells needs a very accurate gate setting because the coexistence of target antigen negative subclone may become the source of recurrence [9–12]. The evaluation of CAR-T products before infusion and MRD detection after CAR-T immunotherapy need to be careful of the target antigen-negative malignant and benign cells [3, 19, 20]. The presence of CAR-T cells may affect the MRD detection of T lymphocytic malignancies. In the identification of CAR-T products and early immunological evaluation after treatment, it is necessary to evaluate the composition and activating status of CAR-positive and CAR-negative cells simultaneously [32–35].

## 2. Tumor or target antigen-expressing cells related assay

### 2.1 Target screening and specificity evaluation

Although the diversity of tumor cells leads to a high tumor escape rate in traditional single-target CAR-T, and new technologies are beginning to use bi-specific targets and even more complex designs, screening of specific target antigens is still the most important part of CAR-T design. MFC is the most important tool to achieve this purpose at present [3, 4, 17, 18]. The ideal CAR-T target should meet the following requirements: a high rate of occurrence in certain diseases (high availability of CAR-T), a high percentage of expression on tumor cells (covering all tumor cells to minimize relapse), a high intensity of expression (the expression intensity of target antigen on tumor cells is related to the efficacy, although there are contradictory results) [36–39], and good specificity (no or little expression in normal cells will not cause serious impact on patients) [1–4]. Target screening is performed on the basis of immunophenotyping or MRD, but with more stringent precautions than routine clinical diagnosis. It is necessary to accurately gate and define tumor cells, especially to cover all heterogeneous tumor cell populations. Otherwise, target-negative tumor cells will become the source of relapse. The detection of potential targets on tumor cells needs to be reported as a percentage. The mean fluorescence intensity (MFI) or median fluorescence intensity (MdFI) of target antigen expression in tumor cells and the ratio of MdFI to control cells may be used to describe the relative expression intensity. Some studies even use fluorescence microbeads for accurate quantitative detection [36, 37]. Standardization of the operation and calibration of the instrument are required for the testing process, as well as a selection of appropriate internal controls.

### *2.1.1 Overview of the CAR-T targets in various tumors*

The target selection of ALL is relatively consistent. Generally, lineage markers with high coverage are preferred, such as CD19 [1–3, 36, 40, 41], CD22 [42], or CD19/CD22 dual targets [37, 43] for B-ALL and CD7-CAR-T by genetic engineering technology [4, 44, 45] for T-ALL. Although some clinical studies have selected markers expressed in subgroups of ALL, such as CD20 [46] and CRLF2 [31] for B-ALL, and TRBC1 and CD1a for T-ALL [47, 48]. As to lymphoproliferative disease (LPD), other studies have tried to select lineage markers expressed by mature lymphocytes beside CD19 and CD22 [6, 37], for example, CD20, CD37, and BAFFR for B-LPD, CD5, CD4, TRBC1 for T-LPD, and CD38, BCMA or other markers for multiple myeloma (MM) [9, 10, 49–51]. Special subtypes of lymphoma have selected corresponding specific antigens as targets, such as CD30 for anaplastic large cell lymphoma (ALCL) and Hodgkin lymphoma (HL) [52–54]. Acute myeloid leukemia (AML) is a highly heterogeneous tumor, and there are a lot of studies on its targets, including CD33, CD123, CLL1 (CD371), CD25, CD117, Tim3, NKG2D, CD44, CD96, and CD38, or the combination of the above targets [5, 12, 17, 18, 55–60]. Although studies on solid tumors have made some achievements, searching for solid tumor-specific or associated antigens is still an interesting field for researchers. Therefore, current researches focus on immunosuppressive TME and modified CAR-T design [9, 10, 61, 62].

### *2.1.2 Standardized evaluation of target antigen expression*

Although some studies have shown that the efficacy of CAR-T is highly dependent on the density of target antigen expression [36, 37], and clinical trials has found that high tumor burden is a high-risk factor to relapse [40, 41], more detailed data remains unclear. For example, the percentage and numbers of antigen expressed on tumor cells and the expression intensity that can activate CAR-T to obtain the best response rate and longest survival rate; the suitable target antigen expression in tumor cells that allows the patient to be enrolled in the CAR-T study; the corresponding relations between absolute counts of target positive tumor cells or antigens on total tumor cells and dose of CAR-T needed for treatment [63, 64], etc. On the other side, the efficacy, stability, and difference of CAR detection antibody, qualitative and quantitative heterogeneity of antigen expression on tumor cells in the same disease, differences in antigen expression intensity caused by different fluorescence, and the influence factors in the process of antibody staining, can lead to significant intra-lab and inter-lab differences. Thus, the accurate relationship between the expression of CAR-T target antigens and the efficacy/side effects/survival rate is not comparable in different studies, which is more obvious in studies of weakly expressed target antigens. Given the diversity of CAR-T products and the multiple factors affecting MFC testing, uniform standard operating procedures (SOPs) may not be available in a short time. However, we hope to make the technique relatively stable and objective by standardizing the process of MFC detection, which will be helpful in exploring the most ideal target, accurately evaluating the efficacy and side effects of CAR-T, studying the complex relapse mechanism and promoting the update of CAR-T products to obtain the best effect for individual study [21–25]. To do this, the same protocol should be used in a study, especially in a multicenter study, including antibody clone and fluorescein combination; titration and inter-batch comparison of the antibodies are required. Use the same instrument as far as possible, accurate comparisons are required if different instruments are used, and daily calibration and regular maintenance is also mandatory; residual normal counterparts in the specimen are good controls to evaluate the expression of target antigen with high or moderate intensity, such as CD19, CD22, and CD7, and we can describe target antigen as dim (dimmer than normal) or bright (brighter than normal) besides percentage; MFI/MdFI or quantitative fluorescence microbeads need to use to determine the expression of target antigen with very low intensity [37–39].

#### *2.1.3 Evaluation of the specificity of target antigen*

The ideal target antigen has been described above, where the specificity is evaluated by the expression of the antigen in normal cells, which is very important for CAR-T target selection. Because CAR-T is a very powerful and specific targeted therapy, most cells expressing the target will be killed, whether normal or malignant. Killing tumor cells is effective, while killing normal cells is toxic, not to say this effect lasts 1–3 months [3, 4, 34–37].

An ideal target is only specifically expressed in tumor cells but not in normal cells, or in normal cells the expression rate is low or the functions of these cells can be replaced by other cells or drugs. Unfortunately, almost no antigen is absolutely specific or low expressed in normal cells [9, 10] except those associated with B cells and plasma cells. Fortunately, with the development of modern life science, more and more gene modification methods and other technologies are overcoming this problem, such as the emergence of gene knockout or selecting CD7-CAR-T [4, 44, 45]. MFC plays an important role during the process. Accurate analysis of the target antigen expression on different cells can predict the toxicity and side effects, and help researchers to modify CAR-Ts.

### 2.2 MRD

MRD is an important indicator for evaluating efficacy and is closely related to prognosis [1–4, 19, 65]. MRD monitoring after CAR-T therapy is difficult due to tumor adaptation and off-target effects. The issues that need to be paid attention to are gating with multiple markers and recognizing malignant or normal cell loss target antigens [3, 19, 20].

#### *2.2.1 Selection of gating markers*

CD19-CAR-T is the most used immunotherapy, and MRD detection after CD19-CAR-T in B-ALL is also the focus of researchers. Because all or part of CD19 expression is lost or weak in 7.4–62.5% of B-cell malignancies after CD19-CAR-T treatment, CD19 gating cannot be the only rough B gating marker [3, 19, 20, 36, 37]. As for the selection of alternative gate markers, some laboratories chose CD22+ and/or CD24+/CD66b− [19], while we and some laboratories chose multiparameter synchronous gate setting by cytoplasmatic (c) CD79a combined with CD19 and lymphoblast markers [1–3, 20]. The reasons are as follows: 10–20% of B-ALL cases do not express CD24, especially in cases with MLL-related fusion genes [3, 19]. After the failure of CD19-CAR-T therapy, the choice of CD19/CD22 bi-specific CAR-T or CD22-CAR-T, coupled with the weak expression of CD22 in B lymphoblasts, all determine that this is not an ideal rough B gating marker [3, 38]. Although studies have found that CD22dim/-MRD did not appear after CD22-CAR-T treatment [37], further studies are needed because of the small number of cases. Therefore, we used cCD79a as the main B marker in MRD detection after CD19-CAR-T or CD19/CD22 combined CAR-T treatment, and achieved good clinical evaluation results [3]. Besides the biggest advantage of cCD79a panel is that we can use the same panel for all MRD detection after any B marker CAR-T treatment in the future because it is an intracellular antigen not for CAR-T target [51].

The same idea was adopted in CD7-CAR-T for T-ALL, other lineage markers are added in the MRD panel, such as cCD3, CD5, and CD2, as well as blast markers, such as TdT, CD34, CD99bri, and CD1a [4].

#### *2.2.2 Changes in phenotype and observation methods*

When selecting cCD79a combined panel to detect MRD after CD19 and/or CD22-CAR-T therapy in B-ALL, the following should be noted: (1) the expression intensity of some antigens may change after the intracellular operation. (2) Recognize the immunophenotype of normal CD19-negative hematogones, most of which are the earliest stage of CD34+ B progenitor cells. They are different from the CD19 positive counterpart in that weaker CD10 expression and larger SSC, and may be misdiagnosed as MRD; (3) in fact, CD19-negative hematogones exist in normal BM but are ignored, because most of them are rare and CD19 is routinely used for gating. A significant decrease in the proportion of CD19 positive B progenitors with CD19-CAR-T results in a relative increase in the proportion of CD19-negative B progenitors, which together with changes in gate setting and most importantly the focus on CD19-negative B cells, made this population prominent [3, 19, 20].

Given that the heterogeneity of tumor cells is obvious after CAR-T therapy, even with the use of alternative gate markers, detection will be difficult, not to say the rare use of cytoplasmatic markers in cerebrospinal fluid (CSF) specimens. After CAR-T, multiple gates by multiple markers will be helpful in MRD detection by MFC. For example, SSC/cCD79a, SSC/CD19, SSC/CD10,SSC/CD34, and SSC/TdT in B-ALL, CD99bri/SSC, cCD3/CD45dim, CD5/CD45dim, CD34and/or CD1a/SSC, and TdT/SSC in T-ALL, CD229/CD45dim and CD138/CD45dim in MM. CD45dim/CD10 positive and/or CD34 positive and/or CD38 positive cells are not present in normal CSF samples, so CD34 and/or CD10 and/or CD38 combined with CD45 gate method was used for identification of CD19-negative B-ALL MRD. See **Figure 1**.

In addition, special attention should be paid to myeloid conversion after CAR-T in ALL patients [66]. After CD7-CAR-T cell therapy, MRD detection may be affected due to interference of CAR-T cells. In the case of targeted therapy with CD38, CD123, and other markers of progenitors, attention should be paid to the phenotypic changes of the normal blast caused by the loss of these markers during MRD detection.

### 2.3 Kinetics of target antigen recovery

After injection, CAR-T cells expand more than 10,000 times *in vivo*. The number of amplifications and duration of presence *in vivo* largely determine the efficacy and side effects of CAR-T. The recovery of cells expressing the target antigen can indirectly reflect the recovery kinetics of CAR-T [3, 19, 20, 34, 35, 67]. Target antigen recovery is not evaluated alone, generally detected as part of MRD or immunoassay [3, 19, 20, 34, 35, 67].

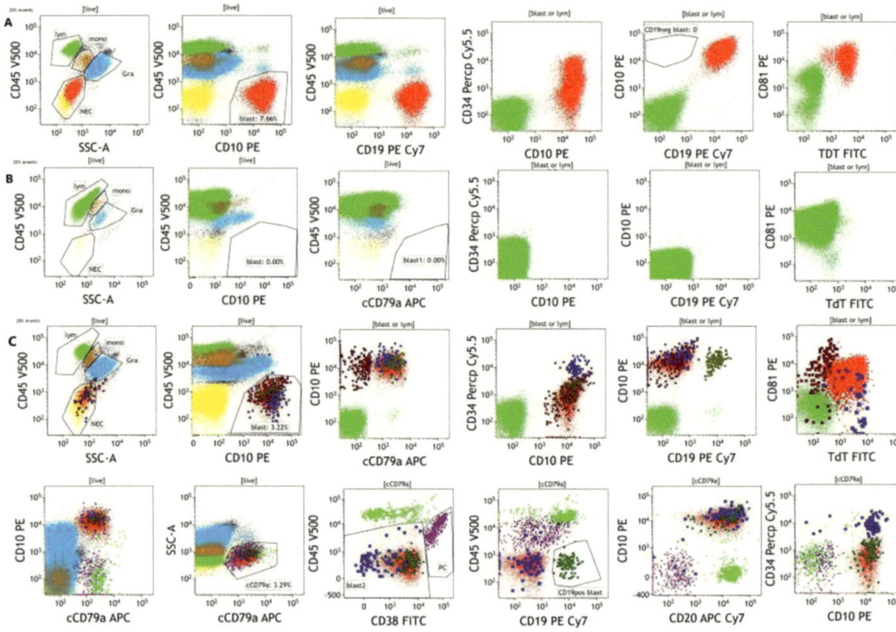


**Figure 1.**
*BM from one B-ALL patient for MRD detection by MFC, the title of each dot plot was the gate where the subplot showed the cell. A, before CD19-CAR-T immunotherapy. The cells in red color were malignant B lymphoblasts with 7.66% of live cells. They were positive for CD19, CD10, CD81, TdT, and CD34part, negative for CD45. B, 30d after CD19-CAR-T. No CD10 or cytoplasmatic (c)CD79a-positive cells were observed. C, relapsed 4 months after CD19-CAR-T. the blast was 3.22% of live cells and consisted of four subsets. The cells in red color were the major subset, positive for CD10, CD38, CD81, TdT, and cCD79a part, negative for CD45, CD34, and CD19. The cells in dark green color were the minor subset 1, positive for CD10, CD19, CD38, and cCD79a, negative for CD45and CD34, not known for CD81 and TdT. The cells in dark brown color were the minor subset 2, positive for CD10, CD38, and CD81, negative for CD45, CD34, TdT, cCD79a, and CD19. The cells in sapphire color were the minor subset 3, positive for CD10, CD34, TdT, and cCD79a, negative for CD38, CD81, CD45, and CD19. Normal B cells (fluorescent green color) and plasma cells (magenta color) were all CD19 partially positive.*

The recovery dynamics decide the choice of detection time points. Besides CAR-T products, the efficacy depends largely on *in vivo* CAR-T cell proliferation. The target expression cells begin to recover 1–3 months after treatment, and commonly BM, CSF, or other involved sites are selected as specimens. BM should ideally be tested once a month for the first 6 months and at least once every 3 months for the first 6 to 12 months [1–4, 19–22, 32]. Generally, PB or CSF of patients is selected as specimens for CAR-T cell assay and cytokines detection. Before infusion on day 0, and after infusion on other time points, PB-related assays are frequent in the first month, such as 4 d, 7 d (optional 10 d or 11 d), 14 d, 28 d, 2 m, 3 m, and 6 m [1–4, 32–37]. The detection of CAR-expressing cells can be stopped after the detected values are lower than the limit of detection (LOD) for two consecutive times. MRD and CAR-T cell detection of CSF are performed at the appropriate time point. PB is selected for immune assay, at least once a month for the first 6 months, and once every 3–6 months after 6 months [32–37].

Taking CD19-CAR-T treatment for B-ALL as an example, the duration of B-cell deficiency varies greatly among different studies, generally lasting 2–3 months. The recovery of B cells in PB is a signal of CD19-CAR-T dysfunction. In pediatric B-ALL, recovery of B cells at 3 months suggests a high risk of relapse, possibly due to CAR-T depletion [36, 37, 40–43].

## 3. Immune-related assays

There will be an overlap of parameters in these assays. The panels are recombined for different time points. For example, in CAR-T product evaluation and samples were drawn at earlier time points after CAR-T, CAR-expressing cells and other immune subsets may be detected in the same panel. If CAR-T cells continuously decrease and are lower than LOD twice in a row, the MFC method will no longer be used to detect CAR-T cells and the protocol will be changed to immune function and cytokine assays without CAR-T cell detection.

### 3.1 Evaluation of lymphocyte activity and function

The detection of lymphocyte activity and function by MFC mainly includes release of cytotoxic proteins (granzyme, perforin), degranulation (CD107a), expression of surface activation markers (PD1, CD25, CD38, HLA-DR, CD69, etc.) [15, 27, 36, 37], killing ability assays through apoptotic cells detection, expression of death signal molecules (Fas-L or TRAIL) [36, 37], new kinds of nuclear dye to stain dead and live cells in a high throughput format [36, 37, 68], and production of various inflammatory cytokines [4, 25–30, 36, 37].

These tests mainly involve the selection of the cell source for CAR-T and the quality evaluation of the product after successful preparation. Each study may apply a different method, and some studies do not choose MFC method. The advantage of MFC is that it can evaluate cell subsets and effector targets simultaneously [4, 25–30, 36, 37].

The choice of autologous or allogeneic cells for CAR-T has its own advantages and disadvantages. Compared to allogeneic CAR-T cells, autologous CAR-T cells are safer. However, CAR-T cell preparation may be compromised when patients have the following conditions: elderly patients, high tumor load, multiple treatments, low number and poor viability of lymphocytes, etc., in which case other immunotherapeutic products may be chosen [4, 41].

After successful CAR-T preparation, not only the proportion of CAR-positive cells affects the efficacy, but also the killing activity of lymphocytes [34–37].

### 3.2 Detection of CAR-positive cells

This test needs to be repeated as it involves CAR-T product quality evaluation and dynamics assay at different time points. After successful preparation of CAR-T, quality evaluation should be carried out before the infusion. The proportion and count of CAR-positive cells are the most important parts of them [1–4, 21–27, 34, 35]. Values detected by MFC and qPCR are well consistent [22]. Compared with the qPCR method, MFC may have a lower sensitivity [34]. However, MFC has unique advantages. Through multicolor and gating technology, MFC can clearly mark the proliferate, activated, or suppressive subgroups of CAR-T cells [36, 37, 69–75]. In rare cases, MFC can identify CAR-positive transduced leukemic cells [76, 77]. In addition, quality testing can also be carried out to detect other cells in the CAR-T product. The high speed, simplicity, and low cost of MFC facilitate its application in CAR-T studies because these assays need to be repeated.

#### *3.2.1 Selection of CAR detection antibodies*

CAR-positive cells can be detected by MFC using direct or indirect fluorescein-labeled antibodies against their extracellular domain (ECD). Initial clinical studies used sheep anti-mice IgG (polyclonal anti-IgG antibodies), which was not suitable for humanized CAR-T. Anti-idiotype monoclonal antibodies, antigen-Fc, protein L-based assays, and anti-linkers antibodies are commonly used CAR detection methods as well. Each method has different properties and shortcomings. For example, the anti-IgG antibodies and protein L have higher reagent stability but lower specificity to CAR, and antigen-Fc and anti-idiotype antibodies can detect CARs with very high specificity [36, 37, 69–75].

At present, most CAR protein detection antibodies are customized by CAR-T companies resulting in a lack of standardization in the assay. Therefore, an extremely strict quality control is needed for MFC. Firstly, since CAR is an unknown antigen and CAR-positive cells may have a high background because CAR-T cells are often large activated cells, the effect of compensation and fluorescence spillover should be eliminated by fluorescence minus one (FMO) in panel design. Secondly, fluorescence with high brightness should also be selected to reduce the possible false negative results caused by dim fluorescence. Third, in addition to the traditional isotype negative control, a group of cells processed with the same method but without transduction should be added as biological control, while successfully constructed CAR-T cells as a positive control, especially for those with low fluorescence intensity or without a gap between negative and positive cells. Fourth, the exclusion of dead cells and nonspecific binding are carried out by different methods, such as using dead/living cell dyes to exclude dead cells, CD14 to exclude monocytes, and Fc receptors blocking reagent or serum/IgG to eliminate nonspecific binding of IgG1 and IgG2a to Fc fragments. Fifth, the performance of new lots/shipments of antibodies and reagents should be compared with old ones to minimize inter-lot and even inter-shipment differences, which is more important for polyclonal antibodies. Sixth, in addition to strict quality control of MFC, it should also be compared with the qPCR method at the beginning of the study. Last but not the least, it is necessary to use the same antibody panel in one study [21–27, 36, 37, 69–75].

#### *3.2.2 Cellular kinetics at different time points*

After infusion, CAR-T kinetic detection is an important indicator to evaluate its effectiveness and safety. Although a big variety exists in different CAR-T and different studies, regular changes in CAR-T kinetics can be observed. For example, CAR-T cells begin to proliferate *in vivo* 4 days after CD19-CAR-T treatment, peak at 7–19 days, and most of them recover around 28–60 days [1–4, 21, 22]. The indicators reflecting CAR-T cell kinetics include direct (the proportion and number of CAR-positive cells, and concentration of corresponding cytokines) and indirect one (the recovery kinetics of target antigens on cells mentioned in 2.3 above).

At present, data from many clinical trials show that CAR-T proliferation *in vivo* is significantly related to the therapy effect. Compared with patients with ineffective treatment, patients with effective treatment have a much higher CAR-T cell proliferation peak and the area under the curve (AUC) within one month of CAR-T infusion [32–37]. CAR-T < LOD is associated with B-cell recovery, and the consistent result of MFC and PCR has been verified in many studies [21–26, 33–37].

#### *3.2.3 Composition of CAR-positive cells*

MFC can detect the subsets of CAR-T cells (CD4 or CD8), including differentiation (naive, memory, and effector), activation (expression of activation markers), and inhibitory receptors (PD1, Tim3, LAG3, CTLA-4, and TIGIT). These markers may correlate with clinical responses. However, the results of testing the proportion and number of CAR-positive cells in patients at different time points vary greatly. Therefore, the panel varies according to them.

Generally, a relatively detailed panel is chosen when the quality of the product is evaluated before infusion and when the proportion of CAR-positive cells is high in the early post-CAR-T infusion period. However, the basic panel may be chosen for the consideration of price, sample size, and the low concentration of CAR-positive cells. Taking CD19-CAR-T as an example, the basic panel may include CD4, CD8, CD3, CD19, CD16 + CD56, CD45, CAR, and CD14, to evaluate the common lymphocyte composition, CD4/CD8 ratio, residual CD19-positive cells, and recovery kinetics, in addition to accurate detection of CAR-positive cells. Further assays include CD25/CD127 for CD25dim/CD127+ regulatory T cells (Treg) and CD25 high-activated cells. The different effector and memory T subsets are evaluated by using CCR7 (CD197) and CD45 RA, such as naive T cells (TN, CD197+/CD45RA+), central memory T cells (TCM, CD197+/CD45RA−), effector memory T cells (TEM, CD197−/CD45RA−), and effector T cells (TEFF, CD197−/CD45RA+).

If further evaluated, CD38/HLA-DR assay for activated T cells will be added, and CD38+ or HLA-DR + or double-positive (DP) activated subsets can be acquired. Stem cell memory-like T cells (TSCM) expressing markers, such as CD45RA, CCR7 (optional CD62L), CD95, CD27, CD28, CD127, CD11adim, and lacking CD45RO, these cells can be detected by simply adding CD95 to CD197/CD45RA panel. Studies have shown that TSCM has the ability to self-renew and differentiate [22–27, 78]. The immune composition of CAR-T products is associated with antitumor efficacy, and CAR-T cells with TN, TSCM, and TCM phenotypes have been found to have longer *in vivo* persistence and higher antitumor efficacy [32–37]. After infusion, CAR-positive cells are mainly TEM in the expansion phase, which will last in a long term, and TN begins to appear later [22].

It has been found that specific populations of the donor T cells identified by MFC can predict the prognosis, especially T subsets that co-express certain suppressive signals. Finney [36] found that increased frequency of LAG-3+/TNF-αlow CD8+ T cells in PB apheresis product was related to relapse of pediatric B-ALL patients treated with anti-CD19 CAR-T.

High expression of target antigens by tumor cells can effectively stimulate CAR T cell proliferation [36, 37], but high tumor load is in turn a poor prognostic factor for CAR-T [40, 41], the paradox may be caused by the expansion of certain CAR-T subpopulations expressing inhibitory signals hindering CAR-T cell expansion *in vivo* [36, 37, 77, 78].

### *3.2.4 Detection of other cells*

At present most CAR-T cells are derived from the patient's own immune cells, and although most patients' tumor cells will die during *in vitro* culture, there will be some cases in which the tumor cells remain alive or even survive off-target [75–77]. Therefore, a rigorous MRD test of tumor cells should be performed in the quality evaluation of the product. The MRD panel and data analysis should be performed according to the method described in 3.2 above.

### *3.2.5 Absolute counts of CAR-positive cells*

Absolute counting of CAR-T cells can be performed using either a single- or dual-platform method, where the single-platform can be done using the volumetric method or the absolute counting microbeads method [79].

The single-platform method is considered to be more accurate than the dual-platform method and requires less sample volume. However, since the single platform method cannot be washed, there may be a high background signal or failure to correctly detect some antibodies or fluorescent dyes. Therefore, any method can be chosen, but use the same method in a total clinical study, including multicenter studies.

The quality control of CAR-T cell enumeration is referenced to that of CD34+ hematopoietic stem cells [15, 79], with a minimum collection of 100 positive cells, and the LOD and lower limit of quantitation (LLOQ) for MRD assays should be verified. Mostly more than 1,000,000 events are recommended to acquire for detailed analysis of CAR-T cells when the percentages are high, and for accurate enumeration at later time points when the percentages may be down to less than $10^{-4}$ [15, 16, 19, 20]. In the lymphocyte ablation phase, as many as possible cells are acquired, and a minimum of 100,000 cells is recommended [15, 22–26].

### 3.3 Immune cell subsets

Immune cell subset detection has many similarities and overlaps with CAR-T cell detection. Therefore CAR-positive cells can be detected along with the immune cell subset detection before infusion and early days after CAR-T treatment. When CAR expression cells cannot be detected twice in a row, immune subset detection will last for a longer time without CAR antibody [15, 22–26].

Because CAR-T is a kind of immunotherapy, including the specific killing of target antigen-positive cells and nonspecific killing of CAR-negative cells, there is a positive and negative regulation balance between efficacy and side effects. Nowadays 8 or more colors panel are recommended to analyze detailed subsets in CAR positive and negative parts with a similar panel [15, 22–26].

The titration of all monoclonal antibodies is highly recommended before performing actual experiments. An isotype control should be used at the same concentration of the antibody of interest. DAPI or 7AAD or other dye to distinguish live or dead cells may be added. In addition, with the development of immunology, the different configuration of instruments, and the intersection of various antigens, the antibody combination to define the same functional subgroups in different studies maybe not the same, and the detection panels are also very heterogeneous [15, 22–26]. Therefore, it is necessary to adopt a consistent panel in a study, especially a multicenter study.

### 3.4 Cytokine detection

#### *3.4.1 Cytokines*

Due to different processes and cell sources of CAR-T, different cytokines may be produced. For example, CAR-T from PB CD3+ T cells may lead to the formation of multiple cytokines. CD4+ T cell-related factors are IL-2, IL-4, IL-5, IL-10, IL −13, and IL-17, while CAR-T from CD8+ T cells mainly produces IFN-γ, TNF-α, perforin, and granzyme B. CAR-T proliferation and efficacy are related to most important cytokines, so cytokine detection is an important assay for quality evaluation of the product in development process and CAR-T efficacy evaluation after the immunotherapy [26–30, 36, 37, 80, 81].

However, the toxicity of CAR-T is always along with its effectiveness. The most common toxic side effects are cytokine release syndrome (CRS). CRS is caused by the release of a large number of inflammatory factors by activated immune cells. IL-6, IL-1, and IFN-γ are all related to CRS. Any CAR-T or other immune cells that cause IFN-γ to elevate will aggravate CRS, which is more obvious in CRS level ≥ 3 [26, 27, 36, 37, 41]. Each CAR-T study uses cytokines to evaluate the activation characteristics of T cells, and basically includes IL-6, IFN-γ, TNF-α, and IL-2. The selection of other cytokines varies from study to study, including IL-1RA, IL-1β, IL-4, IL-5, IL-8, IL-10, IL-12, IL-13, IL-15, IL-17, IL-18, IL-21, IL-22, IL-23, IL-31, IL-36, monocyte chemoattractant protein (MCP)-1, perforin, granzyme B, erythropoietin, granulocyte/macrophage colony-stimulating factor (GM-CSF), soluble CD25, (sCD25), ferritin, CCL20, REG3a, ST-2, TNFRI, and elafin [1, 4, 26–30, 36, 37, 80, 81].

#### *3.4.2 Cytokine detection method*

Although some studies used enzyme-linked immune sorbent assay (ELISA) [31, 34] or ELISpot assay [82], recently MFC has been used in CAR-T cytokine detection with requirements for more cytokines, or subsets that secrete cytokines. Cytometric bead array (CBA) [28] or couple intracellular cytokines staining [29, 30, 36, 37] are two main kinds of cytokines assay methods by MFC, and each has its own advantages and disadvantages. The advantages of CBA are fast, simple, sensitive, repeatable, flexible, and high throughput, which can detect dozens of cytokines in a short time with rare samples [28]. However, the unique advantage of intracellular cytokines staining lies in the simultaneous detection of cellular immunophenotyping and intracellular cytokines, and it is the only one to allocate cytokines to subsets without the help of cell isolation [29, 30, 36, 37].

Clinical studies can choose one of them, but a complete study, especially a multicenter study, should use the same method from beginning to end because there is a lack of comparability between different methods.

### 3.5 Tumor microenvironment and immune checkpoint detection

TME is a complex network of local immune cells, stromal cells, signaling molecules and cytokines secreted by these cells. In the study of solid tumors, signal networks represented by PD1 and PDL1 have achieved remarkable results in mechanism research and immunotherapy [13, 14, 36, 37, 54]. The immune microenvironment of hematologic malignancies is more complicated. MFC can detect a variety of immune cells and immune signals, so it has become the main research tool in this field in recent years [22–27, 36, 37].

The biggest problem of CAR-T is resistance and relapse [1–7], involving a variety of complex mechanisms [8–14, 34, 35, 40, 41, 66, 67, 72–78], among which the study of immune-suppressive signals and immune microenvironment has been the focus of attention in recent years: (1) T-cell exhaustion, effector T-cell reduction, and the increased expression of inhibiting receptors. The high expression of LAG-3 and PD-1 and low expression of TNF-α in CD8+ T cells are associated with CAR-T loss of function, which will reduce the antitumor ability of CAR-T cells and lead to CD19-positive relapse. Target expression cell recovery in PB is a signal of the weakening of CAR-T cell function. CAR-T exhaustion is one of the factors. In some studies, exhaustion-related signals, such as PD1 (CD279), LAG-3(CD223), CTLA-4(CD152), and Tim3 (CD366), are included in the CAR-T detection panel, hoping to find the role of immune checkpoints, and trying to relieve the inhibitory signals by targeted drugs, such as PD1 monoclonal antibody or PDL1-CAR-T, to acquire long-term OS [13, 14, 54, 72–78]. (2) Immune aging and age-related T-cell quality. With the introduction of theories about immune age and immunosenescence, as well as the discovery of age-related CAR-T cell phenotypes, studies begin to include immunosenescence-related markers. Senescent T cells exhibit some phenotypes, including downregulation of CD27, CD28, and upregulation of CD57, KLRG-1, Tim-3, TIGIT, and CD45RA [83]. The emergence of these phenotypes is a signal of the weakening of CAR-T cells [22–27]. (3) Other signaling-related studies on the antagonization of the CAR-T function. When CD19-negative tumor recurrences, tumor cells may have high expression of CD123, and CD123-CAR-T cell therapy may be effective; it may be related to the increased expression of Bcl-2. Thus, monitoring Bcl-2 in tumor cells and Bcl-2 antagonist treatment in Bcl-2 highly expressed patients may be effective [72–78]. (4) Inhibitive BM microenvironment. Myeloid-derived suppressor cells (MDSC), TAMs, and Treg inhibit CAR-T cell proliferation and function. Detecting these inhibitory signals through MFC contributes to the CAR-T mechanism research. Blocking these signals can restore lymphocyte function. Combined CD30-CAR-T and anti-PD-1 therapy have showed promising results in CD30-positive lymphomas [54].

Similar to immune subsets, there are also some differences in the panels of TME and immune checkpoints. CD15/CD33/CD11b/HLA-DR/CD16/CD4/CD14/CD45 is one recommended panel to detect MDSC subgroups, and CD27, CD28, CD57, and PD1 (optional LAG-3, CTLA-4, and Tim3) may be simple supplements to common immune subsets panel for immune checkpoints and immunosenescence [22–27]. CD123 and Bcl-2 should be added to MRD panel. Similar to the previous requirements, it is necessary to perform quality control, stick to same panel, and keep a high degree of standardization, stability, and good reproducibility.

## 4. Advancement in MFC promote CAR-T study

As technology advances, MFC evolves toward more and more channels, of which mass cytometry and full spectral flow cytometry are two major trends [27, 84]. The traditional MFC is limited by fluorescence channels, so the tumor-related and immune-related assays are basically carried out separately. In future, with the introduction of more than 20 or even 40 multiparameter MFC, it will realize one complicated panel to simultaneously finish the above-related assays, saving costs and samples, and more importantly, obtaining geometric growth of big data information [27, 84].

Other MFC-related latest advances, such as single-cell sequencing, high-dimensional data analysis, and artificial intelligence, will also enter the field of CAR-T research with the application of MFC in CAR-T. These new advances will certainly promote the realization of MFC-assisted CAR-T efficacy-related factor analysis and obtain standardized treatment formula.

Therefore, with the improvement of more clinical information and more detailed MFC data, it is possible for us to obtain a formula for the best performance of CAR-T. We can obtain the prediction of each patient by bringing the number of malignant cells in different patients with different tumors, the sum of all tumor antigen expressions, immunosuppressive signals, and the immune-stimulative and immune-suppressive components of CAR-T subsets into the formula. If the corrective strategies of various inhibitory factors are added to the formula, it is expected that in future we will provide a standardized prediction of prognosis and treatment guidance for obtaining the best curative effect of CAR-T therapy.

## 5. Conclusion

MFC plays a pivotal role in every step of the clinical and development process of CAR-T. The repeated validation of MFC assays with clinical efficacy may obtain the best data in future, which will promote the CAR-T study, to obtain the longest *in vivo* proliferation and duration of CAR-T, the best CR rate, the lowest side effects, and the highest survival rate.

## Conflict of interest

The authors declare no conflict of interest.

## Appendices and nomenclature

| | |
|---|---|
| ALCL | anaplastic large cell lymphoma |
| ALL | acute lymphoblastic leukemia |
| allo-HSCT | allogeneic hematopoietic stem cell transplantation |
| AML | acute myeloid leukemia |
| AUC | area under the curve |
| CAR | chimeric antigen receptor |
| CAR-T | chimeric antigen receptor-modified T-cell |
| CBA | cytometric bead array |
| CR | complete remission |
| CRS | cytokine release syndrome |
| CSF | cerebrospinal fluid |
| DP | double positive |
| ECD | extracellular domain |
| ELISA | enzyme-linked immune sorbent assay |
| FMO | fluorescence minus one |
| GM-CSF | granulocyte/macrophage colony-stimulating factor |
| HL | Hodgkin lymphoma (HL) |
| LLOQ | lower limit of quantitation |
| LOD | lower limit of detection |
| LPD | lymphoproliferative disease |
| MdFI | median fluorescence intensity |
| MDSC | myeloid-derived suppressor cells |
| MFC | multiparametric flow cytometry |
| MFI | mean fluorescence intensity |
| MRD | minimal residual/measurable diseases |
| OS | overall survival |
| SOPs | standard operating procedures |
| TCM | central memory T cells |
| TEFF | effector T cells |
| TEM | effector memory T cells |
| TME | tumor microenvironment |
| TN | naive T cells |
| Treg | regulatory T cells |
| TSCM | stem cell memory-like T cells |

## Author details

Hui Wang[1,2*] and Man Chen[1,2]

1 Hebei Yanda Lu Daopei Hospital, Langfang, China

2 Beijing Lu Daopei Hospital, Beijing, China

*Address all correspondence to: ldpwanghui@163.com

## References

[1] Zhang X, Lu XA, Yang J, et al. Efficacy and safety of anti-CD19 CAR T-cell therapy in 110 patients with B-cell acute lymphoblastic leukemia with high-risk features. Blood Advances. 2020;**4**(10):2325-2338. DOI: 10.1182/bloodadvances.2020001466

[2] Zhao YL, Liu DY, Sun RJ, et al. Integrating CAR T-cell therapy and transplantation: Comparisons of safety and long-term efficacy of allogeneic hematopoietic stem cell transplantation after CAR T-cell or chemotherapy-based complete remission in B-cell acute lymphoblastic leukemia. Frontiers in Immunology. 2021;**12**:605766. DOI: 10.3389/fimmu.2021.605766

[3] Chen M, Fu M, Wang A, et al. Cytoplasmic CD79a is a promising biomarker for B lymphoblastic leukemia follow up post CD19 CAR-T therapy. Leukemia & Lymphoma. 2021;**21**:1-9. DOI: 10.1080/10428194.2021.1980214

[4] Lu P, Liu Y, Yang J, et al. Naturally selected CD7 CAR-T therapy without genetic manipulations for T-ALL/LBL: First-in-human phase 1 clinical trial. Blood. 2022;**140**(4):321-334. DOI: 10.1182/blood.2021014498

[5] Marofi F, Rahman HS, Al-Obaidi ZMJ, et al. Novel CAR T therapy is a ray of hope in the treatment of seriously ill AML patients. Stem Cell Research & Therapy. 2021;**12**(1):465. DOI: 10.1186/s13287-021-02420-8

[6] Jain T, Bar M, Kansagra AJ, et al. Use of chimeric antigen receptor T cell therapy in clinical practice for relapsed/refractory aggressive B cell non-Hodgkin lymphoma: An expert panel opinion from the American Society for Transplantation and Cellular Therapy. Biology of Blood and Marrow Transplantation. 2019;**25**(12):2305-2321. DOI: 10.1016/j.bbmt.2019.08.015

[7] Straathof K, Flutter B, Wallace R, et al. Antitumor activity without on-target off-tumor toxicity of GD2-chimeric antigen receptor T cells in patients with neuroblastoma. Science Translational Medicine. 2020;**12**:eabd6169

[8] Keshavarz A, Salehi A, Khosravi S, et al. Recent findings on chimeric antigen receptor (CAR)-engineered immune cell therapy in solid tumors and hematological malignancies. Stem Cell Research & Therapy. 2022;**13**(1):482. DOI: 10.1186/s13287-022-03163-w

[9] Pearson AD, Rossig C, Mackall C, et al. Paediatric strategy forum for medicinal product development of chimeric antigen receptor T-cells in children and adolescents with cancer: ACCELERATE in collaboration with the European medicines agency with participation of the Food and Drug Administration. European Journal of Cancer. 2022;**160**:112-133. DOI: 10.1016/j.ejca.2021.10.016

[10] Wei J, Han X, Bo J, et al. Target selection for CAR-T therapy. Journal of Hematology & Oncology. 2019;**12**(1):62. DOI: 10.1186/s13045-019-0758-x

[11] Xu X, Huang S, Xiao X, et al. Challenges and clinical strategies of CAR T-cell therapy for acute lymphoblastic leukemia: Overview and developments. Frontiers in Immunology. 2021;**11**:569117. DOI: 10.3389/fimmu.2020.569117

[12] Marvin-Peek J, Savani BN, Olalekan OO, et al. Challenges and advances in chimeric antigen receptor

therapy for acute myeloid leukemia. Cancers (Basel). 2022;**14**(3):497. DOI: 10.3390/cancers14030497

[13] Hou AJ, Chen LC, Chen YY. Navigating CAR-T cells through the solid-tumour microenvironment. Nature Reviews. Drug Discovery. 2021;**20**(7):531-550. DOI: 10.1038/s41573-021-00189-2

[14] Lemoine J, Ruella M, Houot R. Born to survive: How cancer cells resist CAR T cell therapy. Journal of Hematology & Oncology. 2021;**14**(1):199. DOI: 10.1186/s13045-021-01209-9

[15] Piccoli S, Mehta D, Vitaliti A, et al. 2019 white paper on recent issues in bioanalysis: FDA immunogenicity guidance, gene therapy, critical reagents, biomarkers and flow cytometry validation (part 3 - recommendations on 2019 FDA immunogenicity guidance, gene therapy bioanalytical challenges, strategies for critical reagent management, biomarker assay validation, flow cytometry validation & CLSI H62). Bioanalysis. 2019;**11**(24):2207-2244. DOI: 10.4155/bio-2019-0271

[16] Riva G, Nasillo V, Ottomano AM, et al. Multiparametric flow cytometry for MRD monitoring in hematologic malignancies: Clinical applications and new challenges. Cancers (Basel). 2021;**13**(18):4582. DOI: 10.3390/cancers13184582

[17] Bras AE, de Haas V, van Stigt A, et al. CD123 expression levels in 846 acute leukemia patients based on standardized immunophenotyping. Cytometry. Part B, Clinical Cytometry. 2019;**96**(2):134-142. DOI: 10.1002/cyto.b.21745

[18] Haubner S, Perna F, Köhnke T, et al. Coexpression profile of leukemic stem cell markers for combinatorial targeted therapy in AML. Leukemia. 2019;**33**(1):64-74. DOI: 10.1038/s41375-018-0180-3

[19] Cherian S, Miller V, McCullouch V, et al. A novel flow cytometric assay for detection of residual disease in patients with B-lymphoblastic leukemia/lymphoma post anti-CD19 therapy. Cytometry. Part B, Clinical Cytometry. 2018;**94**(1):112-120. DOI: 10.1002/cyto.b.21482

[20] Mikhailova E, Semchenkova A, Illarionova O, et al. Relative expansion of CD19-negative very-early normal B-cell precursors in children with acute lymphoblastic leukaemia after CD19 targeting by blinatumomab and CAR-T cell therapy: Implications for flow cytometric detection of minimal residual disease. British Journal of Haematology. 2021;**193**(3):602-612. DOI: 10.1111/bjh.17382

[21] Sarikonda G, Pahuja A, Kalfoglou C, et al. Monitoring CAR-T cell kinetics in clinical trials by multiparametric flow cytometry: Benefits and challenges. Cytometry. Part B, Clinical Cytometry. 2021;**100**(1):72-78. DOI: 10.1002/cyto.b.21891

[22] Peinelt A, Bremm M, Kreyenberg H, et al. Monitoring of circulating CAR T cells: Validation of a flow cytometric assay, cellular kinetics, and phenotype analysis following Tisagenlecleucel. Frontiers in Immunology. 2022;**13**:830773. DOI: 10.3389/fimmu.2022.830773

[23] Maryamchik E, Gallagher KME, Preffer FI, et al. New directions in chimeric antigen receptor T cell [CAR-T] therapy and related flow cytometry. Cytometry. Part B, Clinical Cytometry. 2020;**98**(4):299-327. DOI: 10.1002/cyto.b.21880

[24] Demaret J, Varlet P, Trauet J, et al. Monitoring CAR T-cells using flow cytometry. Cytometry. Part B, Clinical Cytometry. 2021;**100**(2):218-224. DOI: 10.1002/cyto.b.21941

[25] Sarikonda G, Mathieu M, Natalia M, et al. Best practices for the development, analytical validation and clinical implementation of flow cytometric methods for chimeric antigen receptor T cell analyses. Cytometry. Part B, Clinical Cytometry. 2021;**100**(1):79-91. DOI: 10.1002/cyto.b.21985

[26] Blache U, Weiss R, Boldt A, et al. Advanced flow cytometry assays for immune monitoring of CAR-T cell applications. Frontiers in Immunology. 2021;**12**:658314. DOI: 10.3389/fimmu.2021.658314

[27] Michelozzi IM, Sufi J, Adejumo TA, et al. High-dimensional functional phenotyping of preclinical human CAR T cells using mass cytometry. STAR protocols. 2022;**3**(1):101174. DOI: 10.1016/j.xpro.2022.101174

[28] He P, Tan Z, Wei Z, et al. Co-expressing LRP6 with anti-CD19 CAR-T cells for improved therapeutic effect against B-ALL. Frontiers in Oncology. 2020;**10**:1346. DOI: 10.3389/fonc.2020.01346

[29] Xu C, Yin Y. Measuring chimeric antigen receptor T cells (CAR T cells) activation by coupling intracellular cytokine staining with flow cytometry. Methods in Molecular Biology. 2020;**2108**:159-165. DOI: 10.1007/978-1-0716-0247-8_14

[30] Hombach A, Barden M, Hannappel L, et al. IL12 integrated into the CAR exodomain converts CD8+ T cells to poly-functional NK-like cells with superior killing of antigen-loss tumors. Molecular Therapy. 2022;**30**(2):593-605. DOI: 10.1016/j.ymthe.2021.10.011

[31] Qin H, Cho M, Haso W, et al. Eradication of B-ALL using chimeric antigen receptor-expressing T cells targeting the TSLPR oncoprotein. Blood. 2015;**126**(5):629-639. DOI: 10.1182/blood-2014-11-612903

[32] Kansagra AJ, Frey NV, Bar M, et al. Clinical utilization of chimeric antigen receptor T cells in B cell acute lymphoblastic leukemia: An expert opinion from the European Society for Blood and Marrow Transplantation and the American Society for Blood and Marrow Transplantation. Biology of Blood and Marrow Transplantation. 2019;**25**(3):e76-e85. DOI: 10.1016/j.bbmt.2018.12.068

[33] Castella M, Caballero-Baños M, Ortiz-Maldonado V, et al. Point-of-care CAR T-cell production (ARI-0001) using a closed semi-automatic bioreactor: Experience from an academic phase I clinical trial. Frontiers in Immunology. 2020;**11**:482. DOI: 10.3389/fimmu.2020.00482

[34] Maude SL, Frey N, Shaw PA, et al. Chimeric antigen receptor T cells for sustained remissions in leukemia. The New England Journal of Medicine. 2014;**371**(16):1507-1517. DOI: 10.1056/NEJMoa1407222 Erratum in: The New England Journal of Medicine 2016;374(10):998

[35] Faude S, Wei J, Muralidharan K, et al. Absolute lymphocyte count proliferation kinetics after CAR T-cell infusion impact response and relapse. Blood Advances. 2021;**5**(8):2128-2136. DOI: 10.1182/bloodadvances.2020004038

[36] Finney OC, Brakke HM, Rawlings-Rhea S, et al. CD19 CAR T cell product and disease attributes

predict leukemia remission durability. The Journal of Clinical Investigation. 2019;**129**(5):2123-2132. DOI: 10.1172/JCI125423

[37] Spiegel JY, Patel S, Muffly L, et al. CAR T cells with dual targeting of CD19 and CD22 in adult patients with recurrent or refractory B cell malignancies: A phase 1 trial. Nature Medicine. 2021;**27**(8):1419-1431. DOI: 10.1038/s41591-021-01436-0

[38] Rosenthal J, Naqvi AS, Luo M, et al. Heterogeneity of surface CD19 and CD22 expression in B lymphoblastic leukemia. American Journal of Hematology. 2018;**93**(11):E352-E355. DOI: 10.1002/ajh.25235 PMID: 30058145

[39] Pillai V, Muralidharan K, Meng W, et al. CAR T-cell therapy is effective for CD19-dim B-lymphoblastic leukemia but is impacted by prior blinatumomab therapy. Blood Advances. 2019;**3**(22):3539-3549. DOI: 10.1182/bloodadvances.2019000692

[40] Anagnostou T, Riaz IB, Hashmi SK, et al. Anti-CD19 chimeric antigen receptor T-cell therapy in acute lymphocytic leukaemia: A systematic review and meta-analysis. The Lancet Haematology. 2020;**7**(11):e816-e826. DOI: 10.1016/S2352-3026(20)30277-5

[41] Zhang X, Yang J, Li J, et al. Factors associated with treatment response to CD19 CAR-T therapy among a large cohort of B cell acute lymphoblastic leukemia. Cancer Immunology, Immunotherapy. 2022;**71**(3):689-703. DOI: 10.1007/s00262-021-03009-z

[42] Fry TJ, Shah NN, Orentas RJ, et al. CD22-targeted CAR T cells induce remission in B-ALL that is naive or resistant to CD19-targeted CAR immunotherapy. Nature Medicine. 2018;**24**(1):20-28. DOI: 10.1038/nm.4441

[43] Qin H, Ramakrishna S, Nguyen S, et al. Preclinical development of bivalent chimeric antigen receptors targeting both CD19 and CD22. Molecular Therapy - Oncolytics. 2018;**11**:127-137. DOI: 10.1016/j.omto.2018.10.006

[44] Gomes-Silva D, Srinivasan M, Sharma S, et al. CD7-edited T cells expressing a CD7-specific CAR for the therapy of T-cell malignancies. Blood. 2017;**130**(3):285-296. DOI: 10.1182/blood-2017-01-761320

[45] Li S, Wang X, Yuan Z, et al. Eradication of T-ALL cells by CD7-targeted universal CAR-T cells and initial test of Ruxolitinib-based CRS management. Clinical Cancer Research. 2021;**27**(5):1242-1246. DOI: 10.1158/1078-0432.CCR-20-1271

[46] Shah NN, Johnson BD, Schneider D, et al. Bispecific anti-CD20, anti-CD19 CAR T cells for relapsed B cell malignancies: A phase 1 dose escalation and expansion trial. Nature Medicine. 2020;**26**(10):1569-1575. DOI: 10.1038/s41591-020-1081-3

[47] Scherer LD, Brenner MK, Mamonkin M. Chimeric antigen receptors for T-cell malignancies. Frontiers in Oncology. 2019;**9**:126. DOI: 10.3389/fonc.2019.00126

[48] Mamonkin M, Rouce RH, Tashiro H, et al. A T-cell directed chimeric antigen receptor for the selective treatment of T-cell malignancies. Blood. 2015;**126**(8):983-992. DOI: 10.1182/blood-2015-02-629527

[49] Ou Z, Qiu L, Rong H, et al. Bibliometric analysis of chimeric antigen receptor-based immunotherapy in cancers from 2001 to 2021. Frontiers in Immunology. 2022;**13**:822004. DOI: 10.3389/fimmu.2022.822004

[50] Miao L, Zhang J, Zhang Z, et al. A bibliometric and knowledge-map analysis of CAR-T cells from 2009 to 2021. Frontiers in Immunology. 2022;**13**:840956. DOI: 10.3389/fimmu.2022.840956

[51] Mihályová J, Hradská K, Jelínek T, et al. Promising immunotherapeutic modalities for B-cell lymphoproliferative disorders. International Journal of Molecular Sciences. 2021;**22**(21):11470. DOI: 10.3390/ijms222111470

[52] Ramos CA, Ballard B, Zhang H, et al. Clinical and immunological responses after CD30-specific chimeric antigen receptor-redirected lymphocytes. The Journal of Clinical Investigation. 2017;**127**(9):3462-3471. DOI: 10.1172/JCI94306

[53] Ramos CA, Grover NS, Beaven AW, et al. Anti-CD30 CAR-T cell therapy in relapsed and refractory Hodgkin lymphoma. Journal of Clinical Oncology. 2020;**38**(32):3794-3804. DOI: 10.1200/JCO.20.01342

[54] Sang W, Wang X, Geng H, et al. Anti-PD-1 therapy enhances the efficacy of CD30-directed chimeric antigen receptor T cell therapy in patients with relapsed/refractory CD30+ lymphoma. Frontiers in Immunology. 2022;**13**:858021. DOI: 10.3389/fimmu.2022.858021

[55] Maucher M, Srour M, Danhof S, et al. Current limitations and perspectives of chimeric antigen receptor-T-cells in acute myeloid leukemia. Cancers (Basel). 2021;**13**(24):6157. DOI: 10.3390/cancers13246157

[56] Mardiros A, Santos CD, McDonald T, et al. T cells expressing CD123-specific chimeric antigen receptors exhibit specific cytolytic effector functions and antitumor effects against human acute myeloid leukemia. Blood. 2013;**122**(18):3138-3148. DOI: 10.1182/blood-2012-12-474056

[57] Bonifant CL, Szoor A, Torres D, et al. CD123-engager T cells as a novel immunotherapeutic for acute myeloid leukemia. Molecular Therapy. 2016;**24**(9):1615-1626. DOI: 10.1038/mt.2016.116

[58] Qin H, Yang L, Chukinas JA, et al. Systematic preclinical evaluation of CD33-directed chimeric antigen receptor T cell immunotherapy for acute myeloid leukemia defines optimized construct design. Journal for Immunotherapy of Cancer. 2021;**9**(9):e003149. DOI: 10.1136/jitc-2021-003149

[59] Pollard JA, Loken M, Gerbing RB, et al. CD33 expression and its association with Gemtuzumab Ozogamicin response: Results from the randomized phase III Children's oncology group trial AAML0531. Journal of Clinical Oncology. 2016;**34**(7):747-755. DOI: 10.1200/JCO.2015.62.6846

[60] Willier S, Rothämel P, Hastreiter M, et al. CLEC12A and CD33 coexpression as a preferential target for pediatric AML combinatorial immunotherapy. Blood. 2021;**137**(8):1037-1049. DOI: 10.1182/blood.2020006921

[61] Miao L, Zhang Z, Ren Z, et al. Obstacles and coping strategies of CAR-T cell immunotherapy in solid tumors. Frontiers in Immunology. 2021;**12**:687822. DOI: 10.3389/fimmu.2021.687822

[62] Kast J, Nozohouri S, Zhou D, et al. Recent advances and clinical pharmacology aspects of chimeric antigen receptor (CAR) T-cellular therapy development. Clinical and Translational Science. 2022;**15**(9):2057-2074. DOI: 10.1111/cts.13349

[63] Dasyam N, George P, Weinkove R. Chimeric antigen receptor T-cell therapies: Optimising the dose. British Journal of Clinical Pharmacology. 2020;**86**(9):1678-1689. DOI: 10.1111/bcp.14281

[64] Clé DV, Hirayama AV, Alencar AJ, et al. Associação Brasileira de Hematologia, Hemoterapia e Terapia Celular consensus on genetically modified cells. I: Structuring centers for the multidisciplinary clinical administration and management of CAR-T cell therapy patients. Hematology, Transfusion and Cell Therapy. 2021;**43**(Suppl 2):S3-S12. DOI: 10.1016/j.htct.2021.09.001

[65] Hay KA, Gauthier J, Hirayama AV, et al. Factors associated with durable EFS in adult B-cell ALL patients achieving MRD-negative CR after CD19 CAR T-cell therapy. Blood. 2019;**133**(15):1652-1663. DOI: 10.1182/blood-2018-11-883710

[66] Khan M, Maker AV, Jain S. The evolution of Cancer immunotherapy. Vaccines (Basel). 2021;**9**(6):614. DOI: 10.3390/vaccines9060614

[67] Strati P, Varma A, Adkins S, et al. Hematopoietic recovery and immune reconstitution after axicabtagene ciloleucel in patients with large B-cell lymphoma. Haematologica. 2021;**106**(10):2667-2672. DOI: 10.3324/haematol.2020.254045

[68] Rabinovich PM, Zhang J, Kerr SR, et al. A versatile flow-based assay for immunocyte-mediated cytotoxicity. Journal of Immunological Methods. 2019;**474**:112668. DOI: 10.1016/j.jim.2019.112668

[69] Xu Y, Zhang M, Ramos CA, et al. Closely related T-memory stem cells correlate with in vivo expansion of CAR.CD19-T cells and are preserved by IL-7 and IL-15. Blood. 2014;**123**(24):3750-3759. DOI: 10.1182/blood-2014-01-552174

[70] Turtle CJ, Hanaf LA, Berger C, et al. CD19 CAR-T cells of defined CD4+:CD8+ composition in adult B cell ALL patients. The Journal of Clinical Investigation. 2016;**126**(6):2123-2138. DOI: 10.1172/JCI85309

[71] Sommermeyer D, Hudecek M, Kosasih PL, et al. Chimeric antigen receptor-modified T cells derived from defined CD8+ and CD4+ subsets confer superior antitumor reactivity in vivo. Leukemia. 2016;**30**(2):492-500. DOI: 10.1038/leu.2015.247

[72] Locke FL, Rossi JM, Neelapu SS, et al. Tumor burden, inflammation, and product attributes determine outcomes of axicabtagene ciloleucel in large B-cell lymphoma. Blood Advances. 2020;**4**(19):4898-4911. DOI: 10.1182/bloodadvances.2020002394

[73] Yan ZX, Li L, Wang W, et al. Clinical efficacy and tumor microenvironment influence in a dose-escalation study of anti-CD19 chimeric antigen receptor T cells in refractory B-cell non-Hodgkin's lymphoma. Clinical Cancer Research. 2019;**25**(23):6995-7003. DOI: 10.1158/1078-0432.CCR-19-0101

[74] de Azevedo JTC, Mizukami A, Moço PD, et al. Immunophenotypic analysis of CAR-T cells. Methods in Molecular Biology. 2020;**2086**:195-201. DOI: 10.1007/978-1-0716-0146-4_14

[75] Deng Q, Han G, Puebla-Osorio N, et al. Characteristics of anti-CD19 CAR T cell infusion products associated with efficacy and toxicity in patients with large B cell lymphomas. Nature Medicine. 2020;**26**(12):1878-1887. DOI: 10.1038/s41591-020-1061-7

[76] Ruella M, Xu J, Barrett DM, et al. Induction of resistance to chimeric

antigen receptor T cell therapy by transduction of a single leukemic B cell. Nature Medicine. 2018;**24**(10):1499-1503. DOI: 10.1038/s41591-018-0201-9

[77] Song MK, Park BB, Uhm JE. Resistance mechanisms to CAR T-cell therapy and overcoming strategy in B-cell hematologic malignancies. International Journal of Molecular Sciences. 2019;**20**(20):5010. DOI: 10.3390/ijms20205010

[78] Tantalo DG, Oliver AJ, von Scheidt B, et al. Understanding T cell phenotype for the design of effective chimeric antigen receptor T cell therapies. Journal for Immunotherapy of Cancer. 2021;**9**(5):e002555. DOI: 10.1136/jitc-2021-002555

[79] Murugesan M, Nair CK, Nayanar SK, et al. Flow cytometric enumeration of CD34+ hematopoietic stem cells: A comparison between single- versus dual-platform methodology using the International Society of Hematotherapy and Graft Engineering protocol. Asian Journal of Transfusion Science. 2019;**13**(1):43-46. DOI: 10.4103/ajts.AJTS_83_18

[80] Jin J, Cheng J, Huang M, et al. Fueling chimeric antigen receptor T cells with cytokines. American Journal of Cancer Research. 2020;**10**(12):4038-4055

[81] Lee DW, Santomasso BD, Locke FL, et al. ASTCT consensus grading for cytokine release syndrome and neurologic toxicity associated with immune effector cells. Biology of Blood and Marrow Transplantation. 2019;**25**(4):625-638. DOI: 10.1016/j.bbmt.2018.12.758

[82] Ma N, Liu H, Zhang Y, et al. Identification of CD8+ T-cell epitope from multiple myeloma-specific antigen AKAP4. Frontiers in Immunology. 2022;**13**:927804. DOI: 10.3389/fimmu.2022.927804

[83] Lian J, Yue Y, Yu W, et al. Immunosenescence: A key player in cancer development. Journal of Hematology & Oncology. 2020;**13**(1):151. DOI: 10.1186/s13045-020-00986-z

[84] Chen M, Fu M, Zhao W, Wang A, Wu X, Gong M, et al. Full spectral flow cytometry analysis of the bone marrow immune cells in patients with myelodysplastic syndrome. International Journal of Laboratory Hematology. 11 Aug 2022. DOI: 10.1111/ijlh.13945. PMID: 35950633 [Epub ahead of print]

Section 4

# Immune Related Adverse Events in Immunotherapy

Chapter 9

# The Flip of the Coin of Personalized Cancer Immunotherapy: A Focused Review on Rare Immune Checkpoint Related Adverse Effects

*Nabil E. Omar, Hebatalla M. Afifi, Arwa O. Sahal, Rana Mekkawi and Hazem Elewa*

## Abstract

Immune checkpoint inhibitors (ICIs) are a type of cancer immunotherapy that has provided a tremendous breakthrough in the field of oncology. Currently approved checkpoint inhibitors target the cytotoxic T-lymphocyte-associated protein 4 (CTLA4), programmed death receptor-1 (PD-1), and programmed death-ligand 1(PD-L1). One of the most known complications of these advances is the emergence of a new spectrum of immune-related adverse events (irAEs). In this chapter, we will focus on selected rare or very rare irAEs, shedding the light on the other side of the coin of personalized cancer immunotherapy. We will also discuss general management approach of irAEs with an in-depth look on each one of these rare irAEs. The chapter will also cover principles of immunotherapy rechallenge post-occurrence of irAEs, and the impact of irAEs incidence on the efficacy of ICI. We will discuss some of the rare or very rare irAEs including cutaneous irAEs, immune-mediated Hypophysitis, hematological irAEs, ophthalmic irAEs, checkpoint inhibitor pneumonitis (CIP), neurologic irAEs, infectious irAEs, and cardiac irAEs. This chapter tried to highlight the significance of identifying emerging rare and very rare irAEs while considering initial assessments and management approaches identified in various clinical practice guideline and primary literature data.

**Keywords:** immune checkpoint inhibitors, adverse effects, pharmacovigilance, rare, irAEs, cancer immunotherapy

## 1. Introduction

Immune evasion or the ability to evade immune recognition is one of the hallmarks of cancer growth. Cancer cells are able to spread uninhibited by avoiding detection [1] and from that prospective immunotherapy medications were developed and revolutionized the field of oncology. They have been considered the most important development in cancer treatment over the past decade. With recent advancements in immunology and cancer biology, new classes of immunomodulatory therapy have been developed to aid tumor management [2]. Among the most important targeted pathways of this line of therapy is the inhibition of the cytotoxic T-lymphocyte-associated protein (CTLA-4) and programmed death-1 (PD-1) immune checkpoint. Numerous studies have highlighted the significantly improved survival with the use of immunomodulatory therapy in locally advanced and metastatic cancers including melanoma, lung cancer, urothelial cancer, gastric cancer, renal and hepatocellular carcinoma, and other solid tumors. Trials in other malignancies are ongoing, and undoubtedly the number of drugs in this space will grow beyond the drugs currently approved [2].

Current approved immunotherapy agents are nivolumab, pembrolizumab, cemiplimab, and dostarlimab; all which target PD-1. Moreover, atezolizumab, avelumab, and durvalumab, all of which target programmed death lingand-1 (PDL-1). While ipilimumab is the only drug that targets CTLA-4 [3]. One of the most known complication of these advances is the emergence of a new spectrum of immune-related adverse events (irAEs). Such toxicities are known to be distinctly different from classical chemotherapy-induced adverse events [4–7].

## 2. Mechanism of immune-related adverse events

The mechanism of irAEs remains unclear; however, it is believed to be related to the immune dysregulation caused by immune checkpoint inhibitors (ICI) [8]. Four potential mechanisms leading to the development of irAEs have been postulated. Firstly, increasing T-cell activity against antigens that are present in tumors and healthy tissues. Secondly, increasing levels of pre-existing autoantibodies. Thirdly, increasing level of inflammatory cytokines. Finally, the direct binding of an antibody against CTLA-4 with CTLA-4 expressed on normal tissues that results in enhanced complement-mediated inflammation [7, 9].

irAEs occur in nearly 90% of patients who are receiving CTLA-4 inhibitors, 70% of patients who are receiving anti-PD-1 or anti-PD-L1, and approximately all patients treated with combined therapy [10–19]. Severity of most of the reported irAEs is grade 1–2. For patients treated with CTLA-4 inhibitors, irAEs mostly involve the skin (44%), gastrointestinal tract (35%), endocrine system (6%), and liver (5%). Although severe irAEs remain rare, they can become life-threatening if not anticipated and managed appropriately [10–20].

The frequency of treatment-related adverse events in general was classified by the World Health Organization as follow: common toxicities arise at the rate of >1% (>1 in 100), uncommon toxicities of 1–0.1% (1 in 100 to 1 in 1000), rare toxicities at a rate of 0.1–0.01% (1 in 1000 to 1 in 10,000), and very rare toxicities at a rate of less than 0.01% [21].

In this chapter we will focus on selected rare or very rare irAEs, shedding the light on the other side of the coin of personalized cancer immunotherapy. We will also discuss general management approach of irAEs with an in-depth look on each one of these rare irAEs. The chapter will also cover principles of immunotherapy rechallenge post occurrence of irAEs, and the impact of irAEs incidence on the efficacy of ICI.

## 3. General treatment approach of immune-related adverse events

In general, treatment is based on the severity of the observed toxicity defined according to Common Terminology Criteria for Adverse Events Version 5.0, (CTCAEs v5) [22]. For most of patients with moderate (grade 2) irAEs, treatment with ICI should be withheld and should not be resumed until toxicity becomes grade 1 or less. In addition, systemic glucocorticoid should be started if symptoms did not resolve within 1 week. For patients with severe (grade 3) or life-threatening (grade 4) irAEs, treatment with ICI should be permanently discontinued and higher doses of systemic glucocorticoid should be given. Glucocorticoids can be tapered gradually over a minimum duration of 1 month when symptoms subside to grade 1 or less. Use of other immunosuppressive agents such as infliximab, vedolizumab, mycophenolate mofetil can be considered in case of refractory toxicity to glucocorticoids [5, 20].

## 4. Principles of immunotherapy rechallenge post occurrence of immune-related adverse events

Caution should be considered upon resumption of immunotherapy especially after a severe irAE. After rechallenging with ICI, close follow-up should be performed to monitor for symptoms recurrence [23]. Permanent discontinuation of the ICI is warranted if the ICI is re-challenged and toxicity recur [5, 24, 25]. Prior to re-challenge, patient's tumor status should be assessed. Due to risk of toxicity recurrence following the resumption of the ICI, re-challenge can be considered if the response was partially or fully achieved [26]. A consultation with the irAEs designated specialists might be appropriate before immunotherapy re-challenge.

## 5. Association of immunotherapy toxicities with efficacy in patients treated with immune checkpoint inhibitors

After a comparison between patients with and without irAEs, it has been noticed that irAEs are associated with either improved efficacy of immunotherapy in terms of favorable response rates and prolonged survival or similar efficacy [27–29]. The interpretation of this finding is that the immune system is sufficiently activated to target patient's cancer and further cause irAEs [30].

In a retrospective analysis that assessed nivolumab efficacy in melanoma patients, treatment-related adverse events of any grade were associated with higher tumor objective response rate (ORR), but no progression-free survival benefit [31]. In patients receiving anti PD-1 or anti PD-L-1 medications an analysis was done on seven trials including 1747 patients on the association between adverse events and outcome, an increase in overall survival was seen in patients with reported adverse events compared to those with no related immune mediated adverse events [27]. It was also concluded in this trial that the relationship between outcome and reported adverse events did not seem to be due to the increased duration of exposure in responding patients [27]. Nevertheless, in a retrospective multicenter study, cumulative time-adjusted risk of disease progression and cumulative time-adjusted risk of death according to both the early-irAEs ($\leq$12 months) and late-irAEs (>12 months) occurrence revealed no statistically significant differences [29].

While in case of high grade rare irAEs; grade 3 or more rare irAEs were associated with inferior overall survival and no impact on PFS [32].

From our point of view, more studies should be done to have a solid conclusion regarding the correlation between immunotherapy toxicities and their favorable impact on patients.

In this chapter we will discuss some of the rare or very rare irAEs including cutaneous irAEs, immune mediated Hypophysitis, hematological irAEs, ophthalmic irAEs, checkpoint inhibitor pneumonitis (CIP), neurologic irAEs, infectious irAEs and cardiac irAEs.

## 6. Cutaneous immune-related adverse events

Cutaneous irAEs might affect more than half of patients receiving ICI [12]. They are considered the most common toxicity in patients receiving immunotherapy, and out of all irAEs, cutaneous toxicities usually manifest first [33, 34]. The most widely reported dermatological toxicities are inflammatory skin reaction, rash, pruritus, and vitiligo. Rates of cutaneous irAEs were mostly similar in patients receiving anti-PD-1 antibodies and those receiving anti- CTLA-4 antibodies [33]. Severe irAEs were reported more frequently with combination therapy of anti-PD-1 plus anti-CTLA-4 than with monotherapy with either class of agents [35].

The spectrum of irAEs can be categorized into auto-inflammatory and auto-immune responses. Auto-inflammatory side effects are usually nonspecific upregulations of the innate immune system. However, most of the cutaneous irAEs are autoimmune responses. Thus, they represent a more specific activation of adaptive immunity [33]. Cutaneous, autoimmune diseases occur more frequently with anti-PD-1/programmed cell death ligand 1 (PD-L1) than with anti-CTLA-4 therapy [32].

A pooled analysis of mucocutaneous irAEs revealed rare toxicities including urticaria, photosensitivity reactions, xerosis, stomatitis, changes in hair color, alopecia areata and hyperhidrosis [33]. Other reported cutaneous presentations included: ICI-induced dermatomyositis, drug response with eosinophilia and granulomatous, lichenoid, panniculitis-like and lupus-like reactions [36, 37]. For patients with psoriasis, episodes of exacerbation have been reported in patients receiving pembrolizumab, nivolumab or durvalumab [38]. In a single centre experience rare dermatological irAEs were reported as single cases of pemphigoid and bullous dermatitis respectively [32]. Other reported cutaneous irAEs that occurred rarely were vasculitis, neutrophilic dermatosis, erythema nodosum [39–41]. Keratoacanthoma specifically pembrolizumab induced keratoacanthoma type squamous cell carcinoma was reported with a description of eruptive or reactive morphologies [42]. Severe cutaneous irAEs are considered rare. They include Stevens-Johnson syndrome (SJS), toxic epidermal necrolysis (TEN), drug reaction with eosinophilia and systemic symptoms (DRESS), and acute generalized exanthematous pustulosis (AGEP) [43–46].

## 7. Treatment of cutaneous immune-related adverse events

The treatment of cutaneous irAEs follows the standard treatment of irAEs.

Treatment of mild to moderate pruritis or maculopapular rash is topical emollient, oral antihistamine for pruritus, and topical steroids to affected areas. For moderate cutaneous toxicities, if unresponsive to topical steroids within 1 week, prednisone

0.5 mg/kg/day should be considered [38]. Treatment of severe cutaneous irAEs include the administration of topical and systemic steroids and dermatology consultation. For patients with severe pruritis, gabapentinoids and phototherapy can be considered, intravenous immunoglobulin (IVIG) can be given to severe cases of bullous dermatitis, TEN and SJS [5]. Conservative treatment with cryotherapy, intralesional steroids, electrodessication, curettage, and excision were done for patients having keratoacanthoma [42].

Grade 1 and 2 cutaneous irAEs do not require holding the ICI. However, Immunotherapy should be held in case of severe cutaneous toxicities. In case of severe or life-threatening bullous disease, SJS or TEN. ICI should be permanently discontinued [5]. ICI can be re-challenged if the patient's symptoms have resolved to ≤ grade 1. However, permanent discontinuation of immunotherapy should be warranted in the setting of severe or life-threatening bullous disease (grade 3–4), including all cases of SJS and TEN [5].

## 8. Immune mediated hypophysitis

It is not uncommon for patients receiving immunotherapy to suffer from endocrinopathies, the most common is hypothyroidism [4]. Central adrenal insufficiency and autoimmune diabetes mellitus are extremely rare adverse events related to ICI. Central adrenal insufficiency can be life threatening when it is severe as it is associated with severe electrolyte disturbance, dehydration, and hypoglycemia [7, 32, 34, 47, 48]. Another well-known endocrine irAE is hypophysitis. Hypophysitis is the inflammation of the pituitary gland (the anterior lobe of the hypophysis) [49].

Hypophysitis was known to be a rare condition, however, with ICI therapy it has become more common [50]. The incidence of hypophysitis was found to be more in patients receiving anti-CLTA-4 therapy as compared to patients receiving anti-PD-1 therapy [51]. It has been reported that hypophysitis occurs in up to 10% of patients receiving anti-CTLA-4 therapy [50, 51]. This might be because pituitary cells can express CTLA-4, thus, anti-CTLA-4 therapy can cause direct damage to the pituitary gland [52, 53]. Furthermore, the incidence of hypophysitis increases with combination ICI therapy compared to ICI monotherapy [50, 51]. Beside the type of ICI therapy, male gender is another risk factor for hypophysitis mainly with anti-CTLA-4 [54]. The onset of hypophysitis is typically 2–3 months after initiation of ICI therapy, however, it may occur even later, and it has been reported 19 months after initiation of therapy [55].

Hypophysitis is generally manifested with vague symptoms. These symptoms include mild fatigue, arthralgias, and behavioral changes. Severe headache and visual changes may also occur. Because the symptoms are non-specific, hypophysitis might be under-diagnosed [5, 20].

Since enlargement of the pituitary gland is rare, the diagnosis of hypophysitis is recommended to be based on clinical presentation and hormonal evaluation rather than imaging [56]. The main consequence of ICI Hypophysitis is deficiency in one or more pituitary hormones. The most reported deficiencies are central adrenal insufficiency, central hypothyroidism, and hypogonadotropic hypogonadism. Around 80% of patients with ICI-induced hypophysitis present with one or more of these deficiencies [52, 53, 55].

Hypophysitis grading depends on the severity of symptoms and can be divided into asymptomatic or mild, moderate but hemodynamically stable, and severe mass effect or severe hypoadrenalism. Hypophysitis is managed according to the symptoms and hormonal deficiency identified upon presentation. Asymptomatic and mild vague symptoms with no headache does not indicate an interruption of ICI therapy. In such patients, ICI therapy is continued with appropriate hormonal replacement therapy (HRT). On the other hand, patients with mild symptoms (no visual disturbance and no electrolyte imbalance) but hemodynamically stable are recommended to withhold ICI therapy. In addition, oral prednisolone might be initiated. Finally, for severe mass effect symptoms or severe hypoadrenalism, holding ICI therapy and starting IV prednisolone are recommended. In most cases, ICI therapy can be continued. However, most of the patients will require long-term HRT [5, 20, 57].

## 9. Hematological immune-related adverse events

Hematological irAEs are considered rare in patients receiving ICIs, however, a variety of hematological related toxicities have been reported [58]. These include antibody-mediated hemolytic anemia, thrombotic thrombocytopenic purpura, acquired hemophilia A, autoimmune neutropenia, pancytopenia and autoimmune thrombocytopenia [59–64]. Interestingly, cross-reactions that provoke autoimmune thrombocytopenia after sequential treatment with nivolumab and ipilimumab have been described, this might indicate that the same or similar irAEs might re-emerge on subsequent treatment with a different class of agents [64].

A worth mentioning extremely rare adverse effect is hemophagocytic lymphohistiocytosis (HLH) as it is life threating with a high mortality rate and considered to be a serious complication [65]. Therefore, a patient presenting with severe inflammatory syndrome with associated fever, cytopenias and splenomegaly should prompt a full clinical work- up, including analysis of bone marrow aspirates and/or biopsy samples for the presence of hemophagocytic signs [65].

## 10. Ophthalmic immune-related adverse events

Ophthalmic toxicity induced by ICI occur in less than 1% of patients treated with ICI therapy [66]. Ocular irAEs can be divided into ocular inflammation, orbital inflammation, and retinal and choroidal disease [67]. The most common ocular irAEs are dry eyes and uveitis. Dry eye syndrome could be severe enough to cause corneal perforation. Uveitis is a type of ocular inflammation and might be anterior, posterior, or panuveitis. Symptoms of uveitis include eye redness, pain, floaters, photophobia, and blurred vision [68]. In patient treated with ICI therapy, dry eye syndrome occurs at a rate of 1–24%. While the incidence of uveitis caused by ICI therapy is reported to range from less than 1% up to 6% [66, 69].

The risk factors of ocular toxicity induced by ICI agents include the type of ICI and the type of cancer [66]. Clinical cases reported that patients on anti-CTLA-4 agents showed higher incidence and severity of ophthalmic toxicity as compared to patients on PD-1/PDL1 inhibitors [67, 70]. Furthermore, ocular toxicity was found to occur more often in melanoma than other solid cancers. This can be explained by the fact of the presence of cross-reactivity between normal choroidal melanocytes and malignant melanoma [70].

Ocular toxicity should be properly recognized and accurately managed because untreated ocular toxicities may lead to vision loss [71, 72]. The treatment of ocular toxicity depends on the severity of the side effect. Anterior uveitis is treated using topical corticosteroids. While more severe side effects such as ocular inflammation and orbital inflammation are indications for systemic corticosteroids. Artificial tears and other over-the-counter medication can be as symptomatic treatment when it is clinically indicated [5, 68].

## 11. Immune mediated pneumonitis

One of the worrisome irAEs is the checkpoint inhibitor pneumonitis (CIP). CIP is a term used to refer to pneumonitis induced by ICI. CIP is defined as the occurrence of respiratory signs or symptoms related to new emerging inflammatory lesions viewed on chest computed tomography (CT) after ICI treatment and after exclusion of pulmonary infection, tumor progression, and other reasons [73].

The incidence of CIP was reported to be between 3% and 5% with a fatality rate between 10% and 17%. However, a higher incidence of pneumonitis was noted in patients with non-small cell lung cancer (NSCLC) and renal cell carcinoma (RCC) and in patients treated with combination therapy [74, 75]. The median time to the onset of CIP is approximately 2.8 months post-initiation of ICI, and the overall range spans from 9 days to 19.2 months [76].

Some risk factors may predispose patients to develop pneumonitis with ICI therapy. An example of these risk factor is the type of ICI therapy. Patients receiving anti-PD-1 were found to be at increased risk of CIP as compared to patients on anti-CTLA-4 inhibitors. Other risk factors include combination therapy, cancer's primary site, and prior thoracic radiotherapy. In addition, recent literature indicates that a history of asthma and/or smoking may increase the risk of CIP [9, 77].

CIP can manifest as acute, subacute, chronic, and occult. Dyspnea, cough, and decreased activity tolerance are the most common symptoms of CIP. Sometimes, patient may present with chest pain or fever. For patients presenting with fever, the possibility of infectious pneumonia must be excluded. The main signs of CIP include elevation of inflammatory markers such as C-reactive protein and erythrocyte sedimentation rate in most cases. In some patients, velcro crackles can be heard in the lungs on physical examination [73, 74, 76].

The grading of CIP is mainly based on the severity of signs and symptoms. Grade 1 (G1) is referred to asymptomatic or clinically observed CIP only. When common symptoms occur such as shortness of breath and cough, pneumonitis would be graded as grade 2 (G2). While grade (G3) is referred to pneumonitis manifested as severe symptoms that are limiting the activities of daily living. Finally, life-threatening difficulty in breathing would be defined as Grade 4 (G4) pneumonitis [5, 68, 70].

The main therapeutic modality for CIP is corticosteroids as recommended by guidelines on immunotherapy-related toxicity. If no remission is observed after 48 hours, the specific management approach based on the grade should be followed. G1 pneumonitis is managed by delaying the immunotherapy and monitoring symptoms every 2–3 days; in case of worsening, it should be treated as grade 2. While G2 pneumonitis is treated by withholding ICI therapy and initiating an empirical antibiotic in case infection is suspected. If there is no evidence of infection and no improvement occurred within 48 hours, prednisone should be added; if there is no improvement, it should be treated as G3. In G3 and G4 pneumonitis, ICI therapy should be permanently discontinued, and patient should be admitted to the hospital and should be covered with empirical antibiotic. In case there is worsening or no improvement after 48 hours, IV steroids should be continued, and initiation of infliximab (or mycophenolate mofetil in case of hepatic toxicity) is recommended [5, 68, 76, 78, 79].

The decision to reintroduce the same ICI therapy in a patient who has recovered from CIP must be made based on the individual agent, the severity of the reaction, and the availability of alternative therapies. Patients with G2 pneumonitis can be re-challenged with the same ICI therapy once symptoms are resolved. However, these patients must be monitored closely and more frequently. Mainly all patients with history of CIP require careful and close monitoring because recurrent CIP has been observed in some patients even if they have not been re-challenged with ICI therapy [23, 26, 57].

## 12. Neurologic immune-related adverse events

Some irAEs such as neurological toxicities recognition and diagnosis is very challenging [80]. There are limited reported data describing neurological manifestations associated with ICI use, with extrapolated incidence of 1–5% highlighting difficult neurotoxicity recognition and possible underreporting [81, 82].

Commonly reported immune relates neurological or neuromuscular toxicities included myasthenia gravis, peripheral neuropathy, multiple sclerosis, Guillain-Barre syndrome, immune-medicated myopathies and encephalitis/meningitis [62, 63, 81–83]. Early recognition and prompt management of immune related neurotoxicity might prevent severe and/or permanent consequences or uncommonly reported fatalities [84].

A common mechanism of irAEs include T-cell activation by the deactivation of inhibitory regulators. However, there is no clear explanation why some patients develop more immune-related neurotoxicity than others [8, 52].

Median time to onset of serious neurological irAEs, of any grade, was 45 days form ICI initiation in melanoma patients with median time to toxicity resolution of 32 days [82].

### 12.1 Encephalitis

Among neurological manifestations associated with ICI use, encephalitis is considered a rare adverse event with a challenging diagnosis [82, 84]. Although, there is no clear causes of immune mediate encephalitis, around 40–70% of cases were linked to infectious etiologies [85]. On that basis, individualized diagnostic approach to immune associated encephalitis is recommended considering identified clinical presentation. Altered mental status, fever, headache, weakness, neck stiffness, sleepiness, hallucinations or seizure among other neurological sequalae of immune mediate encephalitis were reported by affected patients [82].

With no specified encephalitis grading, initial assessment for suspected immune mediated encephalitis includes neurologist consultation, brain magnetic resonance imaging (MRI), lumbar puncture, electroencephalogram (EEG) to evaluate for subclinical seizures, in addition to complete blood count (CBC), comprehensive metabolic panel (CMP) and autoimmune encephalopathy and paraneoplastic panel [5, 68].

Pertaining to encephalitis associated fatalities, permanent discontinuation of suspected ICI is generally recommended [84]. In-patient admission is warranted for grade 3–4 encephalitis. Corticosteroid trial in the form of methylprednisolone could be administered and then tapered over 4 weeks upon resolving of symptoms. Enhanced symptoms severity or progression over 24 hours, requires higher doses of methylprednisolone for 3–5 days with IVIG or plasmapheresis. Rituximab may be considered if minimal or no symptoms improvement was obtained after 7–14 days or in cases of positive autoimmune encephalopathy antibody [5, 68]. Additional therapy such as empirical antibiotics and antivirals could be utilized as well. Empiric antiepileptics are reasonable to address any seizure concerns [81, 84].

### 12.2 Aseptic meningitis

Immune related meningitis is poorly differentiated from encephalitis, mainly in metastatic cancer patients treated with ICI with newly presented seizures or impaired cognitive functions [86, 87].

Unlike, immune medicated encephalitis that is more associated with anti-PD-1 treatment, meningitis is linked particularly with ipilimumab (CTLA-4 inhibitor) use [86, 87]. National Comprehensive Cancer Network (NCCN) 2022 guideline recommended initial assessment involves brain MRI, with or without contrast, lumbar puncture when feasible while considering neurologist consultation [5]. Management of ICI induced meningitis do not significantly differ from encephalitis. Withholding ICI is recommended in mild to moderate toxicity conditions, while permanent discontinuation is required in severe case as per NCCN guideline. Corticosteroids may be considered after ruling out suspected bacterial or viral infections [5].

Rechallenging of ICI after suffering immune medicated meningitis was suggested in cases of mild to moderate toxicity grades while assuring complete symptoms resolution before re-starting immunotherapy agent [5].

### 12.3 Myasthenia gravis

Immune-mediated myasthenia gravis is an emerging neurologic irAE [88]. Immune-mediated myasthenia gravis induced by ICI use can occur earlier compared to other neurological irAEs (29 vs. up to 80 days) [87].

Concurrent myositis and/or myocarditis are frequently noticed along with immune associated myasthenia gravis, unlike isolated presentation of other immune related neurotoxicity [86, 87].

NCCN 2022 guideline recommend testing for erythrocyte sedimentation rate (ESR), C-reactive protein (CRP), creatinine phosphokinase (CPK), aldolase and anti-striational antibodies, pulmonary function, electromyography (EMG) and considering neurologist consultation while assessing suspected immune-mediated myasthenia gravis. Brain MRI may be considered based on presented symptoms and mainly to rule out central nervous system involvement in disease state. Acetylcholine receptor antibodies testing is not mandated for diagnosis [5].

Upon assessment of toxicity, immune mediated myasthenia graves grading is divided into moderate (grade 2) or severe (grade 3–4).

Regardless of grading, permanent discontinuation of ICI should be carried with immune mediated myasthenia gravis. In-patient care to manage patient symptoms is needed while considering intensive care unit in severe cases. In moderate grade of myasthenia gravis induced by ICI, pyridostigmine and low dose corticosteroids could be initiated. In severe cases or grades 3–4, higher doses of steroids, and initiation of IVIG or plasmapheresis are recommended. Rituximab may be adder in cases of refractory symptoms to IVIG or plasmapheresis [5, 68].

Rechallenging of ICI remains controversial after immune medicated myasthenia gravis, however data of safe re-initiation after complete resolution of symptoms is suggested [89].

## 13. Infectious immune-related adverse events

### 13.1 Mycobacterium tuberculosis activation/reactivation

Extended immune response modulation as a response to ICI therapy in addition to administered corticosteroids and/or other immunosuppressants for irAEs management may increase the risk of opportunistic infections [90]. Moreover, such immune response extended manipulation may augment preexisting chronic infections or mask clinical presentations of serious infections such as cytomegalovirus-enterocolitis, pneumocystis pneumonia, infection by varicella-zoster virus, activation of latent tuberculosis, and pulmonary aspergillosis [90]. In addition to that, atypical mycobacterial infection was reported in association with anti PD-1/anti-PD-L-1 therapy [91].

In a review of metastatic melanoma patients treated with different ICIs either anti-CTLA-4, PD-1, and/or PD-L1; the incidence of immune-medicated serious infections was estimated to be 7.3%, with an average time of onset of 135 days from the start of ICI therapy [92]. Highlighted risk factors for developing serious infections included corticosteroids and infliximab use as well as the combination of CTLA-4 inhibitor and anti-PD-1 (mainly nivolumab) [92]. On the contrary, the authors of a retrospective review of melanoma patients treated with ICI concluded that the use of pembrolizumab, an anti-PD-1, was associated with protection against serious infections [92].

Mycobacterium tuberculosis (Mtb) reactivation is an emerging infectious complication of ICI therapy that has been reported with the use of nivolumab [93], pembrolizumab [94] and atezolizumab [95].

Although there is no clear mechanism of action for Mtb reactivation associated with ICI use, preclinical studies on mice [96] and human who administered anti-PD-1 suggested an increase in CD4 T cells production of interferon alfa (INF-α) leading to further bacterial replication [97, 98]. Moreover, extended immunity response could lead to augmented cytotoxicity or extracellular destruction potentiating the growth of Mtb and facilitate disease transmission [99, 100].

A recent systematic review supported the relation between the use of anti-PD-L-1 and Mtb reactivation. Mtb reactivation was disseminated to multiple organs other than the lungs, with reported fatalities [101]. Testing cancer patients for latent Mtb prior the initiation of ICI and use of Mtb chemoprophylaxis, if tested positive, lack the evidence [95], however, is highly recommended for consideration in high-risk individuals [94].

NCCN 2022 guideline recommends baseline testing for latent/active Mtb in patients treated with anti-tumor necrosis factor alfa (TNF-α) that is indicated for the management of irAEs. Moreover, Mtb testing shall not delay the start of anti- TNF-α [5]. There is lack of evidence for the management of immune mediated Mtb reactivation, however, withholding ICI during active infection to avoid possibly excessive inflammatory response is warranted. After anti-Mtb treatment initiation, the safe timing of ICI resumption is not clearly defined. A two-week duration of anti-Mtb prior re-initiation of immunotherapy was suggested [95].

### 13.2 Hepatitis B reactivation

In relation to PD-1 pathway and hepatitis B virus (HBV), it is previously proven that upregulation of PD-1 is associated with HBV specific T cell dysfunction. In hepatocellular carcinoma patients, PD-L expression was shown to be connected to HBV load [102, 103]. Moreover, it was noted that lung cancer patients with chronic HBV infection have a significantly higher PD-L-1 expression compared to patients lacking HBV infection [104].

Patients with active infections including viral hepatitis B/C or human immunodeficiency virus (HIV) were usually excluded from ICI clinical trials [105]. Considering the possible risk of HBV reactivation for patients with chronic or resolved HBV infections, baseline hepatitis serology should be performed for all patients being treated with ICI with aspartate transaminase (AST)/alanine transaminase (ALT) and HBV deoxyribonucleic acid (DNA) being monitored closely throughout immunotherapy treatment [105–109]. While anti-PD1 was safely administered to lung cancer patient with HBV infection [110, 111], some fatal HBV reactivation associated with durvalumab was reported [105].

## 14. Cardiac immune-related adverse events

ICI cardiotoxicity most reported manifestations included acute coronary syndrome, arrhythmias, cardiomyopathy, and vasculitis, while myocarditis being mostly reported with high morbidity and mortality rates [112–115]. The exact mechanism of ICI cardiotoxicity is not completely understood. In animal models, ICI use shown to make cardiac cells more vulnerable to injury; this was explained that PD 1, and CTLA-4 pathways appeared to have cardioprotective effects against immune-mediated damage due to stress [116, 117].

The prevalence of reported myocarditis, in an international multicenter registry, was 1.14%, while reaching up to 2.4% with the combination of more than one ICI [118]. The median time of onset is 34 days with majority of presentations occur within 3 months of the start of ICI therapy [119]. Despite that, cardiotoxicity can still present at any time during treatment and even after discontinuation of the therapy [120, 121].

Due to the lack of typical clinical symptoms, and challenges in diagnosis and differentiation from other cardiac disease, the incidence of ICI-related myocarditis is underestimated [112, 113, 122]. Moreover, true incidence of smoldering or subclinical myocarditis is underreported as well [114].

The fatality rate of ICI-related myocarditis increases with the combination of anti-CTLA-4 inhibitors with anti-PD-1/anti-PD-L1, compared to monotherapy with anti-PD-1/anti-PD-L1 [114, 119, 123].

Although risk factors for developing ICPI-related cardiotoxicities are not fully understood, underlying autoimmune diseases is thought to be an independent risk factor [124, 125]. Other risk factors identified in an international registry included use of combination therapy of two or more ICP, CTLA-4 inhibitors, diabetes mellitus, and obesity [119, 126]. Moreover, higher prevalence of ICPI-induced myocarditis was highly reported in patients with pre-existing hypertension (60% vs. 48%, $p < 0.009$), tobacco use (48% vs. 17%, $p < 0.001$), of male gender (65% vs. 55%, $p = 0.02$) and patients on statin (39% vs. 29%, $p = 0.04$) and angiotensin-converting enzyme inhibitors/angiotensin receptor blockers (32% vs. 23%, $p = 0.04$) [126].

As per the NCCN 2022 guideline, immediate cardiology assessment along with echocardiogram (ECG) at baseline or with any suspected immune mediated cardiotoxicity, cardiac biomarkers (troponin I or T, creatine kinase (CK), B-type natriuretic peptide (BNP) or N-terminal (NT)-pro hormone BNP (NT pro BNP) and lipid panel), Cardiac MRI (if possible), and inflammatory markers are needed for assessment and grading of cardiovascular irAEs. Cardiac catheterization and/or myocardial biopsy is considered if myocarditis is suspected [5].

Based on the American Society of Clinical Oncology (ASCO) clinical practice guideline, four categorized grading are defined based on the intensity of clinical presentation into: Grade 1 (G1) and G2 for considerably stable or minimally symptomatic patients, and G3 and G4 for unstable or very symptomatic patients [127].

Further grading criteria such as myocarditis versus pericarditis or pericardial effusion, rather than numerical grading, was applied in NCCN guideline [5].

Withholding the ICI when immune mediated myocarditis is suspected is an essential step in management while initiating further necessary workup [5, 115, 127].

Further management of confirmed ICI- induced myocarditis utilizes high dose intravenous (IV) steroids for 3–5 days. Upon follow up, and if the patient is responding and stable, IV steroids could be switched to oral form and then tapered slowly over 6–12 weeks depending on biomarkers improvement and clinical response. If no such improvement was obtained within 24–48 hours after steroids initiation, additional immunosuppressive therapies could be considered such as: mycophenolate mofetil, tacrolimus, alemtuzumab [128], and abatacept [129]. In hemodynamically unstable patients, further options are suggested including anti-thymocyte globulin (ATG), IVIG, and plasmapheresis [5, 115, 127].

It is still controversial and requires an individualized decision by multidisciplinary team to rechallenge patients who developed ICI-induced myocarditis, where single ICI is recommended upon rechallenging [127]. Severity of cardiotoxicity, status of disease, further treatment options and patient preference should be considered for rechallenging decisions [23, 26].

## 15. Summary

It has been proven that the use of immunomodulatory therapy has significantly improved survival in locally advanced and metastatic cancers. However, the use of ICIs was associated with some adverse events. This chapter focused on selected rare or very rare irAEs including cutaneous irAEs, immune mediated hypophysitis, hematological irAEs, ophthalmic irAEs, checkpoint inhibitor pneumonitis (CIP), neurologic irAEs, infectious irAEs, and cardiac irAEs. Immune-mediated T cell activation underlines the efficacy as well as possible explanation of most irAEs. In general, treatment of irAEs is decided based on the severity of the observed toxicity which can be defined according to Common Terminology Criteria for Adverse Events Version 5.0, (CTCAEs v5). After resolution of symptoms associated with irAEs, a consultation with the irAEs designated specialists might be appropriate before deciding to re-challenge or permanently discontinue the immunotherapy.

This chapter tried to highlight the significance of identifying emerging rare and very rare irAEs while considering initial assessments and management approaches identified in various clinical practice guideline and primary literature data.

## Acknowledgements

Open Access funding provided by the Qatar National Library.

## Author details

Nabil E. Omar[1,2*], Hebatalla M. Afifi[1], Arwa O. Sahal[1], Rana Mekkawi[3] and Hazem Elewa[2,4]

1 Pharmacy Department, National Center for Cancer Care and Research, Hamad Medical Corporation, Doha, Qatar

2 College of Pharmacy, Qatar University, Doha, Qatar

3 Independent Researchers, Doha, Qatar

4 College of Pharmacy and Health Science, Butler University, Indiana, USA

*Address all correspondence to: nomar4@hamad.qa

## References

[1] Hanahan D, Weinberg RA. Hallmarks of cancer: The next generation. Cell. Cell. 2011;**144**:646-674. Available from: https://pubmed.ncbi.nlm.nih.gov/21376230/

[2] Stanculeanu DL, Daniela Z, Lazescu A, Bunghez R, Anghel R. Development of new immunotherapy treatments in different cancer types. Journal of Medicine and Life. 2016;**9**:240-248. Available from: /pmc/articles/PMC5154307/

[3] Vaddepally RK, Kharel P, Pandey R, Garje R, Chandra AB. Review of indications of FDA-approved immune checkpoint inhibitors per NCCN guidelines with the level of evidence. Cancers 2020;**12**(3):738. Available from: /pmc/articles/PMC7140028/

[4] Winer A, Nicholas Bodor J, Borghaei H. Identifying and managing the adverse effects of immune checkpoint blockade. Journal of Thoracic Disease 2018;**10**(3):S480–S489. Available from: https://jtd.amegroups.com/article/view/18834/html

[5] Thompson JA, Schneider BJ, Brahmer J, Achufusi A, Armand P, Berkenstock MK, et al. Management of immunotherapy-related toxicities, version 1.2022, NCCN clinical practice guidelines in oncology. Journal of the National Comprehensive Cancer Network. 2022;**20**(4):387-405. Available from: https://pubmed.ncbi.nlm.nih.gov/35390769/

[6] Michot JM, Bigenwald C, Champiat S, Collins M, Carbonnel F, Postel-Vinay S, et al. Immune-related adverse events with immune checkpoint blockade: A comprehensive review. European Journal of Cancer. 2016;**54**:139-148. Available from: https://pubmed.ncbi.nlm.nih.gov/26765102/

[7] Postow MA, Sidlow R, Hellmann MD. Immune-related adverse events associated with immune checkpoint blockade. The New England Journal of Medicine. 2018;**378**(2):158-168. Available from: https://www.nejm.org/doi/10.1056/NEJMra1703481

[8] Stucci S, Palmirotta R, Passarelli A, Silvestris E, Argentiero A, Lanotte L, et al. Immune-related adverse events during anticancer immunotherapy: Pathogenesis and management. Oncology Letters. 2017;**14**(5):5671-5680. Available from: https://pubmed.ncbi.nlm.nih.gov/29113194/

[9] Zhai X, Zhang J, Tian Y, Li J, Jing W, Guo H, et al. The mechanism and risk factors for immune checkpoint inhibitor pneumonitis in non-small cell lung cancer patients. Cancer Biology & Medicine. 2020;**17**(3):599-611. Available from: https://pubmed.ncbi.nlm.nih.gov/32944393/

[10] Linardou H, Gogas H. Toxicity management of immunotherapy for patients with metastatic melanoma. Annals of Translational Medicine. 2016;**4**(14):272. Available from: http://www.ncbi.nlm.nih.gov/pubmed/27563659

[11] Weber JS, Postow M, Lao CD, Schadendorf D. Management of adverse events following treatment with anti-programmed death-1 agents. The Oncologist. 2016;**21**(10):1230-1240

[12] Villadolid J, Amin A. Immune checkpoint inhibitors in clinical practice: Update on management of immune-related toxicities. Translational Lung

Cancer Research. 2015;**4**(5):560-575. Available from: https://pubmed.ncbi.nlm.nih.gov/26629425/

[13] Eggermont AMM, Blank CU, Mandala M, Long GV, Atkinson V, Dalle S, et al. Adjuvant pembrolizumab versus placebo in resected stage III melanoma. The New England Journal of Medicine. 2018;**378**(19):1789-1801. Available from: https://www.nejm.org/doi/full/10.1056/nejmoa1802357

[14] Robert C, Schachter J, Long GV, Arance A, Grob JJ, Mortier L, et al. Pembrolizumab versus ipilimumab in advanced melanoma. The New England Journal of Medicine. 2015;**372**(26):2521-2532. Available from: https://pubmed.ncbi.nlm.nih.gov/25891173/

[15] Robert C, Ribas A, Wolchok JD, Hodi FS, Hamid O, Kefford R, et al. Anti-programmed-death-receptor-1 treatment with pembrolizumab in ipilimumab-refractory advanced melanoma: A randomised dose-comparison cohort of a phase 1 trial. Lancet (London, England). 2014;**384**(9948):1109-1117. Available from: https://pubmed.ncbi.nlm.nih.gov/25034862/

[16] Weber J, Mandala M, Del Vecchio M, Gogas HJ, Arance AM, Cowey CL, et al. Adjuvant nivolumab versus ipilimumab in resected stage III or IV melanoma. The New England Journal of Medicine. 2017;**377**(19):1824-1835. Available from: https://www.nejm.org/doi/full/10.1056/nejmoa1709030

[17] Robert C, Long GV, Brady B, Dutriaux C, Maio M, Mortier L, et al. Nivolumab in previously untreated melanoma without BRAF mutation. The New England Journal of Medicine. 2015;**372**(4):320-330. Available from: https://www.nejm.org/doi/full/10.1056/nejmoa1412082

[18] Weber JS, D'Angelo SP, Minor D, Hodi FS, Gutzmer R, Neyns B, et al. Nivolumab versus chemotherapy in patients with advanced melanoma who progressed after anti-CTLA-4 treatment (CheckMate 037): A randomised, controlled, open-label, phase 3 trial. The Lancet Oncology. 2015;**16**(4):375-384. Available from: https://pubmed.ncbi.nlm.nih.gov/25795410/

[19] Hodi FS, O'Day SJ, McDermott DF, Weber RW, Sosman JA, Haanen JB, et al. Improved survival with ipilimumab in patients with metastatic melanoma. The New England Journal of Medicine. 2010;**363**(8):711-723. Available from: https://www.nejm.org/doi/full/10.1056/nejmoa1003466

[20] Champiat S, Lambotte O, Barreau E, Belkhir R, Berdelou A, Carbonnel F, et al. Management of immune checkpoint blockade dysimmune toxicities: A collaborative position paper. Annals of Oncology. 2016;**27**(4):559-574. Available from: https://pubmed.ncbi.nlm.nih.gov/26715621/

[21] Council for International Organizations of Medical Sciences. Guidelines for preparing core clinical safety information on drugs: report of CIOMS Working Groups III and V: including new proposals for investigator's brochures. 1999. Available from: https://cioms.ch/wp-content/uploads/2018/03/Guidelines-for-Preparing-Core-Clinical-Safety-Info-Drugs-Report-of-CIOMS-Working-Group-III-and-V.pdf

[22] Freites-Martinez A, Santana N, Arias-Santiago S, Viera A. Using the common terminology criteria for adverse events (CTCAE - version 5.0) to evaluate the severity of adverse events of anticancer therapies. Actas Dermo-Sifiliográficas. 2021;**112**(1):90-92. Available from: https://pubmed.ncbi.nlm.nih.gov/32891586/

[23] Takahara Y, Tanaka T, Ishige Y, Shionoya I, Yamamura K, Sakuma T, et al. Efficacy and predictors of rechallenge with immune checkpoint inhibitors in non-small cell lung cancer Thoracic Cancer 2022;**13**(4):624. Available from: /pmc/articles/PMC8841726/

[24] Li M, Sack JS, Rahma OE, Hodi FS, Zucker SD, Grover S. Outcomes following resumption of immune checkpoint inhibitor therapy after high-grade immune-mediated hepatitis. Cancer 2020;**126**(23):5088. Available from: /pmc/articles/PMC7655516/

[25] Abu-Sbeih H, Ali FS, Naqash AR, Owen DH, Patel S, Otterson GA, et al. Resumption of immune checkpoint inhibitor therapy after immune-mediated colitis. Journal of Clinical Oncology. 2019;**37**(30):2738-2745

[26] Nakajima EC, Lipson EJ, Brahmer JR. Challenge of rechallenge: When to resume immunotherapy following an immune-related adverse event. Journal of Clinical Oncology. 2019;**37**(30):2714-2718

[27] Ellen Maher V, Fernandes LL, Weinstock C, Tang S, Agarwal S, Brave M, et al. Analysis of the association between adverse events and outcome in patients receiving a programmed death protein 1 or programmed death ligand 1 antibody. Journal of Clinical Oncology. 2019;**37**(30):2730-2737. Available from: https://pubmed.ncbi.nlm.nih.gov/31116675/

[28] Rogado J, Sánchez-Torres JM, Romero-Laorden N, Ballesteros AI, Pacheco-Barcia V, Ramos-Leví A, et al. Immune-related adverse events predict the therapeutic efficacy of anti–PD-1 antibodies in cancer patients. European Journal of Cancer. 2019;**109**:21-27

[29] Nigro O, Pinotti G, De Galitiis F, Di Pietro FR, Giusti R, Filetti M, et al. Late immune-related adverse events in long-term responders to PD-1/PD-L1 checkpoint inhibitors: A multicentre study. European Journal of Cancer. 2020;**134**:19-28. Available from: https://pubmed.ncbi.nlm.nih.gov/32454395/

[30] Dall'Olio FG, Di Nunno V, Massari F. Immortal time bias question in the association between toxicity and outcome of immune checkpoint inhibitors. Journal of Clinical Oncology. 2020;**38**(1):105-106

[31] Weber JS, Hodi FS, Wolchok JD, Topalian SL, Schadendorf D, Larkin J, et al. Safety profile of nivolumab monotherapy: A pooled analysis of patients with advanced melanoma. Journal of Clinical Oncology. 2017;**35**(7):785-792. Available from: https://pubmed.ncbi.nlm.nih.gov/28068177/

[32] Kuusisalo S, Koivunen JP, Iivanainen S. Association of rare immune-related adverse events to survival in advanced cancer patients treated with immune checkpoint inhibitors: A real-world single-Center cohort study. Cancers (Basel). 2022;**14**(9):2276. Available from: https://pubmed.ncbi.nlm.nih.gov/35565405/

[33] Belum VR, Benhuri B, Postow MA, Hellmann MD, Lesokhin AM, Segal NH, et al. Characterisation and management of dermatologic adverse events to agents targeting the PD-1 receptor. European Journal of Cancer. 2016;**60**:12-25. Available from: https://pubmed.ncbi.nlm.nih.gov/27043866/

[34] Geisler AN, Phillips GS, Barrios DM, Wu J, Leung DYM, Moy AP, et al. Immune checkpoint inhibitor-related dermatologic adverse events. Journal of the American Academy of Dermatology.

2020;**83**(5):1255-1268. Available from: https://pubmed.ncbi.nlm.nih.gov/32454097/

[35] Robert C, Ribas A, Schachter J, Arance A, Grob JJ, Mortier L, et al. Pembrolizumab versus ipilimumab in advanced melanoma (KEYNOTE-006): Post-hoc 5-year results from an open-label, multicentre, randomised, controlled, phase 3 study. Lancet Oncology. 2019;**20**(9):1239-1251. Available from: https://pubmed.ncbi.nlm.nih.gov/31345627/

[36] Trinidad C, Nelson KC, Glitza Oliva IC, Torres-Cabala CA, Nagarajan P, Tetzlaff MT, et al. Dermatologic toxicity from immune checkpoint blockade therapy with an interstitial granulomatous pattern. Journal of Cutaneous Pathology. 2018;**45**(7):504-507. Available from: https://pubmed.ncbi.nlm.nih.gov/29633300/

[37] Tetzlaff MT, Jazaeri AA, Torres-Cabala CA, Korivi BR, Landon GA, Nagarajan P, et al. Erythema nodosum-like panniculitis mimicking disease recurrence: A novel toxicity from immune checkpoint blockade therapy—Report of 2 patients. Journal of Cutaneous Pathology. 2017;**44**(12):1080-1086

[38] Voudouri D, Nikolaou V, Laschos K, Charpidou A, Soupos N, Triantafyllopoulou I, et al. Anti-PD1/PDL1 induced psoriasis. Current Problems in Cancer. 2017;**41**(6):407-412. Available from: https://pubmed.ncbi.nlm.nih.gov/29096940/

[39] Pach J, Moody K, Ring N, Panse G, Zhang M, Deverapalli S, et al. Erythema nodosum-like panniculitis associated with immune checkpoint inhibitor therapy: Two cases reporting a rare cutaneous adverse event. JAAD Case Reports. 2021;**13**:118-120. Available from: http://www.jaadcasereports.org/article/S2352512621003271/fulltext

[40] Ravi V, Maloney NJ, Worswick S. Neutrophilic dermatoses as adverse effects of checkpoint inhibitors: A review. Dermatologic Therapy. 2019;**32**(5):e13074. Available from: https://pubmed.ncbi.nlm.nih.gov/31444856/

[41] Belkaid S, Berger M, Nouvier M, Picard C, Dalle S. A case of Schönlein-Henoch purpura induced by immune checkpoint inhibitor in a patient with metastatic melanoma. European Journal of Cancer. 2020;**139**:169-172. Available from: https://pubmed.ncbi.nlm.nih.gov/32992155/

[42] Freites-Martinez A, Kwong BY, Rieger KE, Coit DG, Colevas AD, Lacouture ME. Eruptive keratoacanthomas associated with pembrolizumab therapy JAMA Dermatology 2017;**153**(7):694. Available from: /pmc/articles/PMC5523926/

[43] Inno A, Metro G, Bironzo P, Grimaldi AM, Grego E, Di NV, et al. Pathogenesis, clinical manifestations and management of immune checkpoint inhibitors toxicity. Tumori. 2017;**103**(5):405-421. Available from: https://pubmed.ncbi.nlm.nih.gov/28497847/

[44] Sibaud V, Meyer N, Lamant L, Vigarios E, Mazieres J, Delord JP. Dermatologic complications of anti-PD-1/PD-L1 immune checkpoint antibodies. Current Opinion in Oncology. 2016;**28**(4):254-263. Available from: https://pubmed.ncbi.nlm.nih.gov/27136138/

[45] Sibaud V. Dermatologic reactions to immune checkpoint inhibitors: Skin toxicities and immunotherapy. American Journal of Clinical Dermatology. 2018;**19**(3):345-361. Available from:

https://pubmed.ncbi.nlm.nih.gov/29256113/

[46] Muntyanu A, Netchiporouk E, Gerstein W, Gniadecki R, Litvinov IV. Cutaneous immune-related adverse events (irAEs) to immune checkpoint inhibitors: A dermatology perspective on management. Journal of Cutaneous Medicine and Surgery. 2021;**25**(1):59-76

[47] Martins F, Sofiya L, Sykiotis GP, Lamine F, Maillard M, Fraga M, et al. Adverse effects of immune-checkpoint inhibitors: Epidemiology, management and surveillance. Nature Reviews Clinical Oncology. 2019;**16**(9):563-580. Available from: https://www.nature.com/articles/s41571-019-0218-0

[48] Zhai Y, Ye X, Hu F, Xu J, Guo X, Zhuang Y, et al. Endocrine toxicity of immune checkpoint inhibitors: A real-world study leveraging US Food and Drug Administration adverse events reporting system. Journal for Immunotherapy of Cancer. 2019;**7**(1):1-11

[49] Darnell EP, Mooradian MJ, Baruch EN, Yilmaz M, Reynolds KL. Immune-related adverse events (irAEs): Diagnosis, management, and clinical pearls. Current Oncology Reports. 2020;**22**(4):1-11. Available from: https://link.springer.com/article/10.1007/s11912-020-0897-9

[50] Barroso-Sousa R, Barry WT, Garrido-Castro AC, Hodi FS, Min L, Krop IE, et al. Incidence of endocrine dysfunction following the use of different immune checkpoint inhibitor regimens a systematic review and meta-analysis. JAMA Oncology. 2018;**4**(2):173-182

[51] De Filette J, Andreescu CE, Cools F, Bravenboer B, Velkeniers B. A systematic review and meta-analysis of endocrine-related adverse events associated with immune checkpoint inhibitors. Hormone and Metabolic Research. 2019;**51**(3):145-156. Available from: https://pubmed.ncbi.nlm.nih.gov/30861560/

[52] Elia G, Ferrari SM, Galdiero MR, Ragusa F, Paparo SR, Ruffilli I, et al. New insight in endocrine-related adverse events associated to immune checkpoint blockade. Best Practice & Research. Clinical Endocrinology & Metabolism. 2020;**34**(1):101370

[53] Wright JJ, Powers AC, Johnson DB. Endocrine toxicities of immune checkpoint inhibitors. Nature Reviews. Endocrinology. 2021;**17**:389-399. Available from: https://pubmed.ncbi.nlm.nih.gov/33875857/

[54] Faje AT, Sullivan R, Lawrence D, Tritos NA, Fadden R, Klibanski A, et al. Ipilimumab-induced hypophysitis: A detailed longitudinal analysis in a large cohort of patients with metastatic melanoma. The Journal of Clinical Endocrinology and Metabolism. 2014;**99**(11):4078-4085. Available from: https://academic.oup.com/jcem/article/99/11/4078/2836487

[55] Paschou SA, Stefanaki K, Psaltopoulou T, Liontos M, Koutsoukos K, Zagouri F, et al. How we treat endocrine complications of immune checkpoint inhibitors. ESMO Open. 2021;**6**(1):100011

[56] Langlois F, Varlamov E V., Fleseriu M. Hypophysitis, the growing Spectrum of a rare pituitary disease. The Journal of Clinical Endocrinology and Metabolism 2022;**107**(1):10. Available from: /pmc/articles/PMC8684465/

[57] Haanen JBAG, Carbonnel F, Robert C, Kerr KM, Peters S, Larkin J,

et al. Management of toxicities from immunotherapy: ESMO Clinical Practice Guidelines for diagnosis, treatment and follow-up. Annals of Oncology. 2017;**28**(suppl_4):iv119-iv142. Available from: https://pubmed.ncbi.nlm.nih.gov/28881921/

[58] Omar NE, El-Fass KA, Abushouk AI, Elbaghdady N, Barakat AEM, Noreldin AE, et al. Diagnosis and management of hematological adverse events induced by immune checkpoint inhibitors: A systematic review. Frontiers in Immunology. 2020;**11**:1354

[59] Kong BY, Micklethwaite KP, Swaminathan S, Kefford RF, Carlino MS. Autoimmune hemolytic anemia induced by anti-PD-1 therapy in metastatic melanoma. Melanoma Research. 2016;**26**(2):202-204. Available from: https://pubmed.ncbi.nlm.nih.gov/26795275/

[60] King J, de la Cruz J, Lutzky J. Ipilimumab-induced thrombotic thrombocytopenic purpura (TTP). Journal for Immunotherapy of Cancer. 2017;**5**(1):1-4. Available from: https://pubmed.ncbi.nlm.nih.gov/28344807/

[61] Delyon J, Mateus C, Lambert T. Hemophilia a induced by ipilimumab. The New England Journal of Medicine. 2011;**365**(18):1747-1748. Available from: https://pubmed.ncbi.nlm.nih.gov/22047582/

[62] Kanbour A, Rasul KI, Albader SB, Sulaiman RJ Al, Melikyan G, Farghaly H, et al. Pancytopenia and limbic encephalopathy complicating immunotherapy for clear cell endometrial cancer with microsatellite instability-high (MSI-H). Oncotargets and Therapy 2019;**12**:9965. Available from: /pmc/articles/PMC6875561/

[63] Omar NE-H, Nasser S, Gasim M, Khanna M, Nashwan AJ, Feilchenfeldt JW, et al. CLO19-045: Safety of immune checkpoint inhibitors in cancer patients with microsatellite instability-high (MSI-H) status: An experience from Qatar. Journal of the National Comprehensive Cancer Network. 2019;**17**(3.5):CLO19-CL045. Available from: https://jnccn.org/view/journals/jnccn/17/3.5/article-pCLO19-045.xml

[64] Shiuan E, Beckermann KE, Ozgun A, Kelly C, McKean M, McQuade J, et al. Thrombocytopenia in patients with melanoma receiving immune checkpoint inhibitor therapy. Journal for Immunotherapy of Cancer. 2017;**5**(1):1-6. Available from: https://pubmed.ncbi.nlm.nih.gov/28239462/

[65] Rajapakse P, Andanamala H. Hemophagocytic Lymphohistiocytosis secondary to immune checkpoint inhibitor therapy. World Journal of Oncology. 2022;**13**(2):49-52. Available from: https://pubmed.ncbi.nlm.nih.gov/35571340/

[66] Zhou L, Wei X. Ocular immune-related adverse events associated with immune checkpoint inhibitors in lung cancer. Frontiers in Immunology 2021;**12**. Available from: /pmc/articles/PMC8421677/

[67] Yu CW, Yau M, Mezey N, Joarder I, Micieli JA. Neuro-ophthalmic complications of immune checkpoint inhibitors: A systematic review Eye and Brain 2020;**12**:139. Available from: /pmc/articles/PMC7648547/

[68] Brahmer JR, Abu-Sbeih H, Ascierto PA, Brufsky J, Cappelli LC, Cortazar FB, et al. Society for Immunotherapy of cancer (SITC) clinical practice guideline on immune checkpoint inhibitor-related adverse events. Journal for Immunotherapy of

Cancer 2021;**9**(6):2435. Available from: /pmc/articles/PMC8237720/

[69] Fang T, Maberley DA, Etminan M. Ocular adverse events with immune checkpoint inhibitors. Journal of Current Ophthalmology 2019;**31**(3):319. Available from: /pmc/articles/PMC6742617/

[70] Sun MM, Kelly SP, Mylavarapu BSAL, Holland GN, Coleman AL, Yu F, et al. Ophthalmic immune-related adverse events after anti-CTLA-4 or PD-1 therapy recorded in the American Academy of ophthalmology intelligent research in sight registry. Ophthalmology. 2021;**128**(6):910-919. Available from: http://www.aaojournal.org/article/S0161642020310423/fulltext

[71] Wilson MA, Guld K, Galetta S, Walsh RD, Kharlip J, Tamhankar M, et al. Acute visual loss after ipilimumab treatment for metastatic melanoma. Journal for Immunotherapy of Cancer. 2016;**4**(1):66. Available from: https://jitc.bmj.com/content/4/1/66

[72] Yeh OL, Francis CE. Ipilimumab-associated bilateral optic neuropathy. Journal of Neuro-Ophthalmology. 2015;**35**(2):144-147. Available from: https://journals.lww.com/jneuro-ophthalmology/Fulltext/2015/06000/Ipilimumab_Associated_Bilateral_Optic_Neuropathy.9.aspx

[73] Wang H, Guo X, Zhou J, Li Y, Duan L, Si X, et al. Clinical diagnosis and treatment of immune checkpoint inhibitor-associated pneumonitis. Thoracic Cancer. 2020;**11**(1):191-197. Available from: https://pubmed.ncbi.nlm.nih.gov/31762218/

[74] Nishino M, Giobbie-Hurder A, Hatabu H, Ramaiya NH, Hodi FS. Incidence of programmed cell death 1 inhibitor-related pneumonitis in patients with advanced cancer: A systematic review and meta-analysis. JAMA Oncology. 2016;**2**(12):1607-1616. Available from: https://pubmed.ncbi.nlm.nih.gov/27540850/

[75] Khunger M, Rakshit S, Pasupuleti V, Hernandez AV, Mazzone P, Stevenson J, et al. Incidence of pneumonitis with use of programmed death 1 and programmed death-ligand 1 inhibitors in non-small cell lung cancer: A systematic review and meta-analysis of trials. Chest. 2017;**152**(2):271-281

[76] Zhang Q, Tang L, Zhou Y, He W, Li W. Immune checkpoint inhibitor-associated pneumonitis in non-small cell lung cancer: Current understanding in characteristics, diagnosis, and management. Frontiers in Immunology. 2021;**12**:1889

[77] Gomatou G, Tzilas V, Kotteas E, Syrigos K, Bouros D. Immune checkpoint inhibitor-related pneumonitis. Respiration. 2020;**99**(11):932-942. Available from: https://www.karger.com/Article/FullText/509941

[78] Ichimura T, Hinata M, Ichikura D, Suzuki S. Safety of immune checkpoint inhibitors in non-small-cell lung cancer patients with idiopathic interstitial pneumonia: A matched case–control study. Cancer Chemotherapy and Pharmacology. 2022;**89**(1):21-30

[79] Haanen JBAG, Carbonnel F, Robert C, Kerr KM, Peters S, Larkin J, et al. Management of toxicities from immunotherapy: ESMO clinical practice guidelines for diagnosis, treatment and follow-up†. Annals of Oncology. 2017;**28**:iv119-iv142. Available from: http://www.annalsofoncology.org/article/S0923753419421534/fulltext

[80] Reynolds KL, Guidon AC. Diagnosis and management of immune checkpoint

inhibitor-associated neurologic toxicity: Illustrative case and review of the literature. The Oncologist 2019;**24**(4):435. Available from: /pmc/articles/PMC6459240/

[81] Kao JC, Brickshawana A, Liewluck T. Neuromuscular complications of programmed cell death-1 (PD-1) inhibitors. Current Neurology and Neuroscience Reports. 2018;**18**(10):1-9. Available from: https://link.springer.com/article/10.1007/s11910-018-0878-7

[82] Larkin J, Chmielowski B, Lao CD, Hodi FS, Sharfman W, Weber J, et al. Neurologic serious adverse events associated with nivolumab plus ipilimumab or nivolumab alone in advanced melanoma, including a case series of encephalitis. The Oncologist. 2017;**22**(6):709-718. Available from: https://pubmed.ncbi.nlm.nih.gov/28495807/

[83] Möhn N, Beutel G, Gutzmer R, Ivanyi P, Satzger I, Skripuletz T. Neurological immune related adverse events associated with nivolumab, ipilimumab, and pembrolizumab therapy—Review of the literature and future outlook. Journal of Clinical Medicine 2019;**8**(11). Available from: /pmc/articles/PMC6912719/

[84] Haugh AM, Probasco JC, Johnson DB. Neurologic complications of immune checkpoint inhibitors. Therapeutic Advances in Neurological Disorders. 2020;**19**(4):479-488. Available from: https://www.tandfonline.com/doi/abs/10.1080/14740338.2020.1738382

[85] Bloch KC, Glaser C. Diagnostic approaches for patients with suspected encephalitis. Current Infectious Disease Reports. 2007;**9**(4):315-322. Available from: https://link.springer.com/article/10.1007/s11908-007-0049-5

[86] Mikami T, Liaw B, Asada M, Niimura T, Zamami Y, Green-LaRoche D, et al. Neuroimmunological adverse events associated with immune checkpoint inhibitor: A retrospective, pharmacovigilance study using FAERS database. Journal of Neuro-Oncology. 2021;**152**(1):135-144

[87] Johnson DB, Manouchehri A, Haugh AM, Quach HT, Balko JM, Lebrun-Vignes B, et al. Neurologic toxicity associated with immune checkpoint inhibitors: A pharmacovigilance study. Journal for Immunotherapy of Cancer. 2019;**7**(1). Available from: https://pubmed.ncbi.nlm.nih.gov/31118078/

[88] Kolb NA, Trevino CR, Waheed W, Sobhani F, Landry KK, Thomas AA, et al. Neuromuscular complications of immune checkpoint inhibitor therapy. Muscle & Nerve. 2018;**58**(1):10-22. Available from: https://onlinelibrary.wiley.com/doi/full/10.1002/mus.26070

[89] Safa H, Johnson DH, Trinh VA, Rodgers TE, Lin H, Suarez-Almazor ME, et al. Immune checkpoint inhibitor related myasthenia gravis: Single center experience and systematic review of the literature. Journal for Immunotherapy of Cancer. 2019;**7**(1):1-11. Available from: https://jitc.biomedcentral.com/articles/10.1186/s40425-019-0774-y

[90] Fishman JA, Hogan JI, Maus MV. Inflammatory and infectious syndromes associated with cancer immunotherapies. Clinical Infectious Diseases. 2019;**69**(6):909-920. Available from: https://pubmed.ncbi.nlm.nih.gov/30520987/

[91] Anand K, Sahu G, Burns E, Ensor A, Ensor J, Pingali SR, et al. Mycobacterial infections due to PD-1 and PD-L1 checkpoint inhibitors. ESMO Open. 2020;**5**(4):866. Available from:

http://www.esmoopen.com/article/S2059702920326661/fulltext

[92] Del Castillo M, Romero FA, Argüello E, Kyi C, Postow MA, Redelman-Sidi G. The spectrum of serious infections among patients receiving immune checkpoint blockade for the treatment of melanoma. Clinical Infectious Diseases. 2016;**63**(11):1490-1493. Available from: https://academic.oup.com/cid/article/63/11/1490/2526208

[93] Fujita K, Terashima T, Mio T. Anti-PD1 antibody treatment and the development of acute pulmonary tuberculosis. Journal of Thoracic Oncology. 2016;**11**(12):2238-2240. Available from: https://pubmed.ncbi.nlm.nih.gov/27423391/

[94] Suliman AM, Bek SA, Elkhatim MS, Husain AA, Mismar AY, Eldean MZS, et al. Tuberculosis following programmed cell death receptor-1 (PD-1) inhibitor in a patient with non-small cell lung cancer. Case report and literature review. Cancer Immunology, Immunotherapy. 2021;**70**(4):935. Available from: /pmc/articles/PMC7979647/

[95] Anastasopoulou A, Ziogas DC, Samarkos M, Kirkwood JM, Gogas H. Reactivation of tuberculosis in cancer patients following administration of immune checkpoint inhibitors: Current evidence and clinical practice recommendations. Journal for Immunotherapy of Cancer. 2019;7(1):1-13. Available from: https://jitc.biomedcentral.com/articles/10.1186/s40425-019-0717-7

[96] Tousif S, Singh Y, Prasad DVR, Sharma P, van Kaer L, Das G. T cells from programmed Death-1 deficient mice respond poorly to mycobacterium tuberculosis infection. PLoS One. 2011;**6**(5):e19864. Available from: https://journals.plos.org/plosone/article?id=10.1371/journal.pone.0019864

[97] Barber DL, Mayer-Barber KD, Feng CG, Sharpe AH, Sher A. CD4 T cells promote rather than control tuberculosis in the absence of PD-1–mediated inhibition. Journal of Immunology. 2011;**186**(3):1598-1607. Available from: https://www.jimmunol.org/content/186/3/1598

[98] Barber DL, Sakai S, Kudchadkar RR, Fling SP, Day TA, Vergara JA, et al. Tuberculosis following PD-1 blockade for cancer immunotherapy. Science Translational Medicine. 2019;**11**(475). Available from: https://pubmed.ncbi.nlm.nih.gov/30651320/

[99] Elkington PT, Bateman AC, Thomas GJ, Ottensmeier CH. Implications of tuberculosis reactivation after immune checkpoint inhibition. American Journal of Respiratory and Critical Care Medicine. 2018;**198**(11):1451-1453. Available from: www.atsjournals.org

[100] Tezera LB, Bielecka MK, Ogongo P, Walker NF, Ellis M, Garay-Baquero DJ, et al. Anti-PD-1 immunotherapy leads to tuberculosis reactivation via dysregulation of TNF-α. eLife. 2020:9

[101] Zaemes J, Kim C. Immune checkpoint inhibitor use and tuberculosis: A systematic review of the literature. European Journal of Cancer. 2020;**132**:168-175. Available from: https://pubmed.ncbi.nlm.nih.gov/32375103/

[102] Peng G, Li S, Wu W, Tan X, Chen Y, Chen Z. PD-1 upregulation is associated with HBV-specific T cell dysfunction in chronic hepatitis B patients. Molecular Immunology. 2008;**45**(4):963-970. Available from: https://pubmed.ncbi.nlm.nih.gov/17868872/

[103] Zhang Z, Zhang JY, Wherry EJ, Jin B, Xu B, Zou ZS, et al. Dynamic programmed death 1 expression by virus-specific CD8 T cells correlates with the outcome of acute hepatitis B. Gastroenterology. 2008;**134**(7)

[104] Zhang X, Tian D, Chen Y, Chen C, He LN, Zhou Y, et al. Association of hepatitis B virus infection status with outcomes of non-small cell lung cancer patients undergoing anti-PD-1/PD-L1 therapy. Translational Lung Cancer Research. 2021;**10**(7):3191-3202. Available from: https://tlcr.amegroups.com/article/view/53682/html

[105] Godbert B, Petitpain N, Lopez A, Nisse YE, Gillet P. Hepatitis B reactivation and immune check point inhibitors. Digestive and Liver Disease. 2021;**53**(4):452-455

[106] Burns EA, Muhsen IN, Anand K, Xu J, Umoru G, Arain AN, et al. Hepatitis B virus reactivation in cancer patients treated with immune checkpoint inhibitors. Journal of Immunotherapy 2021;**44**(3):132. Available from: /pmc/articles/PMC7946380/

[107] Lee PC, Chao Y, Chen MH, Lan KH, Lee IC, Hou MC, et al. Risk of HBV reactivation in patients with immune checkpoint inhibitor-treated unresectable hepatocellular carcinoma. Journal for Immunotherapy of Cancer. 2020;**8**(2):e001072. Available from: https://jitc.bmj.com/content/8/2/e001072

[108] Lin Z, Zhang X, Zhou Y, Chen C, He L, Li H, et al. Hepatotoxicity associated with PD-1 blockade antibodies in cancer patients co-infected with hepatitis B virus. Cancer Immunology, Immunotherapy. 2022;**71**(5):1247-1255. Available from: https://link.springer.com/article/10.1007/s00262-021-03082-4

[109] Ostios-Garcia L, Faig J, Leonardi GC, Adeni AE, Subegdjo SJ, Lydon CA, et al. Safety and efficacy of PD-1 inhibitors among HIV-positive patients with non-small cell lung cancer. Journal of Thoracic Oncology. 2018;**13**(7):1037-1042. Available from: https://pubmed.ncbi.nlm.nih.gov/29631035/

[110] Xu F, Zeng Z, Yan B, Fu Y, Sun Y, Yang G, et al. Safety and efficacy of anti-PD-1 inhibitors in Chinese patients with advanced lung cancer and hepatitis B virus infection: A retrospective single-center study. Translational Lung Cancer Research. 2021;**10**(4):1819-1828. Available from: https://pubmed.ncbi.nlm.nih.gov/34012795/

[111] Kothapalli A, Khattak MA. Safety and efficacy of anti-PD-1 therapy for metastatic melanoma and non-small-cell lung cancer in patients with viral hepatitis: A case series. Melanoma Research. 2018;**28**(2):155-158. Available from: https://europepmc.org/article/med/29406396

[112] Ganatra S, Parikh R, Neilan TG. Cardiotoxicity of immune therapy. Cardiology Clinics. 2019;**37**(4):385-397. Available from: https://pubmed.ncbi.nlm.nih.gov/31587780/

[113] Patel RP, Parikh R, Gunturu KS, Tariq RZ, Dani SS, Ganatra S, et al. Cardiotoxicity of immune checkpoint inhibitors. Current Oncology Reports 2021;**23**(7). Available from: /pmc/articles/PMC8088903/

[114] Moslehi JJ, Salem JE, Sosman JA, Lebrun-Vignes B, Johnson DB. Increased reporting of fatal immune checkpoint inhibitor-associated myocarditis. Lancet (London, England). 2018;**391**(10124):933. Available

from: https://pubmed.ncbi.nlm.nih.gov/29536852/

[115] Escudier M, Cautela J, Malissen N, Ancedy Y, Orabona M, Pinto J, et al. Clinical features, management, and outcomes of immune checkpoint inhibitor-related cardiotoxicity. Circulation. 2017;**136**(21):2085-2087. Available from: https://pubmed.ncbi.nlm.nih.gov/29158217/

[116] Nishimura H, Okazaki T, Tanaka Y, Nakatani K, Hara M, Matsumori A, et al. Autoimmune dilated cardiomyopathy in PD-1 receptor-deficient mice. Science. 2001;**291**(5502):319-322. Available from: https://pubmed.ncbi.nlm.nih.gov/11209085/

[117] Love VA, Grabie N, Duramad P, Stavrakis G, Sharpe A, Lichtman A. CTLA-4 ablation and interleukin-12 driven differentiation synergistically augment cardiac pathogenicity of cytotoxic T lymphocytes. Circulation Research. 2007;**101**(3):248-257. Available from: https://pubmed.ncbi.nlm.nih.gov/17569889/

[118] Salem JE, Manouchehri A, Moey M, Lebrun-Vignes B, Bastarache L, Pariente A, et al. Cardiovascular toxicities associated with immune checkpoint inhibitors: An observational, retrospective, pharmacovigilance study. The Lancet Oncology. 2018;**19**(12):1579-1589

[119] Mahmood SS, Fradley MG, Cohen J V., Nohria A, Reynolds KL, Heinzerling LM, et al. Myocarditis in patients treated with immune checkpoint inhibitors. Journal of the American College of Cardiology. 2018;**71**(16):1755. Available from: /pmc/articles/PMC6196725/

[120] Ghisoni E, Wicky A, Bouchaab H, Imbimbo M, Delyon J, Gautron Moura B, et al. Late-onset and long-lasting immune-related adverse events from immune checkpoint-inhibitors: An overlooked aspect in immunotherapy. European Journal of Cancer. 2021;**149**:153-164. Available from: https://pubmed.ncbi.nlm.nih.gov/33865201/

[121] Couey MA, Bell RB, Patel AA, Romba MC, Crittenden MR, Curti BD, et al. Delayed immune-related events (DIRE) after discontinuation of immunotherapy: Diagnostic hazard of autoimmunity at a distance. Journal for Immunotherapy of Cancer. 2019;**7**(1):1-11. Available from: https://jitc.biomedcentral.com/articles/10.1186/s40425-019-0645-6

[122] Stein-Merlob AF, Rothberg MV, Holman P, Yang EH. Immunotherapy-associated cardiotoxicity of immune checkpoint inhibitors and chimeric antigen receptor T cell therapy: Diagnostic and management challenges and strategies. Current Cardiology Reports. 2021;**23**(3)

[123] Johnson DB, Balko JM, Compton ML, Chalkias S, Gorham J, Xu Y, et al. Fulminant myocarditis with combination immune checkpoint blockade. The New England Journal of Medicine. 2016;**375**(18):1749-1755. Available from: https://pubmed.ncbi.nlm.nih.gov/27806233/

[124] Johnson DB, Sullivan RJ, Ott PA, Carlino MS, Khushalani NI, Ye F, et al. Ipilimumab therapy in patients with advanced melanoma and Preexisting autoimmune disorders. JAMA Oncology. 2016;**2**(2):234-240. Available from: https://pubmed.ncbi.nlm.nih.gov/26633184/

[125] Johnson DB, Sullivan RJ, Menzies AM. Immune checkpoint

inhibitors in challenging populations. Cancer. 2017;**123**:1904-1911, 1911. Available from: https://pubmed.ncbi.nlm.nih.gov/28241095/

[126] Dal'bo N, Patel R, Parikh R, Shah SP, Guha A, Dani SS, et al. Cardiotoxicity of contemporary anticancer immunotherapy. Current Treatment Options in Cardiovascular Medicine 2020;**22**(12):62. Available from: /pmc/articles/PMC7605901/

[127] Brahmer JR, Lacchetti C, Schneider BJ, Atkins MB, Brassil KJ, Caterino JM, et al. Management of immune-related adverse events in patients treated with immune checkpoint inhibitor therapy: American Society of Clinical Oncology clinical practice guideline. Journal of Clinical Oncology 2018;**36**(17):1714. Available from: /pmc/articles/PMC6481621/

[128] Esfahani K, Buhlaiga N, Thébault P, Lapointe R, Johnson NA, Miller WH. Alemtuzumab for immune-related myocarditis due to PD-1 therapy. The New England Journal of Medicine. 2019;**380**(24):2375-2376. Available from: https://pubmed.ncbi.nlm.nih.gov/31189042/

[129] Salem J-E, Allenbach Y, Vozy A, Brechot N, Johnson DB, Moslehi JJ, et al. Abatacept for severe immune checkpoint inhibitor–associated myocarditis. The New England Journal of Medicine. 2019;**380**(24):2377-2379. Available from: https://www.nejm.org/doi/10.1056/NEJMc1901677